Clinical Atlas of Diabetes Mellitus

Clinical Atlas of Diabetes Mellitus

Arturo R Rolla MD
Beth Israel Deaconess Medical Center
Associate Clinical Professor
Department of Medicine
Harvard Medical School
Boston, Massachusetts, USA

Sanjay Agarwal MD FACE
Director, Aegle Clinic - Diabetes Care
Head, Department of Medicine
Ruby Hall Clinic
Sr. Consultant in Diabetes and Medicine
Jehangir Hospital
Pune, Maharashtra, India

JAYPEE

JAYPEE BROTHERS MEDICAL PUBLISHERS

The Health Sciences Publisher

New Delhi | London

Jaypee Brothers Medical Publishers (P) Ltd

Headquarters
Jaypee Brothers Medical Publishers (P) Ltd
EMCA House, 23/23-B
Ansari Road, Daryaganj
New Delhi 110 002, India
Landline: +91-11-23272143,
+91-11-23272703 +91-11-23282021,
+91-11-23245672
Email: jaypee@jaypeebrothers.com

Corporate Office
4838/24, Ansari Road, Daryaganj
New Delhi 110 002, India
Phone: +91-11-43574357
Fax: +91-11-43574314
e-mail: jaypee@jaypeebrothers.com

Overseas Office
Jaypee Brothers Medical Publishers (P) Ltd
4838/24, Ansari Road, Daryaganj
New Delhi 110 002, India
Phone: +91-11-43574357
Fax: +91-11-43574314
Email: jaypee@jaypeebrothers.com

EU GPSR Authorised Representative
Logos Europe, 9 rue Nicolas Poussin
17000, La Rochelle, France
Phone: +33 (0) 6 67 93 73 78
e-mail: contact@logoseurope.eu

Website: www.jaypeebrothers.com
Website: www.jaypeedigital.com

Inquiries for bulk sales may be solicited at: jaypee@jaypeebrothers.com

Clinical Atlas of Diabetes Mellitus

First Edition: 2020, Reprint: **2026**

ISBN: 978-93-5270-519-1

Printed in India

Dedicated to

"All our patients who inspired and taught us"

Contributors

AG Unnikrishnan MD DM DNB NMAMS
CEO and Chief Endocrinologist
Chellaram Diabetes Institute
Pune, Maharashtra, India

Alan Sinclair MSc MD FRCP
Director, Foundation for Diabetes Research in Older People
Diabetes Frail Ltd, and Hon Prof of Metabolic Medicine, Aston University, Birmingham, UK

Anjali Amit Bhatt
MD (Medicine) PDFD MSc (Endocrine)
Consultant Endocrinologist
Chellaram Diabetes Institute
Pune, Maharashtra, India

Aravind R Sosale
MBBS DNB FRCP (Glasgow and Edinburgh)
Director
Diacon Hospital, Bangalore
Bengaluru, Karnataka, India

Arturo R Rolla MD
Beth Israel Deaconess Medical Center
Associate Clinical Professor
Department of Medicine
Harvard Medical School
Boston, Massachusetts, USA

Ashwin Pillai MBBS
Fellow, Department of Medicine
Ruby Hall Clinic
Pune, Maharashtra, India

Bhavana Sosale MBBS MD MRCPS
Consultant Diabetologist and Physician
Diacon Hospital
Visiting Consultant
Columbia Asia Hospital
Bengaluru, Karnataka, India

David R Campbell MD
Vascular Surgeon
Beth Israel Deaconess Medical Center
Associate Professor
Department of Surgery
Harvard Medical School
Boston, Massachusetts, USA

Florence M Brown MD
Assistant Professor
Harvard Medical School
Co-Director
Joslin and Beth Israel Deaconess Medical Center
Diabetes in Pregnancy Program
Senior Staff Physician
Joslin Diabetes Center
Boston, Massachusetts, USA

Jerry D Cavallerano OD PhD
Associate Professor
Department of Ophthalmology
Harvard Medical School
Staff Optometrist and Clinical Investigator
Beetham Eye Institute
Joslin Diabetes Center
Boston, Massachusetts, USA

Jennifer Wyckoff MD
Clinical Assistant Professor
Medical Director, Adult Diabetes Education
Co-Chair, Diabetes Quality Improvement Committee
MEND DF ACU Director
Associate Chief for Clinical Metabolism, Endocrinology, Diabetes (MEND) and Podiatry
Metabolism, Endocrinology and Diabetes
Department of Internal Medicine
University of Michigan, USA

Jothydev Kesavadev MD FRCP FACP
Chairman
Jothydev's Diabetes and Research Center
Thiruvananthapuram, Kerala, India

Karunakaran Indulekha PhD
Post-Doctoral Scientist
Institute of Medical Microbiology, Immunology and Parasitology
Universitats klinikumbonn
Sigmund-Freud-Str. 25
53127-Bonn, Germany

Manish M Bothale MD Fellowship in Diabetes
Consultant Diabetologist
Chellaram Diabetes Institute
Pune, Maharashtra, India

Medha N Munshi MD
Director, Joslin Geriatric Diabetes Programs
Beth Israel Deaconess Medical Center
Associate Professor
Department of Medicine
Harvard Medical School
Boston, Massachusetts, USA

Nandhakumar Vasu MD DNB
Associate consultant Cardiology
The Madras Medical Mission Hospital
Chennai, Tamil Nadu, India

Paolo S Silva MD
Assistant Professor
Department of Ophthalmology
Harvard Medical School
Assistant Investigator
Department of Eye Research
Staff Ophthalmologist and Assistant Chief of Telemedicine
Beetham Eye Institute
Joslin Diabetes Center
Boston, Massachusetts, USA

Parimal Lawate
MD (Medicine) DM (Gastroenterology)
Consultant Gastroenterologist
Jehangir Hospital and Deenanath Mangeshkar Hospital
Pune, Maharashtra, India

Ranjit Mohan Anjana MD PhD Dip Diab (UK) FRCP (Glasgow, Edinburgh, London) FICP FACP
Managing Director and Consultant Diabetologist
Dr Mohan's Diabetes Specialities Centre and
Madras Diabetes Research Foundation
Chennai, Tamil Nadu, India

Ranjit Unnikrishnan MD Dip Diab (UK) FRCP (London, Edinburgh, Glasgow) FICP FACP
Vice Chairman and Consultant Diabetologist
Dr Mohan's Diabetes Specialities Centre and
Madras Diabetes Research Foundation
Chennai, Tamil Nadu, India

Robert C Stanton MD
Chief
Department of Kidney and Hypertension
Joslin Diabetes Center
Associate Professor
Department of Medicine
Harvard Medical School
Boston, Massachusetts, USA

Sanjay Agarwal MD FACE
Director, Aegle Clinic - Diabetes Care
Head, Department of Medicine
Ruby Hall Clinic
Sr. Consultant in Diabetes and Medicine
Jehangir Hospital
Pune, Maharashtra, India

S Mullasari Ajit MD DM
Director Cardiology
The Madras Medical Mission Hospital
Chennai, Tamil Nadu, India

Sunil Sathe MD DM
Senior Consultant Cardiologist
Ruby Hall Clinic
Pune, Maharashtra, India

Viswanathan Mohan
MD FRCP (London, Edinburgh, Glasgow, Ireland) PhD DSc (Hon. Causa) FNASc FASc FNA FACP FACE FTWAS MACP
Chairman and Chief Diabetologist
Dr Mohan's Diabetes Specialities Centre
WHO Collaborating Centre for Noncommunicable Diseases Prevention and Control
IDF Centre of Excellence in Diabetes Care
President and Chief of Diabetes Research
Madras Diabetes Research Foundation
ICMR Center for Advanced Research on Diabetes
Chennai, Tamil Nadu, India

Preface

Writing of this Atlas was started with the idea that most textbooks of diabetes mellitus had too much research and not enough clinical information for the daily work of a physician. For that reason, we, the Editors, tried to find authors who are seeing patients in each one of their specialties everyday. Every chapter was written with the idea of how to explain each particular subject to a busy physician in a clear and concise manner.

We also wanted to give a more universal view to our Atlas, and hence we included authors from different parts of the world or with international know how, because we hope, that this will be of help to many physicians in many countries.

As you all know diabetes mellitus keeps increasing everywhere. At the same time, science and clinical research in parallel runs a more rapid pace than in the past, which may lead to gaps in knowledge for the practicing physician. Having a handy Atlas such as this, we hope, will help to keep them uptodate. Physicians are now under more pressures, many absolutely bureaucratic, and we barely have the time to do our clinical work. It has been said that "Time is money". For practicing physicians and doctors "Time is health" and being able to solve clinical problems rapidly with an Atlas like ours should be of help.

We had many challenges in the preparation of the Atlas, but our authors overcame all of them, and we are honored to be able to present it to you today. It is only the first one. We hope to publish in the future other similar, practical textbooks to cover the entire subject of diabetes. At the same time, based on the response that we will certainly receive from many readers, we are planning to have subsequent edition of this Atlas in future.

We invite the readers to let us know their comments, ideas, suggestions, additions and critics of our work at the email "agarwalclinic@gmail.com; arolla@comcast.net". It will certainly help us to better prepare the future editions.

Arturo R Rolla
Sanjay Agarwal

Acknowledgments

Clinical Atlas of Diabetes Mellitus has been a memorable journey. It was a pleasure to work on the book during the entire course of its compilation.

It all began with my meeting over dinner with Dr Arturo R Rolla on a windy night in Boston. During our friendly banter, we realized that there were very few books which taught diabetes through pictures and algorithms. The idea to compile such a book germinated from the meeting and we promised to look at our own archives to see whether we could write one.

It is always difficult to put together such a book because very few clinicians take pictures of clinical conditions and catalog them. To add tables, flow diagrams and points of view are difficult because you need to have an in-depth knowledge of the subject. We were very fortunate to be joined by our contributing authors, who authorities in their areas of expertise, have written brilliant chapters. The book is a must read by any practicing clinician who treats diabetes. The ideas and concepts have been written with great clarity and learning has been facilitated with pictures where possible. We thank all the authors for their humongous effort and time to write these chapters.

I would like to thank Dr Arturo R Rolla, who has been the soul of the book and with his direction and vision this book has been made possible to publish.

I would also like to thank all our families for giving us time to write every chapter of this book. They are our inspiration.

My final acknowledgement goes to the entire team of M/s Jaypee Brothers Medical Publishers (P) Ltd, New Delhi, India, who worked very hard to put together such an attractive compilation. The book will be proudly kept on our table for reference.

Contents

CHAPTER 1

Diabetes: Diagnosis and Classification

Arturo R Rolla

When Aretaeus of Cappadocian described and coined the term "diabetes", he was describing excessive urination (*"...it is impossible to put any restraint to the patient's drinking or making water")*. Nowadays diabetes means increased levels of blood glucose, the marker of many different diseases with different etiologies and mechanisms that have in common hyperglycemia and, in many cases, the long-term consequences of the disease. By now, high levels of blood sugar are easily treated and it is very rare to die directly from it, but the consequences of uncontrolled diabetes and its associated problems result in a large number of blindness, renal failure, amputations, and especially cardiovascular problems. Diabetes is bad because it is diabetes but it is worse because of the bad companies it keeps!

The diagnosis of diabetes mellitus-1 (DM-1) is usually straight forward because the blood sugar levels are quite high, has a rapid onset, and the patients are symptomatic. DM-2, on the other hand, has an insidious onset, mostly asymptomatic, and frequently is an incidental finding during a routine physical examination (Box 1.1). The transition from normal to pre-diabetes and then to established diabetes is slow and may have improvements and aggravations over the years. During this gradual aggravation of the metabolic process, some of the complications including the cardiovascular may have already started even though the diagnostic glycemic levels may not have been reached, or have not been found. These diagnostic criteria are general

Box 1.1: Diagnostic criteria for the diagnosis of diabetes (ADA).

- A1c equal or above 6.5%, performed with a method standardized to the DCCT assay

or

- Fasting blood glucose equal or above 126 mg/dL (7.0 mmol/L) with no caloric intake for at least 8 hours

or

- 2 hour post-prandial blood glucose equal or above 200 mg/dL (11.1 mmol/L) during an oral glucose tolerance test, after a glucose load of 75 g of anhydrous glucose dissolved in water

or

- In a patient with classic symptoms of hyperglycemia or hyperglycemic crisis, a random plasma glucose of more than 200 mg/dL (11.1 mmol/L)
- In the absence of unequivocal hyperglycemia the results should confirmed by repeat testing.

guidelines indicating important steps in the pathogenesis of diabetes but the patient has to be considered as a whole—not just an isolated blood glucose value—contemplating also past medical and family history, associated conditions, and cardiovascular risk factors (Box 1.2). In patients at risk the time for medical intervention should be much earlier that in the past.

The diagnostic criteria at the present time are based on the determination of fasting plasma glucose level, glycohemoglobin A1c, and/or less common, an oral glucose tolerance test (OGTT). Each one of these methods has advantages and disadvantages, with variable clinical acceptance depending on their availability and reliability in different parts of the world. Thiazide diuretics, glucocorticoids and atypical antipsychotic medications should be taken into consideration while performing these tests.

Fasting plasma glucose can be obtained with dependable results in most of the world, but note that for diagnostic purposes the plasma glucose must be measured in a laboratory with well calibrated instruments. Home glucose meters measure whole blood glucose and have a variability range of 10–15% or more in the same sample so that they are absolutely not recommended for diagnosis, and they should be used only for glycemic control. It may sound redundant but we urge you to find the best available laboratory to do these tests, and it is always wise to repeat the test on a different day - and may be in a different laboratory. The fasting plasma glucose is a direct indication of the hepatic glucose production that occurs during the night and with the "Dawn phenomenon", which are exaggerated because of insulin resistance at the level of the liver.

The advantages and disadvantages of fasting plasma glucose are listed in the Table 1.1.

Glycohemoglobin A1c: Initially, after its standardization, it seemed to be a better and more simple test to diagnose diabetes but it was later found to be not as sensitive as the fasting plasma glucose determination. There are about 30% of patients with elevated fasting plasma glucose

Box 1.2: Criteria for testing in individuals at increased risk (Modified from American Diabetes Association).

- Overweight (BMI > 25 kg/m^2 or >23 kg/m^2 in Asians)
- Sedentary life
- First degree relative with diabetes
- High-risk ethnicity (Asians, African Americans, Latinos, Pacific islanders)
- Women who delivered a baby weighing > 9 lb (4 kg)
- Women with history of gestational diabetes
- Hypertension or therapy for hypertension
- HDL cholesterol < 35 mg/dL (0.90 mmol/L)
- Fasting triglycerides > 250 mg/dL (2.82 mmol/L)
- Women with polycystic ovaries
- Previous A1c > 5.7%, impaired glucose tolerance or impaired fasting glucose
- Conditions associated with insulin resistance (Obesity, acanthosis nigricans)
- History of cardiovascular disease
- Peripheral neuropathy of unknown cause
- For all individuals, particularly if they are overweight or obese, testing would began at age 45 years. If the results are normal, testing should be repeated at a minimum of 3 years
- Individuals with prediabetes or at high-risk should be tested yearly along with a re-evaluation of their risk factors and lifestyle

Table 1.1: Advantages and disadvantages of fasting plasma glucose.

Advantages	*Disadvantages*
▪ Technically very simple ▪ Extensive experience and standardization ▪ Availability all over the world ▪ Inexpensive ▪ Criteria are well known and accepted ▪ Correlations with complications are well established	▪ Requires fasting for at least 8 hours (Not always done by the patients) ▪ May need an extra visit ▪ Value reflects only one metabolic moment ▪ Acute illness may increase values ▪ Many technical variables (Time to perform, intra-specimen and day to day variations) ▪ Does not represent prandial values

Table 1.2: Advantages and disadvantages of glycohemoglobin A1c.

Advantages	*Disadvantages*
▪ Standardized by the diabetes control and complication trial (DCCT) ▪ May be obtained at any time of the day ▪ Does not require fasting ▪ Less biological variability ▪ More stable in a vial ▪ An index of 3 months of previous glycemic control ▪ Represents both fasting and post-prandial levels ▪ Not affected by acute illness ▪ Criteria well known and accepted ▪ Proven association with control and complications	▪ Not available in certain parts of the world ▪ More expensive ▪ Not reliable with some hemoglobinopathies, anemias, transfusions, and variable half-life of red blood cells in circulation ▪ Hypo and hyper "glycators", higher values in African-Americans ▪ Lower levels in advanced renal disease ▪ Not validated for children and adolescents

who have a hemoglobin A1c less than 6.5%. On the other hand, it is quite specific, and in most clinical situations it has very rare false positives. One advantage is that it represents the previous glycemic levels of about three months. This becomes very useful in situations of hyperglycemias found in acutely ill patients (Infections, acute myocardial infarctions, surgery, trauma etc.) who were not known to have diabetes (Table 1.2). The differential diagnosis is between an unknown diabetes of longer duration, or an acute "stress" diabetes. If the level of hemoglobin A1c is elevated it indicates that the patient has had diabetes in the past. If the level of A1c is normal it becomes a clear indication of acute "stress" diabetes. But, there are some disadvantages also which are listed in the Table 1.2.

The process of hemoglobin glycation is non-enzymatic and depends on the level of hyperglycemia, time, and a less known factor that is the rate of glycation of each protein. The longer the red cells stay in circulation and the higher the glycemic levels, the higher the A1c. The attachment of glucose to the hemoglobin seem to be different in some individuals, and there "High Glycators" (Highher A1c levels for the same levels of glycemia) and "Low Glycators" (Table 1.3).

Table 1.3: Higher levels and lower levels of glycohemoglobin A1c.

Higher levels	*Lower levels*
▪ "High glycators", African-Americans ▪ Increasing age ▪ Some hemoglobinopathies ▪ Iron and B_{12} deficiency anemias ▪ Post-splenectomy because of more prolonged half-life of the red cells. Note that this is very common after a pancreatectomy because frequently it is necessary to remove the spleen during this surgery ▪ Systemic inflammation (CRP, neutrophil and monocyte elevations) ▪ Alcoholism ▪ Chronic renal failure ▪ Hyperbilirubinemia ▪ Large doses of aspirin ▪ Chronic opiate use	▪ "Low glycators", probably genetic ▪ Shortened red blood cell half-life, hemolytic anemias ▪ Acute anemias with high reticulocyte count ▪ Erythropoietin administration ▪ Some hemoglobinopathies ▪ Antiretrovirals and dapsone ▪ Hipertriglyceridemia (Technical problem in the assay)

Oral Glucose Tolerance Test (OGTT): It is still used in some parts of the world as the gold standard for the diagnosis of DM-2, and is routinely used for the diagnosis of gestational diabetes (Although with a different technique). Again, the measurements should be as plasma glucose, and done with laboratory equipment. It is very sensitive, and gives a very good idea of both fasting and post-prandial levels but it requires a prolonged visit, at least two venipunctures and the ingestion of a standardized glucose load of 75 g. Usually two samples are obtained, fasting and two hours. Plasma glucose levels at one hour are usually not necessary since they are highly variable according to the rate of gastric emptying. Blood sugar levels two hours after a glucose load are mostly related to the prandial insulin secretion of the beta cells, particularly to the first phase that normally prepares the cells to take up the carbohydrates coming from the intestinal absorption. Occasionally, patients become nauseated and are unable to drink the entire volume, or they start vomiting. In these cases, the test should be stopped and repeated two or three weeks later.

Each test has advantages, disadvantages and pitfalls so that they have to be utilized according to the patient and their availability and reliability in every part of the world (Table 1.4). With any of the tests if the results are inconclusive or the patient is at high-risk, it is important to repeat the same test or obtain another one to confirm or not the diagnosis. Even with one positive diagnostic test, it is recommended to obtain a confirmation with the same or one of the other tests.

PREDIABETES

DM-1 is preceded by a prediabetic state that may last for several years, and is only diagnosed by checking the specific autoantibodies. Not all the individuals with positive antibodies will develop this form of diabetes. The more positive antibodies, the more the likelihood of developing DM-1.

Table 1.4: Advantages and disadvantages of the oral glucose tolerance test.

Advantages	***Disadvantages***
▪ Well standardized ▪ Very sensitive ▪ Measures both fasting and postprandial levels ▪ May be positive even when the fasting plasma glucose is normal (Abnormal Glucose Tolerance)	▪ Requires fasting- More inconvenience for the patient, (Prolonged visit, repeated venipunctures, nausea or vomiting with the glucose drink) ▪ Day-to-day variability ▪ More expensive ▪ Gastrointestinal factors (Gastrectomy, gastroparesis, malabsorption, etc.)

Box 1.3: Diagnostic criteria for prediabetes.

- Fasting plasma glucose: 100–125 mg/dL (5.6–6.9 mmol/L) (Impaired fasting glucose)
- Two hour plasma glucose: 140–199 mg/dL (7.8–11 mmol/L)
- Glycohemoglobin: 5.7–6.4%

DM-2 also has a very prolonged and asymptomatic prediabetic stage that is characterized by insulin resistance and beta cell hypersecretion initially completely euglycemic. The progression from normoglycemia to dysglycemia may be faster for certain ethnic groups like Asian-Indians. Once the process of beta cell fatigue ensues—usually starting with the loss of the first phase of prandial secretion—progressive increases in glycemic levels appear. There are fluctuations in these metabolic parameters but, if there are no lifestyle or therapeutic interventions, the glycemic levels slowly increase to attain diagnostic levels. Lifestyle modifications, especially weight loss, at this stage can prevent the progression towards diabetes, but they are not easy to implement and maintain over the years. Earlier screening and diagnose permits better results in prevention and in future treatments. Also, the higher the levels of any of these tests there is a continuous increase in the risk of new diabetes.

Diagnostic criteria for prediabetes are discussed in the Box 1.3.

IMPAIRED GLUCOSE TOLERANCE

Impaired glucose tolerance is a prediabetic stage characterized by a 2-hour plasma glucose level between 140 and 199 mg/dL (7.8 and 11 mmol/L) during an OGTT. It indicates a failure of the beta cell secretion after a meal, particularly a decrease or absence in the first phase, and accompanied also by delayed hypersecretion due to the persistent post-prandial hyperglycemia.

WARNING

DM-2 attracts and potentiates cardiovascular risk factors—even before it is diagnosed!

Impaired fasting glucose is diagnosed when the fasting levels are between 100 and 125 mg/dL (5.6-6.9 mmol/L) and it represents mostly inappropriately increased hepatic glucose production during an overnight fast. It is not uncommon for patients with DM-2 after the disease has been diagnosed to have fasting glucose levels that are higher than during the rest of the day ("Reverse diabetes"). This explains why the determination of fasting glucose levels is so sensitive for the diagnosis of diabetes. Individuals with impaired fasting or glucose tolerance have a risk of developing new diabetes at a rate of 5–10% per year. The risk is even greater when both abnormalities are present. Nevertheless, impaired glucose tolerance tends to be more frequent, and has a greater association with cardiovascular mortality later on.

Increased glycohemoglobin A1c: Prediabetes may also be diagnosed with levels of A1c between 5.7 and 6.4%, with the risk increasing with values closer to 6.5%. Again, the determination of A1c is not as sensitive as the other methods for the diagnosis of prediabetes.

Our scientific knowledge has progressed enormously with the new tools of genetics and molecular biology in the last few years but we still have a lot to learn. With the discovery of the genomic sequence many of us thought that we soon will be able to understand the predisposition, causes and mechanisms of many common conditions. So far, only very few, uncommon, usually monogenic, diseases have been elucidated leaving the majority of the common clinical problems we see daily in our clinics and hospitals still without clear explanations. We desperately need ways to understand the different types and etiologies of the diabetes that today we simply classify as type 1 and type 2. In particular, we urgently need simple methods to quantify insulin resistance and beta cell mass in our patients to be able to direct our treatments according to the particular mechanisms that are abnormal in each patient.

An important stimulus to try to diagnose diabetes earlier has to do with the protection of the beta cells. Blood glucose control is much better and easier when there is a considerable residual mass of beta cells in the pancreatic islets able to secrete variable amounts of insulin. The more functioning beta cells the less hyper- and hypoglycemia our patients will have. Aging, glucose toxicity, chronic hypersecretion, fatigue and apoptosis keeps decreasing the viable beta cells in the pancreas day by day. In DM-1, we have to add the autoimmune attack or insulitis. The earlier we intervene to normalize the blood glucose levels and avoid the fatigue caused by the constant hypersecretion the more beta cells that we save for the future. At the same time—even though we still do not know exactly the mechanisms—euglycemia improves insulin resistance, which in turn helps to put the beta cells to rest decreasing their tendency to fatigue. Recent epidemiological studies in Europe have shown that earlier diagnosis and intervention are more important than the improvements later obtained in glycemia, blood pressure and lipid control.

Prevention and early diagnosis: We all know that the best treatment is prevention but at the present time we are still waiting too long to diagnose and treat DM-2. It is relatively easy for an experienced physician to forecast the appearance of hyperglycemia in an obese, sedentary individual with a strong family history of diabetes, several components of the metabolic syndrome, polycystic ovaries, or with a past history of gestational diabetes. Approximately, 50% of persons with DM-2 around the world are undiagnosed. Why do we have to wait for the blood glucose or the glycohemoglobin A1c to increase above an arbitrary level when we know that at the time of the diagnosis of type 2 diabetes half of the patients (in developed countries where they have more frequent medical encounters and interventions) already have signs and symptoms of chronic complications and the blood vessels show already changes of arterio-sclerosis?

WARNING

We desperately need a simple method to measure the beta cell mass and insulin resistance in our patients

BIBLIOGRAPHY

1. American Diabetes Association: Classification and diagnosis of diabetes. Diabetes Care. 2015;38 (Suppl 1):S8.
2. Anjana RM, Shanthi Rani CS, Deepa M, et al. Incidence of diabetes and prediabetes and predictors of progression among Asian Indians: 10 year follow-up of the Chennai Urban Rural Epidemiology Study (CURES). Diabetes Care. 2015:38:1441-8.
3. Gallagher EM, Le Roith D, Bloomgarden Z. Review of hemoglobin A1c in the management of diabetes. J of Diabetes. 2009;1(1):9-17.
   An excellent review of all the technical and biological variations in the measurement of A1c
4. Herman WH, Ye W, Griffin SJ, et al. Early detection and treatment of type 2 diabetes reduce cardiovascular morbidity and mortality: A simulation of the results of the Anglo-Danish-Dutch Study of Intensive Treatment in people with screen-detected diabetes in primary care (ADDITION-Europe). Diabetes Care. 2015;38:1449-55.
5. Higgins T. HbA1c for screening and diagnosis of diabetes mellitus. Endocrine. 2013;43:266.
6. Inzucchi SE. Diagnosis of diabetes. N Engl J Med. 2012;367(6):542-50.
   A complete review of the tests and criteria of the diagnosis.
7. Lotta LA, Gulati P, Day FR, et al. Integrative genomic analysis implicates limited peripheral adipose storage capacity in the pathogenesis of human insulin resistance. Nat Genet. 2017;49(1):17-26.
   A genome-wide study of a very large population looking for insulin resistance.
8. Rockl S, Brinks R, Baumert J, et al. All-cause mortality in adults with and without type 2 diabetes: Findings from the national health monitoring in Germany. BMJ Open Diabetes Res Care. 2017;5(1):e000451.
9. Venkat Narayan KM, Gujral UN. Evidence tips the scale toward screening for hyperglycemia. Diabetes Care. 2015;38:1399-401.

CHAPTER 2

Type 2 Diabetes: Pathogenesis

Arturo R Rolla

INTRODUCTION

Diabetes type 2 is a multifactorial, complex, heterogeneous, both hereditary and acquired, and progressive disease associated with many cardiovascular risk factors. The main clinical characteristic is hyperglycemia but the most serious long-term complication is increased cardiovascular mortality. In a way, we could say that type 2 diabetes is a cardiovascular disease that starts with high blood sugar levels. This concept is very important to understand the basics of the treatment of this condition that requires "Multicontrol" (Lipids, weight and blood pressure) above and beyond the glycemic control.

"Type 2 diabetes is bad because it is hyperglycemic but it is worse because of the bad companies it keeps" (*Cardiovascular Risk factors*)

PATHOGENESIS

The two most important pathogenic factors are: Insulin resistance and Islet cell dysfunction (Beta and alpha cells). Both factors are sine-qua-non to develop diabetes type 2, but the pathogenic contribution of both factors vary in each patient. There are patients that have more insulin resistance, and others that have more islet cell dysfunction (Fig. 2.1). The problem in identifying these pathogenic varieties is that, at this time, we do not have simple clinical ways of measuring insulin resistance and islet cell function in each patient, even though this knowledge could influence the type of treatment we could use in different patients with type 2 diabetes. Measurements of serum insulin or C-peptide levels are usually not helpful in the diagnosis of an individual patient.

Insulin Resistance

It has both hereditary and acquired factors, but the most important one is obesity. We can even consider type 2 diabetes as a frequent complication of obesity. At the same time, we should remember that obesity also has hereditary and acquired factors that are not completely

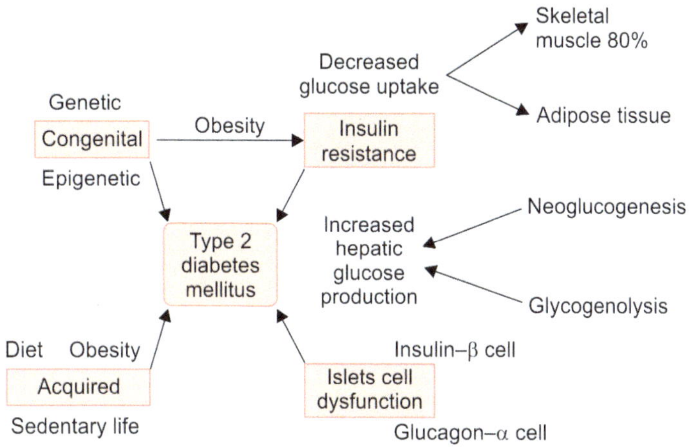

Fig. 2.1: Pathogenesis of diabetes type 2.

understood. Both the prevention and treatment of obesity have a great impact in type 2 diabetes. The great majority of cases of insulin resistance we see clinically are multifactorial and mostly associated with obesity. A very small percentage of patients have single pathogenic factors, most of them congenital (Leprechaunism, Rabson Mendenhall syndrome, lipodystrophies, etc.) but some may be acquired (Type B severe insulin resistance syndrome caused by antibodies against the insulin receptor). Another form of acquired insulin resistance with lipodystrophy may be seen in patients with HIV infection taking antiretroviral medications.

There are no simple clinical methods to determine the presence and severity of insulin resistance in our patients at the present time. On the other hand, there are two skin signs that are indicative of chronic insulin resistance: Acanthosis nigricans and skin tags (Ver chapter on Skin Lesions). Unfortunately, they are not always present in all the insulin-resistant individuals, especially in those with very light skin.

> "In biology everything is both hereditary and acquired"
>
> **Arturo R Rolla** MD

There is no linear relationship between the severity of obesity (Body weight, IMC and even fat mass) and the development of type 2 diabetes. The impact of obesity on insulin resistance in each person can be quite variable. There are obese individuals who are not insulin resistant ("Fat but fit"), and there are individuals that are of normal or moderately increased weight that may develop type 2 diabetes because they have increased insulin resistance, usually on a hereditary basis (Fig. 2.2). And not every obese individual with insulin resistance will develop type 2 diabetes; only those with the second pathogenic factor, islet cell dysfunction, will do so.

The influence of obesity on insulin resistance depends on the adipose distribution and the translocation of the fatty acids outside of the adipocytes. Many epidemiological studies over the years have shown that accumulation of fat in abdomen and trunk—as opposed to the subcutaneous tissue—has a more deleterious effect on the insulin effect ("Abdominal or truncal obesity"), usually determined as "abdominal girth". Not only the fat distribution is a diabetic pathogenic factor of obesity but also the "capacitance" of the adipose mass is important.

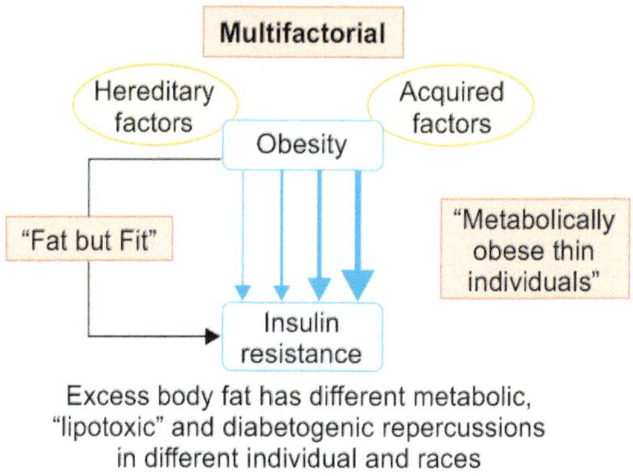

Fig. 2.2: Variable relationship between obesity and insulin resistance.

Adipose capacitance depends on the number and "distensibility" of the fat cells in the body. The larger the capacity of the adipocytes to store fatty acids, the lesser the translocation of fatty acids to non-adipocytic tissues, like the liver and skeletal muscle, the two main target organs of the insulin effect. When the adipose capacitance is overpassed by the amount of fatty acids accumulated, there is a translocation (or "overflow") to non-adipose tissues that makes them less sensitive to the insulin effect. Unknown hereditary factors that predispose to a decreased adipose capacitance will increase the fatty acid translocation to non-adipose tissues and will cause insulin resistance even with a normal body weight.[1] The best example of this is the patients with lipoatrophic diabetes. The opposite happens in individuals who are obese but do not have a marked increase in insulin resistance ("Fat but Fit"), probably because of better adipose capacitance and distribution.

The factors that determine the number and "distensibility" (capacity of each cell of storing more fatty acids) of the adipocytes are not well known but most likely are also determined by hereditary factors. An individual with a decreased adipose capacitance may then develop insulin resistance and type 2 diabetes at a much lower body weight. Again, at the present time, we do not have simple clinical ways of measuring fat mass and its distribution, although the BMI and waist circumference may give us a good approximation.

Another characteristic of the adipose tissue that may predispose or not to insulin resistance is the presence and activity of brown fat. There are several factors that determine the "protective" effect of brown fat, but the most important seem to be the hereditary ones. In general, the more brown fat in the body the less tendency to obesity and type 2 diabetes. Increased amounts of body fat also tend to cause a chronic inflammation of the adipose tissue (Adipositis), completely asymptomatic that tends to increase the adipocytic lipolysis and translocation of fatty acids to other organs. This adipositis also tends to cause a systemic inflammatory state through the liberation of cytokines to the circulation. Both effects of this adipositis lead to increase the resistance to insulin and the blood sugar levels (Table 2.1).

Some congenital factors for both type 2 diabetes and obesity may also be epigenetic. Low birth weight for gestational age, and probably infantile malnutrition, cause changes in the chromatin methylation that alters the expression of the DNA that predispose to adiposity and diabetes later on life, especially if the individual is later exposed to a hypercaloric environment.

Table 2.1: Factors that may influence the impact of obesity on insulin resistance.

- Genetics
- Epigenetics and low birth weight
- Number and activity of mitochondrias
- Types of adipocytes (Brown, white, transformation to beige)
- Adipose tissue distribution (Subcutaneous vs. abdominal)
- Adipocytic capacitance and translocation of Fatty Acids to non-adipocytic cells
- Inflammation: Adipositis
- Adipokines' secretion and effect

The dietary influence on top of the hereditary (and epigenetic) factors became more evident in a recent study where they administered a high fat, hypercaloric diet to similar weight Indian and Dutch young men. Insulin resistance appeared only in the Indian individuals.[2]

The exact mechanism of the induction of insulin resistance by the fatty acid translocation is not completely clear at the present time. It has been clearly shown that in most cases it is not at the level of the insulin receptor GLUT4 ("Post Receptor Resistance"), and it seems to be caused by an accumulation of di-acyl glycerol and ceramide in the insulin target cells. Decreased glucose uptake in the muscle due to ectopic fatty acid accumulation appears to be the first mechanism. It diverts glucose to the liver resulting in hepatic insulin resistance, increased de novo lipogenesis and dyslipidemia.[3,4]

Both fatty acid translocation to non-adipocytic tissues and the systemic effects of the adipositis contribute to cause insulin resistance but the fact is that the most severe cases of insulin resistance seen clinically are in patients with generalized lipoatrophy where the adipocytic mass and capacitance are severely diminished with massive ectopic accumulation of fatty acids and there is no adipositis. Of course, any other cause of increased insulin resistance, like infections, endocrinopathies or corticoid therapy, chronically may also cause insulin resistance, or acutely aggravate it.

The consequences of insulin resistance that lead to hyperglycemia are decreased glucose uptake, mostly in muscle and adipose tissue, and increased hepatic glucose production. Other consequences are encompassed as the Metabolic Syndrome, and include abdominal obesity, fatty liver, hypertension, dyslipidemia, polycystic ovaries and acanthosis nigricans (Fig. 2.3). An important clinical aspect is that both the lipotoxicity from the translocation of fatty acids and the glucotoxicity from the hyperglycemia increase the islet cell dysfunction and the insulin resistance. Weight loss by any method improve both, islet cell dysfunction and insulin resistance.[5] From an strictly clinical point of view, insulin resistance have three main pathogenic components: Genetic, obesity, and glucotoxicity once diabetes type 2 appears (Fig. 2.4). Insulin resistance may be improved with weight loss (Diet and exercise or bariatric surgery), insulino-mimetic drugs (Metformin and thiazolidinediones) and glycemic control (Decreasing glucotoxicity).

Islet Cell Dysfunction

Both beta and alpha cells are involved in the pathogenesis of type 2 diabetes, with the decrease in beta cell function being most important, and the increased glucagon secretion from the

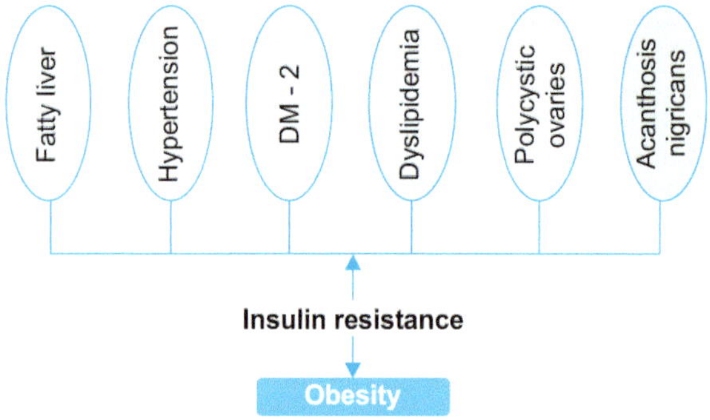

Fig. 2.3: Metabolic syndrome.

The Three "Clinical" Components of Insulin Resistance

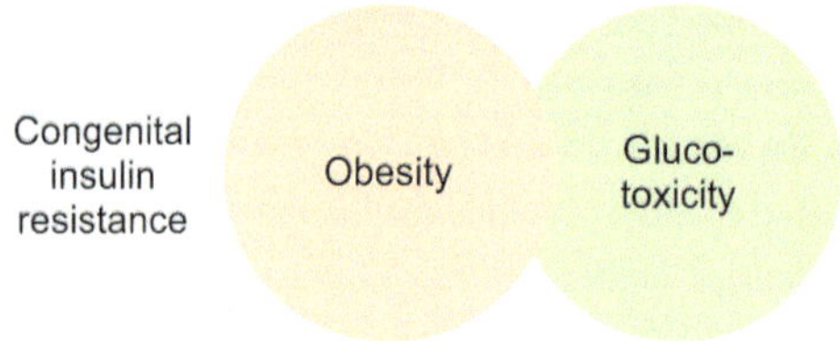

Fig. 2.4: Clinical components of insulin resistance.

alpha cells having a complementary importance. During the years of progressively increasing insulin resistance there is an increase in the beta cell mass with a compensatory increase in insulin secretion. In some individuals (not all) a "second hit" occurs after years of hypersecretion when the beta cells decrease the compensatory hypersecretion, and start becoming progressively more "fatigued". The time of lack of compensatory hypersecretion usually marks the beginning of hyperglycemia, usually in the postprandial period ("Glucose intolerance"). From then on there is a slowly progression of the hyperglycemia, while the insulin resistance increases less in severity. Pathological studies in humans have shown that initially the beta cell mass is increased, but later a progressive decrease appears, which is due to an increased rate of beta cell apoptosis and dedifferentiation plus an inappropriate rate of beta cell regeneration.[6,7]

> "Type 2 diabetes is a progressive disease that becomes more and more hyperglycemic every year because of the increasing fatigue of the beta cells"

Eventually the decrease in beta cell mass and function goes from relative deficiency (insulin levels more or less normal but unable to compensate for the insulin resistance) to an absolute deficiency with insulinopenia that requires insulin administration (Fig. 2.5). For this reason, it is important to tell the patients at the time of the diagnosis that their type 2 diabetes will be able to be controlled with diet, exercise and oral agents but eventually they will require insulinotherapy. In this way, when the time comes, the patients do not have feelings of guilt or of "end of the road" with the new treatment.

The earlier changes in beta cell dysfunction can only be shown in experimental settings, and are the loss of the first phase of postprandial insulin secretion, decrease in the normal

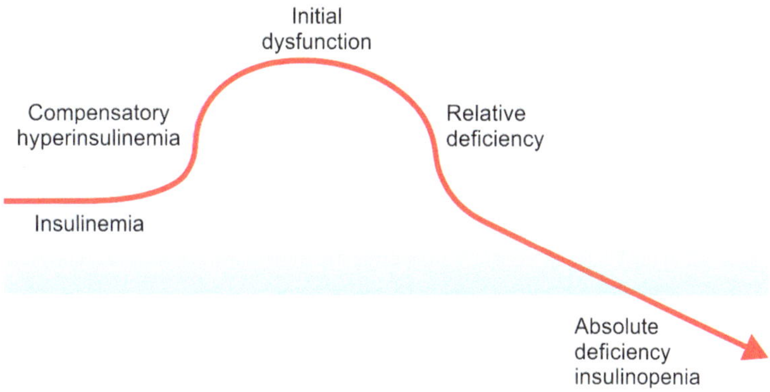

Fig. 2.5: Beta cell dysfunction and progressive fatigue.

secretory pulses, and an increase in the proportion of C-peptide secreted. Decreased first phase of postprandial insulin secretion may also be found in nondiabetic relatives. For years, it was thought that the loss of this first phase of postprandial secretion was irreversible in these patients. With the advent of bariatric surgery and other methods of weight loss it was found that it may reappear almost back to normal.

- Chronic insulin resistance sets the stage but hyperglycemia does not start until beta cell dysfunction starts
- From then on, the "tempo" of the progression of the type 2 diabetes depends on the mass and function of the beta cells

The concept of beta cell mass or function is clinically very important because as the years pass it continues to diminish, and type 2 diabetes becomes more hyperglycemic, requires more treatments, and eventually it goes on to require insulin treatment. The more functioning beta cells the easier the glycemic control with less hyper- and hypoglycemias. A corollary of these pathophysiologic concepts is that we should try to preserve the beta cell mass as much as possible, and this is achieved by earlier diagnosis of type 2 diabetes and glucose intolerance states, weight loss and glycemic control to prevent the glucotoxic effect on the beta cells. Insulin hypersecretion seems to accelerate the beta cell "fatigue" so medications that decrease insulin resistance (and decrease the compensatory insulin hypersecretion), like metformin and the thiazolidinediones tend to maintain glycemic control longer than oral agents that increase insulin secretion, like the sulfonylureas.

Hyperglycemia begets more hyperglycemia because the glucotoxicity increases both insulin resistance and beta cell fatigue in a *"hyperglycemic vicious cycle"*

It was known for many years that significant weight loss during the initial stages of type 2 diabetes was able to normalize the glycemic levels for as long the weight loss lasted. Several surprises appeared later, especially with bariatric surgeries. After gastric bypass surgery, before any weight loss is obtained there is a marked improvement in beta cell function with normalization of the blood glucose levels in patients with type 2 diabetes of short duration

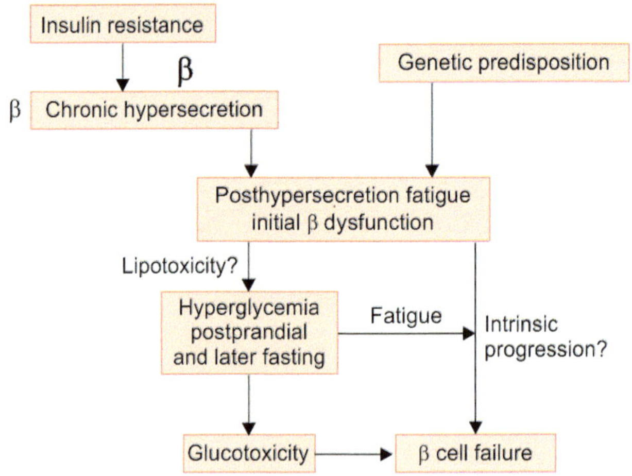

Fig. 2.6: Algorithmic approach to type 2 diabetes progression.

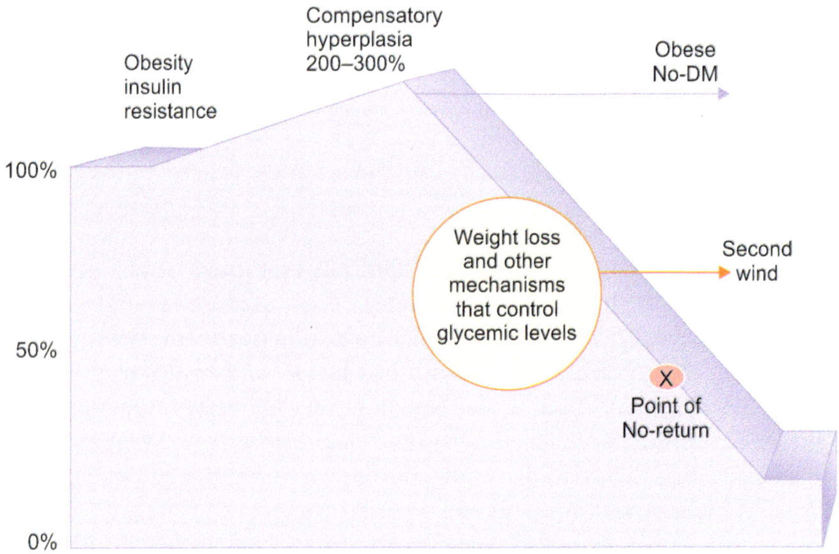

Fig. 2.7: β cell mass and function recovery in type 2 diabetes.

(around three years). In many of them there is reappearance of the first phase of prandial insulin secretion and an increase in overall beta cell secretion as well. The exact mechanisms of this "Second Wind" is still unclear.[8,9] It was also shown to occur after weight loss obtained with severe caloric restriction,[10,11] and in Chinese patients with short-term intensive glucose control with insulin and oral agents. If the weight loss is obtained later on in the course of the disease, when the beta cell mass or function is severely limited the "Second Wind" does not appear, or is very attenuated indicating that there appears to be a "Point of no return" in the recovery of the beta cells (Fig. 2.7).

The differential diagnosis of type 2 diabetes must always be kept in mind, especially at the time of the initial diagnosis. Maturity onset diabetes of the young (MODY), latent autoimmune diabetes of adults (LADA), and secondary forms of DM should be considered, and the appropriate tests should be obtained when there is a clinical suspicion of them. Older literature used to mention the presence of ketoacidosis as an unlikely finding in type 2 diabetes. At the present time, it is clear there are many clinical situation in which that can happen ("Flatbush diabetes", atypical antipsychotic agents, inhibitors of the SGLT-2, etc.)

REFERENCES

1. Yajnik CS, Yudkin JS. The Y-Y paradox. The Lancet. 2004;363:163.
2. Baker LE, Van Schinkel LD, Guigas B, et al. A 5-day high-fat, high-calorie diet impairs insulin sensitivity in healthy, young South Asian men but not in Caucasian men. Diabetes. 2014;63:248-58.
3. Samuel VT, Shulman GI. Mechanisms for insulin resistance: Common threads and missing links. Cell. 2012;148:852. *(Both articles from VT Samuels and GI Shulman are very clear and have great drawings to teach these mechanisms)*
4. Samuel VT, Shulman GI. The pathogenesis of insulin resistance: integrating pathways and substrate flux. J Clin Invest. 2016;126:12.
5. Lim EL, Hollingsworth KG, Aribisala BS, et al. Reversal of type 2 diabetes: normalization of beta cell function in association with decreased pancreas and liver triacylglycerol. Diabetologia. 2011;54:2506-14.
6. Butler A, Janson J, Bonner-Weir S, et al. Beta cell deficit and increased beta cell apoptosis in humans with type 2 diabetes. Diabetes. 2003;52:102.
7. White MG, Shaw JA, Taylor R. Type 2 diabetes: The pathological basis of reversible beta cell dysfunction. Diabetes Care. 2016;39:2080-8.
8. Goldfine AB, Patti ME. Diabetes improvement following Roux-en-Y gastric bypass: understanding dynamic changes in insulin secretion and action. Diabetes. 2014;63:1454.
9. Knop FK, Taylor R. Mechanism of metabolic advantages after bariatric surgery. Diabetes Care. 2013;36:S287.
10. Rehackova L, Arnott B, Araujo-Soares V, et al. Efficacy and acceptability of very low energy diets in overweight and obese people with type 2 diabetes mellitus: a systematic review and meta-analyses. Diabet Med. 2016;33:580-91.
11. Steven S, Hollingsworth KG, Small PK, et al. Weight loss decreases excess pancreatic triacylglycerol specifically in type 2 diabetes. Diabetes Care. 2016;39:158-65.

CHAPTER 3

Treatment of Type 2 Diabetes: Oral Agents

Bhavana Sosale, Aravind R Sosale

INTRODUCTION

Type 2 diabetes mellitus is a progressive disease, and attempts to achieve normal or near normal glycemia often requires multiple oral and or injectable agents. A strong link exists between glycemic control and prevention or reduction in progression of diabetes related complications.[1-10]

The aims of antidiabetic therapy are to:

1. Achieve glycemic targets while minimizing hypoglycemia and other adverse effects.
2. Reduce glycemic variability over time.
3. Prevent or delay the onset and progression of complications of hyperglycemia.

Classification of oral agents and the factors influencing the selection of an oral agent will be discussed in this chapter.

CLASSIFICATION OF ORAL ANTIDIABETIC DRUGS

Oral antidiabetic agents (OADs) achieve normoglycemia by addressing the different pathophysiological defects of type 2 diabetes: increasing insulin secretion, improving sensitivity to insulin, reducing hepatic glucose output, delaying and reducing carbohydrate absorption or by increasing urinary glucose excretion. The different classes are described below and have been summarized in Tables 3.1 and 3.2.[11-18]

Table 3.1: A summary of the mechanism of action and pathophysiological targets of oral antidiabetic drugs.

Class	*Mechanism of action*	*Target pathophysiology*
Biguanides	AMP kinase mediated pathways	Decrease hepatic gluconeogenesis
Thiazolidinediones	Activate PPAR gamma receptor	Improve insulin sensitivity
DPP4 inhibitors	Inhibit DPP4 enzyme, increase physiological GLP 1 levels	Increase glucose dependent insulin secretion, reduce hepatic glucagon production

Contd...

Contd...

Class	Mechanism of action	Target pathophysiology
Sulfonylureas	Close the potassium channels on the beta cell membrane	Stimulate insulin secretion
SGLT 2 inhibitors	Inhibit SGLT 2 in the proximal convoluted tubule	Block glucose reabsorption in the kidney
Alpha glucosidase inhibitors	Inhibit alpha glucosidase	Slows intestinal carbohydrate absorption and digestion
Meglitinides	Close the potassium channels on the beta cell membrane	Stimulate insulin secretion

(DPP 4: Dipeptidyl peptidase 4; SGLT 2: Sodium glucose co-transporter 2; AMP: Adenosine mono-phosphate; PPAR gamma: Peroxisome proliferator-activated receptor gamma; GLP 1: Glucagon like peptide 1)

Table 3.2: A summary of the different classes of oral antidiabetic drugs.

Class	Drugs	HbA1c reduction	Benefits	Side effects
Biguanides	Metformin	1–2%	Extensive experience Weight loss No hypoglycemia Cost Effective	Nausea Diarrhea
Thiazolidinediones	Pioglitazone	1–1.6%	No hypoglycemia Durable action	Weight gain Fluid retention Osteoporosis
DPP4 inhibitors	Sitagliptin Vildagliptin Saxagliptin Linagliptin Alogliptin Teneligliptin	0.5–0.8%	Weight Neutral NO hypoglycemia	Joint pains, Possible risk of heart failure with saxagliptin
Sulfonylureas	Glyburide Gliclazide Glipizide Glimiperide	1–2%	Extensive experience Cost effective Widely available	Weight gain Hypoglycemia
SGLT 2 inhibitors	Canagliflozin Dapagliflozin Empagliflozin	0.5–1%	Weight Loss No hypoglycemia Lowering of blood pressure Cardiovascular benefits	Genital mycotic infections, UTIs Risk of fractures Euglycemic DKA
Alpha glucosidase inhibitors	Acarbose Voglibose Miglitol	0.5–0.8%	Reduces postprandial hyperglycemia	Nausea Flatulence
Meglitinides	Repaglinide Nateglinide	0.5–1%	Reduces postprandial hyperglycemia	Hypoglycemia Weight gain

(UTI: Urinary tract infection; DKA: Diabetic ketoacidosis; HbA1c: Hemoglobin A1c; DPP 4: Dipeptidyl peptidase 4; SGLT 2: Sodium glucose co-transporter 2)

Biguanides

Metformin forms the corner stone of the treatment for type 2 diabetes in the absence of a specific contraindication. It is the preferred agent while initiating pharmacotherapy. It decreases hepatic gluconeogenesis and improves insulin resistance. Its mechanism of action involves adenosine monophosphate (AMP) kinase mediated pathways and several other mechanisms which even today are yet to be completely unraveled. Its efficacy and safety is evident from long-term studies and decades of use in patient care. The expected decrease in hemoglobin A1c with metformin monotherapy is 1–2%.

It can be initiated at a dose of 500 mg once a day and up titrated to a maximum of 2000 mg per day in divided doses. Gastrointestinal side effects like nausea and diarrhea are known. Patients experiencing these effects may be given a lower dose of the drug, switched over to a sustained release preparation, and if still intolerant may be given a drug from a different class. Even though there has been no increase in lactic acidosis with the metformin, it must be discontinued prior to use of radio contrasts and if the glomerular filtration rate (GFR) falls below 45 mL/min/1.73 m^2. It may be used with caution in patients with a GFR between 30 and 45 mL/min/1.73 m^2.

Metformin can be used in combination with any other OADs or injectable therapy. Tolerability, efficacy, lack of hypoglycemia, weight loss, availability and cost effectiveness makes this drug a universal choice.[11-20]

Thiazolidinediones

Pioglitazone improves insulin sensitivity at the level of the liver, muscle and adipocyte. It acts on the peroxisome proliferator activator receptor-gamma (PPAR-γ), reduces the production of adipocytokines. In addition to reducing insulin resistance, it may also help in preserving of the pancreatic beta cell by reducing visceral fat. It improves cardiovascular risk factors like inflammatory markers, endothelial dysfunction, and carotid intima thickness and reduces the progression of atherosclerosis. Action on the PPAR-alpha receptor is minimal and may have beneficial effects on lipid metabolism, may reduce levels of serum triglyceride, low density cholesterol; improve high density cholesterol in addition to HbA1c reduction.[21]

The efficacy of pioglitazone is similar to that of metformin when used as monotherapy. Its dosing ranges from 15 mg to 45 mg per day. It reduces hemoglobin A1c by 1–1.6% from baseline when compared to placebo. Efficacy, durability, lack of hypoglycemia, cost effectiveness and the ability to target a core pathophysiologic defect in type 2 diabetes favor the use of pioglitazone in diabetes management. It can be combined with all other treatment options for diabetes.[11-18,22-26]

Side effects such as weight gain, fluid retention and fracture risk are concerns associated with this drug. The weight gain is dose dependent and due to the activation of the PPAR gamma receptor in the central nervous system. Fluid retention, increase in subcutaneous fat stores and increased food intake contribute to weight gain. The risk of increase in heart failure seen with rosiglitazone, is not seen with this drug. Researchers in observational studies report an increase in the cases of bladder cancer in patients who are exposed to high cumulative doses of pioglitazone. Hence, this drug should not be used in patients with active bladder cancer or with a previous history of bladder cancer.[27]

Alpha Glucosidase Inhibitors

Acarbose, miglitol and voglibose are drugs that reduce blood glucose by delaying and modifying intestinal carbohydrate absorption. They inhibit the alpha glucosidase enzyme which converts polysaccharides into monosaccharides and reduce postprandial glycemic excursions.

Studies report improvement in HbA1c by 0.5 to 0.8% with these agents. They are less efficacious than the other antidiabetic medications that they are often combined with. Acarbose may be initiated at 50 mg thrice a day and up titrated to 100 mg thrice a day. Voglibose can be up titrated from 0.2 mg to 0.3 mg thrice a daily. They are weight neutral; but cost, frequency of dosing and gastrointestinal side effects like nausea, flatulence and diarrhea are barriers to patient acceptance.[11-18,28-34]

Cardiovascular events were lesser with the use of acarbose in the Study to Prevent Non-Insulin-Dependent Diabetes Mellitus (STOP-NIDDM) trial. This study involved patients with impaired glucose tolerance and the findings are attributed to cardiovascular protection offered by postprandial control.[35]

Incretin-based Therapy

Oral incretin based therapies include dipeptidyl peptidase 4 inhibitors (DPP4 i) like sitagliptin, vildagliptin, saxagliptin, alogliptin, linagliptin and teneligliptin. The dipeptidyl peptidase 4 enzyme deactivates glucagon-like peptide-1 (GLP 1), a gut hormone secreted by the L cells of the small intestine in response to a meal. The addition of a DPP4 inhibitor blocks this degradation and prolongs the action of naturally occurring GLP 1; which in turn acts by enhancing glucose dependent insulin release, delays gastric emptying and inhibits glucagon release.[11-18,36-38]

All DPP4 inhibitors have modest glucose lowering ability and have shown similar efficacy in a few head to head trials and meta-analysis. This class of drugs can lower HbA1c by 0.5 to 0.8%. They are weight neutral and do not cause hypoglycemia unless when used in combination with insulin or an insulin secretagogue. Hypoglycemia has been reported rarely when used as an add on to metformin. They may be used as monotherapy or add on therapy in combination with other drugs. The dose of sitagliptin is 100 mg once a day, vildagliptin 50 mg twice a day, saxagliptin 2.5 to 5 mg once a day, alogliptin 25 mg once a day, linagliptin 5 mg once a day and teneligliptin 20 mg once a day. The dose needs to be halved in patients with renal insufficiency, with the exception of linagliptin, which needs no dosage adjustment based on the renal or hepatic function.[39-45]

Commonly reported side effects include headache and nasopharyngitis. Recent reports of increase in joint pain after the initiation of DPP4 inhibitors have led to further enquiries on the long-term safety and effect on the immune system. Effects of other DPP4 substrates are implicated in the pathogenesis of these adverse effects. Increase in bradykinin and substance P levels, form the basis of the hypothesis behind rare adverse events like angioneurotic edema, Steven Johnson syndrome and anaphylaxis. Acute pancreatitis is a reported side effect though a causal relationship has not been well established. DPP4 inhibitors must not be initiated in patients with known hypersensitivity reactions or pancreatitis and must be discontinued in patients who exhibit hypersensitivity or have an episode of acute pancreatitis.[46]

Results from long-term cardiovascular outcome trials have shown no increase in cardiac events in patients on DPP4 inhibitors. Researchers from the SAVOR TIMI-53 reported a nonsignificant increase in hospital admission due to heart failure with saxaglitpin. The TECOS study with sitagliptin showed non-inferiority compared to placebo with respect to cardiac outcomes in patients with type 2 diabetes and ischemic heart disease. Sitagliptin was thus found to be safe in patients with high cardiac risk.[47-49]

Several newer drugs belonging to this class are being studied and may soon be available across different countries. Teneligliptin and gemigliptin are other gliptins available today. Omaragliptin a DPP4 inhibitor with a longer half-life and once a week dosing regimen is currently being studied in Japan. Long-term studies to assess the safety and efficacy parameters of these newer molecules are needed.

Insulin Secretagogues

Sulfonylureas and meglitinides are two classes of glucose lowering agents, which stimulate insulin secretion. Sulfonylureas bind to the sulfonylurea receptor (SUR1), an ATP dependent potassium channel receptor present on the cell membrane of the beta cell. This binding depolarizes the cell membrane, closes the potassium channel, causes influx of calcium and stimulates insulin secretion. These drugs release insulin in a non-glucose dependent manner and are dependent on the residual beta cell function. Meglitinide analogs are structurally different from sulfonylureas. They bind to the sulfonylurea receptor at a different site and have a similar mechanism of action. They are shorter acting and have a stimulatory effect less than that of sulfonylureas.[50]

Glyburide or glibenclamide, glipizide, gliclazide and glimepiride are second generation sulfonylureas. They differ in metabolism; glyburide, gliclazide and glimepiride have longer half-lives and can be prescribed once a day. The dosing of different drugs is as follows:

- Glyburide or Glibenclamide—2.5–20 mg per day
- Glipizide—5–20 mg per day
- Gliclazide—80–360 mg per day immediate release; 30–120 mg per day extended release
- Glimepiride—1–8 mg per day.

The glucose lowering effect increases with increase in the dose and plateaus at half the maximum dose. As the maximum doses increase the risk of hypoglycemia without providing additional glycemic benefits, these higher doses are best avoided. Sulfonylureas are effective drugs, which can be used as monotherapy or in combination with other antidiabetic drugs. The expected HbA1c reduction is 1–2%. The durability lasts for a few years and most patients require additional oral medications or insulin after the initial few years. The dose of the drugs needs to be reduced in patients with mild to moderate renal impairment. Their use is contraindicated in severe renal impairment.

Meglitinide analogs or glinides like repaglinide and nateglinide may be used in patients in whom longer acting sulfonylureas are contraindicated. These drugs need to be dosed three times a day and the expected HbA1c reduction is 0.5–1%. Repaglinide is initiated at a dose of 0.5 mg before each meal and can be increased up to 4 mg. Nateglinide is given at a dose of 120 mg before each meal.

The main side effect of insulin secretagogues is hypoglycemia and weight gain. This is of concern in the elderly and in those with hepatic and renal compromise. The hypoglycemic effect in longer-acting agents like glyburide can persist for more than 24 hours. Hypoglycemia is usually shorter and less severe with meglitinides.[11-18,51-58]

Some studies have raised concerns that the use of sulfonylureas is associated with poorer outcomes due to interference with ischemic preconditioning after a myocardial infarction. Though head to head randomized trials have not been performed, newer sulfonylureas specific to the pancreatic sulfonylurea receptors (like gliclazide and glimepiride) appear to be safe and there is insufficient evidence to suggest that they may be associated with higher cardiovascular mortality. There are no long-term studies on the cardiovascular safety of glinides. The availability, efficacy and cost make sulfonylureas a mainstay of treatment in several countries.[59]

SGLT 2 Inhibitors

Sodium glucose co-transporter 2 (SGLT2) inhibitors are drugs which block the reabsorption of the filtered glucose load. They act on the SGLT 2 receptors located in the proximal convoluted tubule of the kidney and cause glycosuria. The extraglycemic benefits extend to include blood pressure lowering of 2–4 mm Hg, weight loss of 2–5 kg due to osmotic diuresis and caloric loss, visceral fat loss, decrease in uric acid and microalbuminuria. They work independently of the beta cell; can be used at any stage of diabetes provided the renal function is above a certain threshold, below which the efficacy of the drug is reduced.

Canagliflozin (100 mg and 300 mg), dapagliflozin (5 mg and 10 mg) and empagliflozin (10 mg and 25 mg) can be used as monotherapy or in combination with other glucose lowering agents. The HbA1c lowering reduction expected with the use of these drugs is 0.5–1%. Canagliflozin should be taken before the first meal of the day as it is a weak inhibitor of the SGLT1 receptor in the intestine and can reduce galactose absorption; the others can be taken at any time of the day and are dosed once a day.

Side effects such as genital mycotic infections, urinary tract infections, increased frequency of micturition, dizziness, postural hypotension, increased hunger and thirst are known. Genital mycotic infections are more common in women: treatment includes topical antifungal agents, relapses are rare. These agents are known to cause euglycemic ketoacidosis when used in patients with type 1 diabetes, patients in the postoperative period and if insulin is abruptly discontinued. These are not approved for use in patients with type 1 diabetes and must be avoided in those with recurrent urinary tract infections, genital mycotic infections and other contraindications. Some studies report a reduction in bone densitometry and an increased risk of fractures with the use of canagliflozin, due to increase in phosphate reabsorption.

The results of the cardiovascular outcome study with empagliflozin and canagliflozin showed a significant reduction in death from cardiovascular causes in the group on empagliflozin versus placebo. There was a reduction in the hospitalization rates due to heart failure. These changes were attributed to the weight loss, osmotic diuretic effect, blood pressure lowering and possible changes in endothelial dysfunction with empagliflozin. The cardiovascular safety trials of dapagliflozin is underway and the results will indicate if the cardiac benefits can be considered to be a class effect.[11-18,60-70]

CHOOSING THE ORAL ANTIDIABETIC AGENT

Pharmacological therapy should be initiated at the time of diagnosis of type 2 diabetes. A patient, centric approach, which incorporates the following, must be considered while choosing glucose lowering agents[11-18,71-77] (Table 3.3).

Combination Therapy

There are very few head-to-head trials which compare the effect of different drugs as add on to metformin. Results from meta-analysis suggest that the addition of each new group of drugs reduces HbA1c by 0.9 to 1.1%. A second drug may be added after 3 months of monotherapy if the HbA1c target is not reached. Initiation of dual therapy or triple therapy may be considered if the HbA1c is > 7.5% and > 9 % respectively. Insulin may be considered when the HbA1c is > 9%; if the patient has symptoms of hyperglycemia or when immediate glycemic control is needed (Flowchart 3.1). Therapy may later be down titrated to maintain normoglycemia as the blood sugar levels decrease. The selection of the antidiabetic drug for combination therapy should be based on the patient-centric approach discussed earlier. This is supported by the clinical practice recommendations of the American Diabetes Association, the European Association for the Study of Diabetes (ADA/EASD Position Statement) and the American Association of Clinical Endocrinologists (AACE).[11-18,77-80]

The pathophysiology of type 2 diabetes involves multiple core defects: the ominous octet (Fig. 3.1) describes the defects beyond beta cell deficiency and insulin resistance. It includes defects in the adipocytes, gastrointestinal tract, alpha cell, kidneys and the brain. Targeting different mechanisms can help in achieving more effective glycemic control. Early aggressive treatment that is moving away from a beta cell centric approach can reduce the progressive beta cell decline. Hence, a pathophysiologic approach to treatment of diabetes has today largely replaced the classical stepwise up titration of drugs.[81]

Table 3.3: A patient-centric approach to treatment of diabetes.

Clinical judgment + Patient preference		
Drug characteristics	***Patient characteristics***	***Disease characteristics***
Expected HbA1c reduction	Age	Duration of diabetes
Fasting and postprandial glucose lowering ability	Individualized targets	Predominant pathophysiology involved
Ability to address the pathophysiology	Life expectancy	Complications of diabetes
Durability	Comorbidities	
Cardiovascular safety		
Side effects including hypoglycemia and weight gain		
Extraglycemic benefits		
Cost effectiveness		

Flowchart 3.1: Approach to combination therapy.

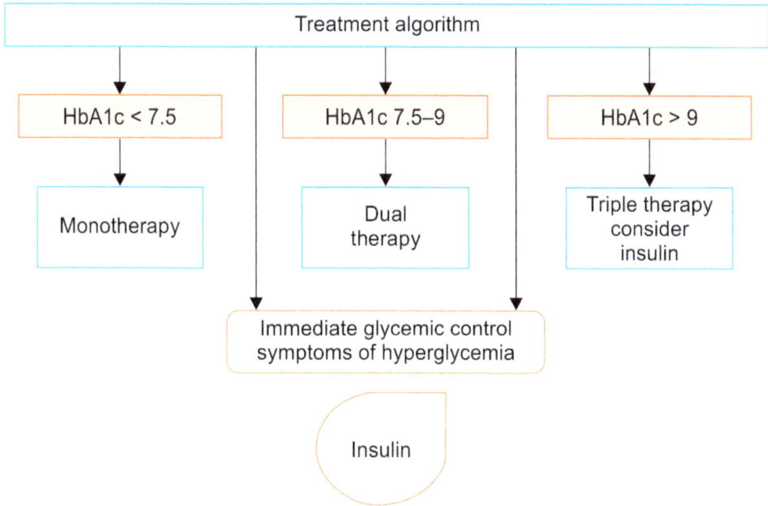

(HbA1c: Hemoglobin A1c)

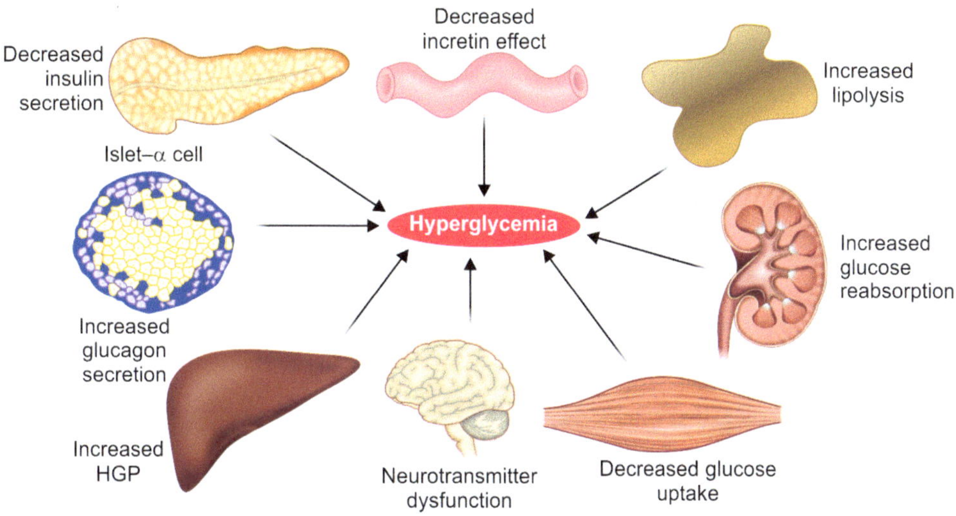

Fig. 3.1: Ominous octet of type 2 diabetes.

Source: Defronso RA. Banting Lecture from Triumvirate to Ominous Octet: a new paradigm shift for the treatment of T2DM. Diabetes. 2009;58:773-95.

CONCLUSION

Treatment of diabetes often requires constant up titration of antidiabetic drugs due to progressive beta cell decline that occurs as a natural history of the disease. The goals of treatment should be achieved with multiple drugs to ensure safe and adequate glycemic control, with minimal side effects of therapy.

CLINICAL SUMMARY FOR PRACTICE

The choice of an agent largely depends on the following:

- The duration of diabetes
- HbA1c reduction required and the ability of the drug to provide that reduction
- The durability of the drug
- The ability of the drug to address the pathophysiology of the disease
- The ability to address the components (fasting and postprandial) of glycemia
- The ability to minimize hypoglycemia and weight gain
- Safety in variety of clinical situations including cardiovascular safety
- Adverse events associated with the drug
- Cost-effectiveness of therapy
- Effects beyond glycemia
- Route of medication delivery preferred by the patient.

REFERENCES

1. Intensive blood-glucose control with sulphonylureas or insulin compared with conventional treatment and risk of complications in patients with type 2 diabetes (UKPDS 33). UK Prospective Diabetes Study (UKPDS) Group. Lancet. 1998;352:837.
2. UK Prospective Diabetes Study (UKPDS) Group. Effect of intensive blood-glucose control with metformin on complications in overweight patients with type 2 diabetes (UKPDS 34). Lancet. 1998;352:854-65.
3. The Diabetes Control and Complications Trial Research Group. The effect of intensive treatment of diabetes on the development and progression of long-term complications in insulin dependent diabetes mellitus. N Engl J Med. 1993;329:977-86.
4. Holman RR, Paul SK, Bethel MA, et al. 10-year follow-up of intensive glucose control in type 2 diabetes. N Engl J Med. 2008;359:1577.
5. Duckworth W, Abraira C, Moritz T, et al. Glucose control and vascular complications in veterans with type 2 diabetes. N Engl J Med. 2009;360:129-39.
6. Hayward RA, Reaven PD, Wiitala WL, et al. Follow-up of glycemic control and cardiovascular outcomes in type 2 diabetes. N Engl J Med. 2015;372:2197-206.
7. ACCORD Study Group, Gerstein HC, Miller ME, et al. Long-term effects of intensive glucose lowering on cardiovascular outcomes. N Engl J Med. 2011;364:818-28.
8. Look AHEAD Research Group, Wing RR, Bolin P, et al. Cardiovascular effects of intensive lifestyle intervention in type 2 diabetes. N Engl J Med. 2013;369:145.
9. ADVANCE Collaborative Group, Patel A, MacMahon S, et al. Intensive blood glucose control and vascular outcomes in patients with type 2 diabetes. N Engl J Med. 2008;358:2560.
10. Action to Control Cardiovascular Risk in Diabetes Study Group, Gerstein HC, Miller ME, et al. Effects of intensive glucose lowering in type 2 diabetes. N Engl J Med. 2008;358:2545.
11. Bennett WL, Odelola OA, Wilson LM, et al. Evaluation of guideline recommendations on oral medications for type 2 diabetes mellitus: a systematic review. Ann Intern Med. 2012;156:27.
12. Bennett WL, Maruthur NM, Singh S, et al. Comparative effectiveness and safety of medications for type 2 diabetes: an update including new drugs and 2-drug combinations. Ann Intern Med. 2011;154:602.
13. Inzucchi SE, Bergenstal RM, Buse JB, et al. Management of hyperglycaemia in type 2 diabetes: a patient-centered approach. Position statement of the American Diabetes Association (ADA) and the European Association for the Study of Diabetes (EASD). Diabetologia. 2012;55(6):1577-96.

14. American Diabetic Association. Approaches to Glycemic Treatment. Diabetes Care. 2016;39(S1):S52-S59.
15. Inzucchi SE, Bergenstal RM, Buse JB, et al. Management of hyperglycemia in type 2 diabetes, 2015: a patient-centered approach. Update to a position statement of the American Diabetes Association and the European Association for the Study of Diabetes. Diabetes Care. 2015;38:140-9.
16. Handelsman Y, Bloomgarden ZT, Grunberger G, et al. American Association of Clinical Endocrinologists and American College of Endocrinology: clinical practice guidelines for developing a diabetes mellitus comprehensive care plan--2015. Endocr Pract. 2015;21(Suppl 1):1-87.
17. Madhu SV, Saboo B, Makkar MB, et al. On behalf of the Guideline Development Group. RSSDI Clinical Practice Recommendations for Management of Type 2 Diabetes Mellitus, 2015. Int J Diabetes Dev Ctries. 2015;35:S1-S71.
18. Garber JA, Abrahamson MJ, Barzilay JI, et al. Consensus statement by the American Association of Clinical Endocrinologists and American College of Endocrinology on the Comprehensive type 2 Diabetes Management Algorithm – 2016 executive summary. Endocr Pract. 2016;22(Suppl 1):84-113.
19. Saenz A, Fernandez-Esteban I, Mataix A, et al. Metformin monotherapy for type 2 diabetes mellitus. Cochrane Database Syst Rev. 2005;CD002966.
20. Kooy A, de Jager J, Lehert P, et al. Long-term effects of metformin on metabolism and microvascular and macrovascular disease in patients with type 2 diabetes mellitus. Arch Intern Med. 2009;169:616.
21. Sosale A, Saboo B, Sosale B. Saroglitazar for the treatment of hypertriglyceridemia in patients with type 2 diabetes: current evidence. Diabetes, Metab Syndr Obesity: Targets and Therapy. 2015;8:189-96.
22. Kahn SE, Haffner SM, Heise MA, et al. Glycemic durability of rosiglitazone, metformin, or glyburide monotherapy. N Engl J Med. 2006;355:2427.
23. Nathan DM. Thiazolidinediones for initial treatment of type 2 diabetes? N Engl J Med. 2006;355:2477.
24. Kipnes MS, Krosnick A, Rendell MS, et al. Pioglitazone hydrochloride in combination with sulfonylurea therapy improves glycemic control in patients with type 2 diabetes mellitus: a randomized, placebo-controlled study. Am J Med. 2001;111:10.
25. Charbonnel B, Schernthaner G, Brunetti P, et al. Long-term efficacy and tolerability of add-on pioglitazone therapy to failing monotherapy compared with addition of gliclazide or metformin in patients with type 2 diabetes. Diabetologia. 2005;48:1093.
26. Dormandy JA, Charbonnel B, Eckland DJA, et al. Proactive Investigators. Secondary prevention of macrovascular events in patients with type 2 diabetes in the PROactive Study (PROspective pioglitAzone Clinical Trial In macroVascular Events): a randomised controlled trial. Lancet. 2005;366:1279-89.
27. Panikar V. Pioglitazone and bladder cancer: the pros and cons. Journal of Association of Physicians of India. 2012;(60):72-3.
28. Meneilly GS, Ryan EA, Radziuk J, et al. Effect of acarbose on insulin sensitivity in elderly patients with diabetes. Diabetes Care. 2000;23:1162.
29. Chiasson JL, Josse RG, Hunt JA, et al. The efficacy of acarbose in the treatment of patients with non-insulin-dependent diabetes mellitus. A multicenter controlled clinical trial. Ann Intern Med. 1994;121:928.
30. Johnston PS, Coniff RF, Hoogwerf BJ, et al. Effects of the carbohydrase inhibitor miglitol in sulfonylurea-treated NIDDM patients. Diabetes Care. 1994;17:20.
31. Johnston PS, Lebovitz HE, Coniff RF, et al. Advantages of alpha-glucosidase inhibition as monotherapy in elderly type 2 diabetic patients. J Clin Endocrinol Metab. 1998;83:1515.
32. Johnston PS, Feig PU, Coniff RF, et al. Long-term titrated-dose alpha-glucosidase inhibition in non-insulin-requiring Hispanic NIDDM patients. Diabetes Care. 1998;21:409.
33. Van de Laar FA, Lucassen PL, Akkermans RP, et al. Alpha-glucosidase inhibitors for patients with type 2 diabetes: results from a Cochrane systematic review and meta-analysis. Diabetes Care. 2005;28:154.
34. Hoffmann J, Spengler M. Efficacy of 24-week monotherapy with acarbose, metformin, or placebo in dietary-treated NIDDM patients: the Essen-II Study. Am J Med. 1997;103:483.

35. Chiasson JL, Josse RG, Gomis R, et al. Acarbose treatment and the risk of cardiovascular disease and hypertension in patients with impaired glucose tolerance: the STOP-NIDDM trial. JAMA. 2003;290:486.
36. Amori RE, Lau J, Pittas AG. Efficacy and safety of incretin therapy in type 2 diabetes: systematic review and meta-analysis. JAMA. 2007;298:194-206.
37. Koliaki C, Doupis J. Incretin-based therapy: a powerful and promising weapon in the treatment of type 2 diabetes mellitus. Diabetes Ther. 2011;2:101.
38. Lee YS, Jun HS. Anti-diabetic actions of glucagon-like peptide-1 on pancreatic beta-cells. Metabolism. 2014;63:9.
39. Raz I, Hanefeld M, Xu L, et al. Efficacy and safety of the dipeptidyl peptidase-4 inhibitor sitagliptin as monotherapy in patients with type 2 diabetes mellitus. Diabetologia. 2006;49:2564.
40. Aschner P, Kipnes MS, Lunceford JK, et al. Effect of the dipeptidyl peptidase-4 inhibitor sitagliptin as monotherapy on glycemic control in patients with type 2 diabetes. Diabetes Care. 2006;29:2632.
41. Nowicki M, Rychlik I, Haller H, et al. Long-term treatment with the dipeptidyl peptidase-4 inhibitor saxagliptin in patients with type 2 diabetes mellitus and renal impairment: a randomised controlled 52-week efficacy and safety study. Int J Clin Pract. 2011;65:1230.
42. Kothny W, Shao Q, Groop PH, Lukashevich V. One-year safety, tolerability and efficacy of vildagliptin in patients with type 2 diabetes and moderate or severe renal impairment. Diabetes Obes Metab. 2012;14:1032.
43. McGill JB, Barnett AH, Lewin AJ, et al. Linagliptin added to sulphonylurea in uncontrolled type 2 diabetes patients with moderate-to-severe renal impairment. Diab Vasc Dis Res. 2014;11:34.
44. Pi-Sunyer FX, Schweizer A, Mills D, Dejager S. Efficacy and tolerability of vildagliptin monotherapy in drug-naïve patients with type 2 diabetes. Diabetes Res Clin Pract. 2007;76:132.
45. Richter B, Bandeira-Echtler E, Bergerhoff K, Lerch CL. Dipeptidyl peptidase-4 (DPP-4) inhibitors for type 2 diabetes mellitus. Cochrane Database Syst Rev. 2008:CD006739.
46. Grouzmann E, Livio F, Buclin T. Angiotensin Converting Enzyme and Dipeptidyl Peptidase IV Inhibitors: An increased risk of angioedema. Hypertension. 2009;54:468-70.
47. Green JB, Bethel MA, Armstrong PW, et al. TECOS Study Group. Effect of sitagliptin on cardiovascular outcomes in type 2 diabetes. N Engl J Med. 2015;373:232-42.
48. Scheen AJ, Charpentier G, Ostgren CJ, et al. Efficacy and safety of saxagliptin in combination with metformin compared with sitagliptin in combination with metformin in adult patients with type 2 diabetes mellitus. Diabetes Metab Res Rev. 2010;26:540.
49. Zannad F, Cannon CP, Cushman WC, et al. Heart failure and mortality outcomes in patients with type 2 diabetes taking alogliptin versus placebo in EXAMINE: a multicentre, randomised, double-blind trial. Lancet. 2015;385:2067.
50. Fuhlendorff J, Rorsman P, Kofod H, et al. Stimulation of insulin release by repaglinide and glibenclamide involves both common and distinct processes. Diabetes. 1998;47:345.
51. Wolffenbuttel BH, Landgraf R. A 1-year multicenter randomized double-blind comparison of repaglinide and glyburide for the treatment of type 2 diabetes. Dutch and German Repaglinide Study Group. Diabetes Care. 1999;22:463.
52. Repaglinide for type 2 diabetes mellitus. Med Lett Drugs Ther. 1998;40:55.
53. Moses R, Slobodniuk R, Boyages S, et al. Effect of repaglinide addition to metformin monotherapy on glycemic control in patients with type 2 diabetes. Diabetes Care. 1999;22:119.
54. Hollander PA, Schwartz SL, Gatlin MR, et al. Importance of early insulin secretion: comparison of nateglinide and glyburide in previously diet-treated patients with type 2 diabetes. Diabetes Care. 2001;24:983.
55. Hermann LS, Scherstén B, Bitzén PO, et al. Therapeutic comparison of metformin and sulfonylurea, alone and in various combinations. A double-blind controlled study. Diabetes Care. 1994;17:1100.

56. Holstein A, Plaschke A, Egberts EH. Lower incidence of severe hypoglycaemia in patients with type 2 diabetes treated with glimepiride versus glibenclamide. Diabetes Metab Res Rev. 2001;17:467.
57. Gangji AS, Cukierman T, Gerstein HC, et al. A systematic review and meta-analysis of hypoglycemia and cardiovascular events: a comparison of glyburide with other secretagogues and with insulin. Diabetes Care. 2007;30:389.
58. Shorr RI, Ray WA, Daugherty JR, Griffin MR. Incidence and risk factors for serious hypoglycemia in older persons using insulin or sulfonylureas. Arch Intern Med. 1997;157:1681.
59. Schramm TK, Gislason GH, Vaag A, et al. Mortality and cardiovascular risk associated with different insulin secretagogues compared with metformin in type 2 diabetes, with or without a previous myocardial infarction: a nationwide study. Eur Heart J. 2011;32:1900.
60. Vasilakou D, Karagiannis T, Athanasiadou E, et al. Sodium-glucose cotransporter 2 inhibitors for type 2 diabetes: a systematic review and metaanalysis. Ann Intern Med. 2013;159:262-74
61. Nauck MA, Del Prato S, Meier JJ, et al. Dapagliflozin versus glipizide as add-on therapy in patients with type 2 diabetes who have inadequate glycemic controlwithmetformin: a randomized, 52-week, double-blind, active-controlled noninferiority trial. Diabetes Care. 2011;34:2015-22.
62. Rosenstock J, Seman LJ, Jelaska A, et al. Efficacy and safety of empagliflozin, a sodium glucose cotransporter 2 SGLT2) inhibitor, as add-on to metformin in type 2 diabetes with mild hyperglycaemia. Diabetes Obes Metab. 2013;15:1154-60.
63. Monami M, Nardini C, Mannucci E. Efficacy and safety of sodium glucose co-transport-2 inhibitors in type 2 diabetes: a meta-analysis of randomized clinical trials. Diabetes Obes Metab. 2014;16:457-66.
64. Abdul-Ghani MA, Norton L, Defronzo RA. Role of sodium-glucose cotransporter 2 (SGLT 2) inhibitors in the treatment of type 2 diabetes. Endocr Rev. 2011;32:515-31.
65. Zinman B, Wanner C, Lachin J, et al. For the EMPA REG OUTCOME investigators. Empagliflozin, Cardiovascular Outcomes, and Mortality in Type 2 Diabetes. NEJM, 2015.
66. Garber AJ, Abrahamson MJ, Barzilay JI, et al. AACE/ACE comprehensive diabetes management algorithm. 2015. Endocr Pract. 2015;21:438-47.
67. Lavalle-Gonzalez FJ, Januszewicz A, Davidson J, et al. Efficacy and safety of canagli- flozin compared with placebo and sitagliptin in patients with type 2 diabetes on background metformin monotherapy: a randomised trial. Diabetologia. 2013;56:2582-92.
68. Wilding JP, Charpentier G, Hollander P, et al. Efficacy and safety of canagliflozin in patients with type 2 diabetes mellitus inadequately controlled with metformin and sulphonylurea: a randomised trial. Int J Clin Pract. 2013;67:1267-82.
69. Taylor, Blau, Rother. SGLT2 inhibitors may predispose to ketoacidosis.J Clin Endocrinol Metab. 2015;100(8):2849-52.
70. Taylor, Blau, Rother. Possible adverse effects on SGLT2 inhibitors on bone. The Lancet Diabetes and Endocrinology. 2015;3:8-10.
71. Vijan S, Sussman JB, Yudkin JS, Hayward RA. Effect of patients' risks and preferences on health gains with plasma glucose level lowering in type 2 diabetes mellitus. JAMA Intern Med. 2014;174:1227-34.
72. Rayappa PH, Raju KNM, Kapur A, et al. The impact of socio-economic factors on diabetes care. Int J Diab Dev Countries. 1999;19:7-16.
73. Moghissi E, Ismail-Beigi F, Devine RC. Hypoglycemia: minimizing its impact in type 2 diabetes. Endocr Pract. 2013;19:526-35.
74. Hauber AB, Mohamed AF, Johnson FR, Falvey H. Treatment preferences and medication adherence of people with type 2 diabetes using oral glucose-lowering agents. Diabet Med. 2009;26:416-24.
75. Akram K, Pedersen-Bjergaard U, Borch-Johnsen K, Thorsteinsson B. Frequency and risk factors of severe hypoglycemia in insulin-treated type 2 diabetes: a literature survey. J Diabetes Complications. 2006;20:402-8.

76. Udell JA, Cavender MA, Bhatt DL, et al. Glucose lowering drugs or strategies and cardiovascular outcomes in patients with or at risk of type 2 diabetes: a meta analysis of randomized controlled trials. The Lancet Diabetes & Endocrinology. 2015;3(5):356-66.
77. Desai NR, Shrank WH, Fischer MA, et al. Patterns of medication initiation in newly diagnosed diabetes mellitus: quality and cost implications. Am J Med. 2012;125:302.
78. Brown JB, Nichols GA, Perry A. The burden of treatment failure in type 2 diabetes. Diabetes Care. 2004;27:1535.
79. Shah BR, Hux JE, Laupacis A, et al. Clinical inertia in response to inadequate glycemic control: do specialists differ from primary care physicians? Diabetes Care. 2005;28:600.
80. Lingvay I, Legendre JL, Kaloyanova PF, et al. Insulin-based versus triple oral therapy for newly diagnosed type 2 diabetes: which is better? Diabetes Care. 2009;32:1789.
81. Defronso RA. Banting Lecture From Triumvirate to Ominous Octet : a new paradigm shift for the treatment of T2DM. Diabetes. 2009;58:773-95.

CHAPTER 4

Monitoring Glycemic Control: Focus on Alternate Markers of Glycemia

Anjali Amit Bhatt, Manish M Bothale, AG Unnikrishnan

INTRODUCTION

One of the most important pillars of effective diabetes management is monitoring of diabetes to assess the glycemic control. The major of treatment of diabetes is to prevent the occurrence and to slow down the rate of progression of debilitating microvascular complications like retinopathy, nephropathy and neuropathy. Significant, though a lesser degree of association also exists between glycemic control and macrovascular complications like myocardial infarction and cerebrovascular accidents in patients with diabetes.[1,2] Glycosylated hemoglobin (HbA1c) is currently the most effective, reproducible and evidence-based glycemic monitoring tool and has also been shown to correlate with the risk of developing diabetes related vascular as well as non-vascular complications. In situations where validity of HbA1c is questioned, end products of glycation of other biomolecules like fructosamine, glycated albumin and 1,5-anhydroglucitol (1,5-AG) may be considered as markers of glycemic control. This chapter will focus on HbA1c, 1,5-AG and similar markers, and will not cover continuous glucose monitoring and self-monitoring of blood glucose.

EVIDENCE FOR UTILITY OF HbA1c—MEAN PLASMA GLUCOSE AND VASCULAR COMPLICATIONS OF DIABETES

Though the concept of HbA1c is known since 1960s,[3] the first major evidence of utility of HbA1c came from DCCT (Diabetes Control and Complications Trial).[4,5] Firstly, the 6 ½ years' follow-up of 1500 odd patients made it possible to relate 25,000 odd readings of self-monitoring of blood glucose with serial reports of HbA1c.[6] This analysis found a linear relationship between mean plasma glucose and HbA1c. The relationship, controversially described by the equation —"Mean plasma glucose (mg/dL) = (35.6 × HbA1c) - 77.3"—is still utilized by clinicians and other healthcare providers to explain the meaning of HbA1c value to patients with diabetes. Some reports have questioned this linearity of the relationship, which is also thought to change according to absolute value of HbA1c. In other words, the same equation may not be applicable to HbA1c of 7% as well as 11%.[6] Additionally HbA1c loses its linearity in patients who have extreme excursions in glucose levels with recurrent hypoglycemia and hyperglycemia. However, currently the evidence in favor of utility of HbA1c as an important predictor of mean plasma glucose is stronger than the evidence otherwise.[7]

Secondly, DCCT[5] also cemented the utility of HbA1c which was further agreed upon by results of UKPDS[8] trial in predicting microvascular complications in patients with type 1 and type 2 diabetes respectively. Indeed on long-term follow-up it was shown that achieving a lower HbA1c during initial period after diagnosis also translates in better long-term outcomes irrespective of subsequent glycemic status - a phenomenon termed as 'metabolic memory or legacy effect'.[9]

Later, three landmark trials ACCORD,[10] ADVANCE[11] and VADT[12] confirmed the beneficial effect of lowering of HbA1c on reduction in onset as well as progression of microvascular complications. But these landmark trials also showed no significant reduction in CVD outcomes with stricter targets of HbA1c.

METHODOLOGICAL CONSIDERATIONS

In the initial phases of discovery using ion-exchange chromatography, five sub-fractions of normal adult hemoglobin (HbA) were demonstrated namely HbA1a, HbA1b, HbA1c, HbA1d and HbA1e based the order of elution.[13] Later, combination of demonstration of a simple biochemical concept of elevated glycosylation product of hemoglobin and a genuine clinical demand led to use of a variety of analytic principles for the measurement of HbA1c. Most notably ion-exchange high-performance liquid chromatography systems are utilized to separate these fractions based on their charge difference. But methods like affinity chromatography and immunochemical methods which identify difference in molecular structure are becoming widely available. It is mandatory to standardize the test results according to the International Federation of Clinical Chemistry (IFCC) Reference Measurement Procedure (RMP) in harmony with the efforts of the National Glycohemoglobin Standardization Program (NGSP).[14]

As the average lifespan of RBC is 120 days, HbA1c logically represents mean glucose levels over the preceding three months. But practically, recent glycemia influences the result largely. It is shown that in a patient with stable glycemic control, HbA1c values have 50% contribution from the glycemic status in the month prior to sampling, 25% in the month before that, and the remaining 25% from the earlier month.[15]

LIMITATIONS IN USE OF HbA1c

Conditions Interfering with Formation of HbA1c

As discussed earlier the normal form of hemoglobin on high performance liquid chromatography (HPLC) is Hemoglobin A (HbA). A glycated product of HbA is recorded on HPLC as HbA1c. People with abnormal hemoglobin, which is different from HbA logically, have an abnormal glycated product. A classical example of this condition is sickle cell anemia in which patients have HbS hemoglobin, which form HbS1c. A similar process occurs in patients with HbC and so on. The proportion of abnormal glycated product to HbA1c depends on severity of the disease but is difficult to predict in a given individual. With advances in the analyzers, it is now possible to detect the non-glycated portion of the abnormal fractions of hemoglobin but it is still difficult to predict HbA1c had it not been a patient with abnormal hemoglobin.[16] Another advantage of the advanced glycosylated hemoglobin analyzers is their ability to account for fetal hemoglobin (Hb) which may persist in few subjects even in adulthood and may interfere with HbA1c formation.

Being a chromatographic representation of hemoglobin, HbA1c values are directly affected by red blood cells (RBCs) survival. In conditions resulting in decreased turnover of RBCs, HbA1c can be falsely elevated losing its relationship with mean blood glucose concentrations. Classical example of this condition is anemia due to deficiency of iron, vitamin B_{12} or folic acid. Conversely, with excellerated hematopoiesis HbA1c values can be lower than that estimated from mean plasma glucose. This condition includes anemia due to blood loss, hemolytic anemia, hyperdynamic circulation like pregnancy, or patients recovering from nutrient deficiency anemia.[17]

Conditions Interfering with the Interpretation of HbA1c

Apart from the glycemic variability making HbA1c difficult to correlate with mean plasma glucose, some health conditions make use of HbA1c less reliable as a marker of glycemic control. HbA1c is less useful as a marker of glycemic control and as a tool for diagnosis of diabetes during pregnancy.

HbA1c values may be unpredictable in various phases of chronic kidney disease including those on dialysis due to multiple factors like iron deficiency, hemolysis, altered RBC survival. Methodologically carbamylated hemoglobin formed by compounding of hemoglobin by urea-derived isocyanate which is difficult to distinguish from HbA1c.[18] Liver disease and chronic malaria have also shown to cause a falsely lowered HbA1c level. Drugs, which cause hemolysis, may theoretically interfere with interpretation of HbA1c, e.g. aspirin but this effect does not seem to be clinically relevant.

Some studies have suggested a racial and ethnic effect on A1c[19] but, the evidence is not strong enough to result in change in recommendations of different interpretations of A1c in different ethnic populations.

RECOMMENDATIONS FOR CLINICAL USE OF HbA1c

Currently, it is recommended to perform HbA1c in all patients with diabetes as an initial assessment and as well as a part of continued monitoring. Measurement should be done every three months to evaluate whether glycemic targets are reached or not. The frequency may change on clinical scenario, intensity of change in medications and choice of clinician as well as patient. Generally patients with unstable control of diabetes require more frequent testing than those with stable control.[20]

The recommended target of HbA1c for most non-pregnant adults with no severe comorbidity is <7% (53 mmol/mol). The target may be higher (up to 8%) in patients with long-standing diabetes with established vascular complications (especially coronary artery disease), multiple associated comorbidities with a reduced life expectancy. The targets are higher in patients with tendency to develop hypoglycemia due to any reason. Antagonistically a stricter target may be recommended in newly detected, otherwise healthy and motivated young patient with availability of resource and support system.[20] HbA1c can be used to diagnose diabetes—a value of more than or equal to 6.5% indicates diabetes, and a value that is between 5.7% and 6.4% is akin to prediabetes, indicating a high risk state of predisposition to diabetes.

ALTERNATIVE BIOMARKERS FOR ASSESSING GLYCEMIC CONTROL IN DIABETES

Due to the knowledge of certain conditions and specific population making HbA1c a less reliable test for assessment of diabetes, there has been increasing interest in developing non-traditional glycemic markers as alternatives to HbA1c. Three such most important biomarkers include fructosamine, glycated albumin, and 1,5-anhydroglucitol.[21,22] Recently evidence has shown those fructosamine and glycated albumin are strongly associated with fasting glucose.[23]

Fructosamine

Contemporary to binding of hemoglobin to glucose, binding of fructose to serum protein results in a ketoamine termed as Fructosamine. The term fructosamine includes end products of glycosylation of all proteins. Though, fructosamine assays are cheaper and easier they are less standardized than HbA1c assays. Fructosamine assays are useful as markers of recent short-term changes in glycemic status as they reflect mean plasma glucose over a period of previous two to three weeks due to much shorter half-life of albumin compared to RBCs. The higher within-subject variation and effect of change in serum protein (especially albumin) are the limitations in widespread utility of fructosamine.[24]

Glycated Albumin

It is the ratio of glycated albumin to total serum albumin. Unlike fructosamine, this product is not affected by serum albumin levels. The value of glycated albumin is approximately three times that of HbA1c. Similar to fructosamine, glycated albumin reflects glycemic control over preceding two to three weeks. Clinical utility of glycated albumin lies in monitoring for glucose control in patients with abnormal RBC lifespan or variant hemoglobin and conditions in which glycemia changes rapidly such as in fulminant type I DM. Limitations of this test include abnormal values in diseases that result in abnormal albumin metabolism including obesity.[25]

1,5-anhydroglucitol

The 1-deoxy form of glucose known as 1,5-anhydroglucitol. It is a dietary compound, which is reabsorbed by renal tubules in an euglycemic subject. A competitive fall in serum levels of Serum 1,5-anhydroglucitol suggests increase serum glucose to >180 mg/dL. Hence, lower serum 1,5-anhydroglucitol levels reflect high circulating glucose over the past 1 to 2 weeks.[26] This test is affected by alteration in renal hemodynamic as well as use of drugs altering the glucose excretion through kidney like SGLT-2 inhibitors. This test is not widely utilized.

CONCLUSION AND FUTURE DIRECTIONS

Monitoring of glycemic status is one of the most important aspects of continued diabetes care. Markers of glycemic control have shown a strong association with onset and progression of microvascular complications and to a certain extent on macrovascular complications. Currently HbA1c is the most preferred method of evaluating long-term status of glycemic status in people with diabetes. In conditions and populations where HbA1c is less reliable, alternative tests like fructosamine, glycated albumin, and 1,5-anhydroglucitol. New research would focus on markers that are related to glucose, but more predictive of complications. It is known that HbA1c is formed by glycation of hemoglobin. It is well known that according to the glycation theory, some advanced glycation products may predict both glucose control and diabetes complications. N-1-(Deoxyfructosyl) valine (DFV) β-hemoglobin (β-Hb), commonly referred as HbA1c, is as mentioned above, a widely used marker of hyperglycemia—and is thought that it also indicates glycation to some extent. However, arguing that HbA1c is still not as advanced a glycation end product, researchers have tried to identify molecules in later stage of glycation, which may reflect hyperglycemia, but also improve accuracy in complication detection. Such carboxy-ethyl and carboxy-methyl variants of glycated hemoglobin have been recently discovered and may predict hyperglycemia and its complications to a better extent.[27] However, they are still under research and if clinical studies prove their relevance, the future may have another new tool to detect diabetes and its complications.[27]

REFERENCES

1. Xu L, Chan WM, Hui YF, Lam TH. Association between HbA1c and cardiovascular disease mortality in older Hong Kong Chinese with diabetes. Diabet Med J Br Diabet Assoc. 2012;29:393-8.
2. Zhao W, Katzmarzyk PT, Horswell R, et al. HbA1c and coronary heart disease risk among diabetic patients. Diabetes Care. 2014;37:428-35.
3. Huisman TH, Dozy AM. Studies on the heterogeneity of hemoglobin. V. Binding of hemoglobin with oxidized glutathione. J Lab Clin Med. 1962;60:302-19.
4. Association AD. Diabetes Control and Complications Trial (DCCT): Results of Feasibility Study. The DCCT Research Group. Diabetes Care. 1987;10:1-19.
5. Control TD, Group CTR. The effect of intensive treatment of diabetes on the development and progression of long-term complications in insulin-dependent diabetes mellitus. N Engl J Med. 1993;329:977-86.
6. Kilpatrick ES, Rigby AS, Atkin SL. Variability in the relationship between mean plasma glucose and HbA1c: Implications for the assessment of glycemic control. Clin Chem. 2007;53:897-901.
7. Makris K, Spanou L. Is there a relationship between mean blood glucose and glycated hemoglobin? J Diabetes Sci Technol. 2011;5:1572-83.
8. Intensive blood-glucose control with sulphonylureas or insulin compared with conventional treatment and risk of complications in patients with type 2 diabetes (UKPDS 33). UK Prospective Diabetes Study (UKPDS) Group. Lancet Lond Engl. 1998;352:837-53.
9. Association AD. Epidemiology of Diabetes Interventions and Complications (EDIC). Design, implementation, and preliminary results of a long-term follow-up of the Diabetes Control and Complications Trial cohort. Diabetes Care 1999;22:99-111.
10. Ismail-Beigi F, Carven T, Banerji MA, et al. Effect of intensive treatment of hyperglycaemia on microvascular outcomes in type 2 diabetes: an analysis of the ACCORD randomised trial. Lancet Lond Engl. 2010;376:419-30.
11. ADVANCE Collaborative Group, et al. Intensive blood glucose control and vascular outcomes in patients with type 2 diabetes. N Engl J Med. 2008;358:2560-72.
12. Duckworth, W, Abraira C, Moritz T, et al. Glucose control and vascular complications in veterans with type 2 diabetes. N Engl J Med. 2009;360:129-39.

13. Allen DW, Schroeder WA, Balog J. Observations on the chromatographic heterogeneity of normal adult and fetal human hemoglobin: a study of the effects of crystallization and chromatography on the heterogeneity and isoleucine content. J Am Chem Soc. 1958;80:1628-34.
14. Weykamp C, Garry John W, Mosca A. A review of the challenge in measuring hemoglobin A1c. J Diabetes Sci Technol. (Online) 2009;3:439-45.
15. Tahara Y, Shima K. Kinetics of HbA1c, glycated albumin, and fructosamine and analysis of their weight functions against preceding plasma glucose level. Diabetes Care. 1995;18:440-7.
16. Lee ST, Weykamp CW, Lee YW, et al. Effects of 7 hemoglobin variants on the measurement of glycohemoglobin by 14 Analytical Methods. Clin Chem. 2007;53:2202-5.
17. NGSP: Factors that Interfere with HbA1c Test Results. Available at: http://www.ngsp.org/factors.asp. (Accessed: 17th May 2016)
18. Ly J, Marticorena R, Donnelly S. Red blood cell survival in chronic renal failure. Am J Kidney Dis Off J Natl Kidney Found. 2004;44:715-9.
19. Buse JB, Kaufman FR, Linder B, et al. Diabetes screening with hemoglobin A1c versus fasting plasma glucose in a multiethnic middle-school cohort. Diabetes Care. 2013;36:429-35.
20. Association AD. 5. Glycemic Targets. Diabetes Care. 2016;39:S39-S46.
21. Lee JE. Alternative biomarkers for assessing glycemic control in diabetes: fructosamine, glycated albumin, and 1,5-anhydroglucitol. Ann Pediatr Endocrinol Metab. 2015;20:74-8.
22. Juraschek SP, Steffes MW, Miller ER, Selvin E. Alternative markers of hyperglycemia and risk of diabetes. Diabetes Care. 2012;35:2265-70.
23. Juraschek SP, Steffes MW, Selvin E. Associations of alternative markers of glycemia with hemoglobin A1c and fasting glucose. Clin Chem. 2012;58:1648-55.
24. Narbonne H, Renacco E, Pradel V, et al. Can fructosamine be a surrogate for HbA(1c) in evaluating the achievement of therapeutic goals in diabetes? Diabetes Metab. 2001;27:598-603.
25. Koga M, Haslimoto K, Murai J, et al. Usefulness of glycated albumin as an indicator of glycemic control status in patients with hemolytic anemia. Clin Chim Acta Int J Clin Chem. 2011;412:253-7.
26. Yamanouchi T, Minoda S, Yabuuchi M, et al. Plasma 1,5-anhydro-D-glucitol as new clinical marker of glycemic control in NIDDM patients. Diabetes. 1989;38:723-9.
27. Jagadeeshaprasad MG, Batkulwar KB, Meshram NN, et al. Targeted quantification of N-1-(carboxymethyl) valine and N-1-(carboxyethyl) valine peptides of β-hemoglobin for better diagnostics in diabetes. Clin Proteomics. 2016;13:7. doi: 10.1186/s12014-016-9108-y.

CHAPTER 5

Insulin Pump Therapy

Jothydev Kesavadev, Viswanathan Mohan, Ranjit Unnikrishnan, Ranjit Mohan Anjana

INTRODUCTION

All patients with type 1 diabetes and a significant number with type 2 diabetes require insulin therapy for achieving glycemic targets. Insulin delivery has been conventionally achieved through with the use of syringes, insulin pens, etc., which have various shortcomings such as the pain of needle prick and less physiological mode of insulin delivery leading to unpredictable and distressing hypo- and hyperglycemic fluctuations in blood glucose levels. This chapter explains both the two secretory patterns of the beta cells (basal and prandial) and the two types of infusion rates of the pump—*basal and bolus*; and the third type of infusion, i.e. *correction* [Mnemonic "BBC" = Basal, Bolus, Correction]. The insulin pump or continuous subcutaneous insulin infusion (CSII) is an attractive alternative mode of insulin delivery that has the potential to overcome many of these shortcomings, improve glycemic control and improve the quality of life of the patients. With the wider use of CSII in routine practice in the 1980s, there were several reports of severe hypoglycemias, diabetic ketoacidosis because of interruption of insulin infusion, site infections and pump malfunctions. Many of the initial technical problems were improved with subsequent technologies.

THE INSULIN PUMP

Insulin pump use regained momentum at the wake of positive results of the Diabetes Control and Complications Trial (DCCT) which favored intensive insulin therapy and strict glycemic control.[1] Insulin pumps subsequently underwent tremendous technological innovation and bioengineering to precisely mimic the delivery from a healthy human pancreas. "Smart" insulin pumps integrated and augmented with glucose biosensors to provide blood sugars in real-time were followed by features for early detection of hypoglycemia and prevention of occurrence of hypoglycemia. The dream of 'closing the loop' with an artificial pancreas is close to reality with encouraging results from recent trials using the modified control algorithms and bionic pancreas.

WHAT ARE INSULIN PUMPS?

The durable insulin pumps consist of a reservoir, a pump, and an infusion set. The reservoir holds a 2–3 days supply of insulin and is connected to a battery-powered pump. The infusion set consists of a tubing that connects the reservoir to a soft plastic cannula that is inserted under the skin. A small piece of adhesive holds the cannula in place at the insertion site. The durable pumps are designed to last several years. The infusion set and reservoir must be changed every 2–3 days. The common infusion sites are abdomen and thighs. Alternative sites include the flanks and top of the buttocks.

The patch pumps are attached directly to the body (pod) with a small length of plastic tubing going directly from the base of the pump into the subcutaneous tissue. The pod houses the insulin reservoir and motor. It is controlled by a separate controller known as Personal Digital Assistant (PDA). Patch pumps can also be applied to the upper arms.

Insulin Delivery

Pump delivers insulin as low 0.025 units or 0.05 unit increments, which make it the best insulin delivery device mimicking the physiology of a human pancreas. In contrast, the lowest dose a syringe can deliver accurately is 0.5 units.

BASAL RATE INFUSIONS

The insulin pump provides exogenous insulin to cover both the between meals (basal) and after meals (prandial or bolus) requirements of the body. The pump is unique in that the same type of insulin (rapid-acting analog) is used to provide both basal and bolus coverage with insulin. The right basal rate is obtained initially by checking blood glucose levels more frequently and at appropriate times. In the majority of patients, these basal rates found will stay stable for long periods of time.

Variable Basal Rate

The pump uses only rapid-acting insulin and even though all rapid insulin analogs may be used in a pump, aspart insulin seems to have an advantage in chemical and physical stability in the tubings, providing lower rates on occlusions (9.2%) in comparison with lispro (15.7%) and glulisine (40.9%).

A variable basal infusion rate during the day is more physiological because it is similar to the normal secretion of the beta cells do during the day. Multiple basal rates help avoid high and low glucose levels and are especially useful in patients experiencing dawn phenomenon, hypoglycemia unawareness or gastroparesis and in those with variable lifestyle. Each patient needs to find, with the help of the medical team, their own program of basal rate infusions according to meal and activity times.

Multiple Basal Patterns

Multiple basal rate patterns can be set in the pump to meet the varying insulin requirements during weekdays versus weekends, work shift days, dialysis day versus normal days in a chronic kidney disease patient, frequent travelers, etc.

Temporary Basal Rate Changes

Temporary changes in basal rate infusion may be necessary during exercise, sick days, or delayed meals.

BOLUS INFUSIONS

Bolus insulin calculators became available in insulin pumps in 2002. The pump bolus calculator makes bolus doses more accurate, provides bolus recommendations to match the carbs the patient eats, brings down high glucose levels and minimizes insulin stacking. For the bolus calculator to provide appropriate bolus doses, accurate settings for the insulin to carbohydrate ratio, insulin sensitivity factor, correction target, etc. are required.[3]

Corrections

The pump has the ability to correct a high blood glucose following a meal using the bolus calculator, which also takes into account the bolus on board, i.e. insulin left from an already administered bolus.

Varied Infusions Options

Insulin pump may be set to deliver as high as 48 different basal profiles a day and varied infusions patterns to suit the diet and lifestyle of the individual on insulin pump therapy.

Normal, square wave and dual wave boluses are the common bolus options available with an insulin pump. The normal (standard) bolus is the most frequently used bolus pattern for meals that contain average fat and carbohydrate content. It is also used for correction bolusing. In a square wave bolus, the bolus amount delivers evenly over the period of time it is set for. It is useful when eating small amounts of carb over an extended period of time or for people who have delayed digestion (gastroparesis). The dual-wave bolus delivers a combination of an immediate normal pre-meal insulin bolus (approximately 3 min) followed by an extended (or square-wave) bolus that is evenly delivered over several hours as set. It is primarily used for meals that are both high in carbs and fat, which may delay digestion. In patients with prolonged postprandial hyperglycemia, dual wave has been identified to be an effective and potential option to improve glycemic control especially in patients with type 1 diabetes.[4-5]

ADVANCED FEATURES IN NEWER PUMPS

SmartGuard Technology

Sensor augmented pump therapy (SAPT) integrates real-time continuous glucose monitoring (RT-CGM) with CSII. The Sensor-Augmented Pump Therapy for A1c Reduction (STAR) 3 study, a multicenter randomized controlled trial comparing the efficacy of SAPT to that of MDI in subjects with type 1 diabetes suggests that SAPT reduces glycemic variability and reduced the number and severity of glycemic excursions.[17] Moreover, it was also associated with significant improvement in glycated hemoglobin levels when compared to MDI.[18] The INTERPRET Study, a 12-month observational study in patients with type 1 diabetes treated with CSII, upon the introduction of CGM, documented the real-life use of SAP, and assessed the variables associated with its improvements in type 1 diabetes management. There was significantly less hospitalization, increased personal satisfaction, and reduced fear of hypoglycemia after 12 months of SAP.[19]

The new insulin pumps with SmartGuard technology (Fig. 5.1) are considered a breakthrough toward an artificial pancreas because they are able to suspend temporarily the insulin infusion

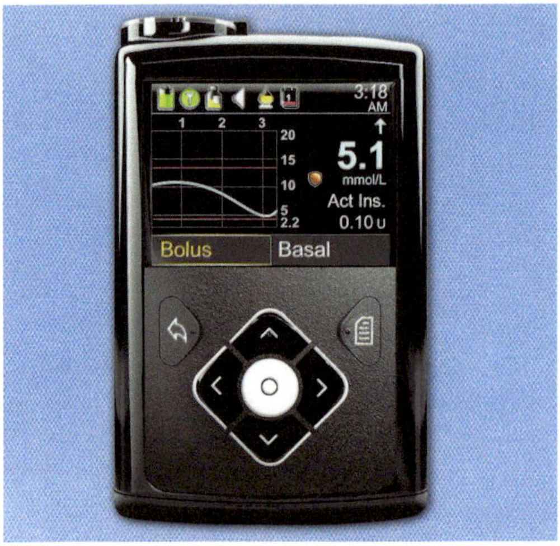

Fig. 5.1: SmartGuard insulin pump.

when the blood glucose levels in the connected continuous sensors are reaching low levels (programmable). Once the blood glucose levels raise to more normal levels the insulin delivery is automatically resumed.

The older version insulin pumps such as the Veo (530G) insulin pump comes with a low-glucose suspend (LGS) feature which recognizes a dangerously low glucose level and acts quickly to suspend insulin delivery for two hours, helping to prevent the hypoglycemic event from becoming any more harmful.

Integrated Glucometer and Remote Control

The 640G insulin pump comes with a glucose meter which automatically transmit blood glucose results into the Bolus Wizard(TM) calculator to help ensure that patients do not have a manual entry error, and to calibrate the Enhanced Enlite sensor. It also allows patients to discreetly give a bolus of insulin remotely from the meter. The meter provides added convenience to help patients manage their diabetes effectively.

Waterproof

The newer insulin pumps are waterproof up to 12 feet of water for 24 hours at a time. Convenient new features include a simpler menu, full-color, light-adjusting screen, customizable alerts and alarms, etc.

EVIDENCES FAVORING INSULIN PUMP THERAPY

The first large randomized controlled trial (RCT) of CSII in T2DM patients by Raskin et al.,[7] demonstrated no statistical difference between the CSII and MDI groups to reach HbA1c targets. However, 93% of the patients in CSII group preferred it over their previous insulin injection regimen for reasons of convenience, flexibility, ease of use, and overall preference.

In a subsequent RCT of CSII among older adults with type 2 diabetes by Herman et al.,[8] both groups achieved a similar mean HbA1c levels at 12 months below the recommended target of

7.0%. Though the superiority of CSII over MDI was not established, the change in treatment satisfaction from baseline was statistically significant for both groups but not statistically significant between groups.

The results of published smaller control studies showed mean HbA1c reductions in favor of CSII. A cross over study by Wainstein et al.[9] demonstrated reduction in mean HbA1c favoring CSII over MDI in type 2 diabetes patients. These positive results indicate that CSII may be clinically effective in T2DM when using the correct treatment regimen. The results of a multicenter pilot study assessing Insulin Pump Therapy in Patients with Type 2 Diabetes suboptimally controlled with MDI showed that glycemic control improved significantly after 16 weeks.[10] In yet another 16-week multicenter pilot study, patients experienced limited weight gain, no severe hypoglycemic episodes, and overall treatment satisfaction improved significantly.[11]

In one of the largest randomized controlled trial (OpT2mise) comparing the efficacy of pump treatment and multiple daily injections in T2DM, mean glycated hemoglobin decreased by 1.1% in the pump treatment group and 0.4% in the multiple daily injection group resulting in a between-group treatment difference of –0.7% ($p < 0.0001$). The mean total daily insulin dose was 97 units (SD 56) with pump treatment versus 122 units (SD 68) for multiple daily injections ($p < 0.0001$), with no significant difference in body weight change between the two groups (1.5 kg [SD 3.5] vs 1.1 kg [3.6], $p = 0.322$) proving pumps to be a safe and valuable treatment option in T2DM.[12]

Another study by Kesavadev et al.[13] demonstrated a mean HbA1c reduction by 0.5% after 6 months in 46 type 2 diabetes patients on CSII. This outcome was statistically significant ($p < 0.0063$; 95% confidence interval, 0.161–0.921%). However, there was no statistically significant change in body weight or total insulin daily dose. Subjects reported high satisfaction with CSII and low interference with daily activities. Patients were also asked to assess how CSII affected the sexual function and peripheral neuropathic pain. After 6 months of CSII, 83% of subjects noted an improvement in sexual function as opposed to when they were on MDI. 87% of subjects reported that they experienced significant reduction in peripheral neuropathic pain after 6 months of CSII.[13] In another study, 90% of the patients expressed satisfaction that pump met their expectations.[14]

A study in India by Mohan[15] with patients with recalcitrant diabetes demonstrated a significant reduction in HbA1c after initiating CSII. The study demonstrated statistically significant reduction in HbA1c after initiating CSII. The study also stressed the importance of regular follow-up of insulin pump patients after being on CSII since the greatest reduction in HbA1c levels occurred in the first 6 months and a slight deterioration thereafter possibly because some patients "relaxed" the control after the initial success with pumps. An extra advantage of insulin pumps is that it obliged the patients to control better and learn more about their diabetes.

INDICATIONS OF INSULIN PUMP THERAPY

The literature and various International scientific organizations[21,22] recommend insulin pump therapy in the following situations:

1. High HbA1c despite multiple daily doses (MDI)
2. Severe insulin resistance

3. Brittle diabetes
4. Frequent and/or severe hypoglycemias
5. Patients seeking improved quality of life (QOL) while on insulin therapy
6. Chronic kidney disease on dialysis or post-renal transplant patients
7. Untimely or variable meal times
8. In patients who can learn how to use the advantages of the pumps
9. Presence of micro- or macrovascular complications where intensive glycemic control may be beneficial in the long-term
10. Continuous glucose monitoring patterns strongly suggesting the need for a variable basal insulin infusion rate
11. Women with poor diabetes control in the childbearing age group contemplating starting a family or who are currently pregnant
12. Hypoglycemia unawareness
13. Recurrent diabetic ketoacidosis (DKA)
14. Marked dawn phenomenon, difficult to control otherwise
15. Gastroparesis
16. Ramadan fasting.[23]

The compelling indications of insulin pump therapy include:[21]

1. Frequent travelers with varied and untimely food habits
2. Post-renal transplant patients/chronic kidney disease patients on dialysis
3. Coronary artery disease patients seeking improved quality of life
4. Women with poor glycemic control planning for pregnancy
5. In some patients with severe neuropathy.

ADVANTAGES AND DISADVANTAGES OF INSULIN PUMP[20]

Advantages	*Disadvantages*
Allows variable meal and exercise times improving quality of life	
Predictable and precise insulin delivery	Risk of diabetic ketoacidosis (DKA) due to pump malfunction
Ability to deliver miniscule doses of insulin	Missed boluses
Stringent blood glucose control, while reducing the risk of low blood glucose	Requires more frequent self-monitoring of blood glucose
Reduces episodes of severe hypoglycemia	Weight gain if used for luxury
Helps manage the "dawn phenomenon"	Having a gadget attached to the body
Helps prevent glycemic variability	Expensive and the recurring cost of accessories ▪ Pump senescence after 4–6 years
	Requires more instructions and continuous attention from medical team and service from the pump manufacturers

CONTRAINDICATIONS TO INSULIN PUMP THERAPY

1. Patients with unrealistic expectations about insulin pump
2. Non educable, not motivated or not responsible patients and/or caregivers caregiver and patients who lack time to attend the pump training sessions
3. Patients with psychiatric problems
4. Patients who work in very hot places
5. Patients with rapidly progressing ischemic or proliferative retinopathy before laser treatment
6. Patients exposed to high magnetic fields (MRI's).

Though CSII is more than 40 years old, there still exists a stigma associated with insulin pump therapy. The apprehensions of having a device attached to the body, scepticism about its benefits and indications and inappropriate beliefs about dangers associated with its use such as pump malfunction.[24] There are also attitudes from non-diabetologists toward CSII mostly from lack of experience, and unavailability of a multidisciplinary diabetes team. Costs and lack of reimbursements are other factors that decrease the use of these pumps.

ARTIFICIAL PANCREAS

Artificial pancreas (AP) combines a glucose sensor, an associated algorithm, and an insulin pump thus fulfilling the dream of a fully closed loop system for diabetes management. Two configurations of AP have been proposed: single-hormone (insulin alone) and dual-hormone (insulin and glucagon).

Bionic Pancreas

"Bionic pancreas" is the name given specifically to the dual-chambered investigational device that comprises two separate pumps for delivering both insulin and glucagon, a continuous glucose monitor (CGM), and a control algorithm built into an iPhone app.

The device is the first and only one of its kind until now to also integrate glucagon delivery. The latest version of the Bionic Pancreas known as the 'iLET' has not only a combo insulin and glucagon infusion pump, but also has the CGM receiver built in, and is the same size as a standard smartphone but about two-and-a-half times as thick. It has a touchscreen interface and an LED screen. It uses two pre-filled cartridges where one contains glucagon (Fig. 5.2).

Future improvements in insulin pumps will consist in better continuous glucose monitoring, the infusion of both insulin and glucagon (in cases de hypoglycemia), with improved algorithms for the integration of glycemic levels and the "bihormonal" infusion.[25-27]

CONCLUSION

Although the concept behind insulin pumps is more than 4 decades old, its use has gained rapid momentum only in the last 10 years, thanks to advancements in biomedical engineering and emergence of rapid-acting insulin analogs. Unlike conventional delivery devices, insulin pumps use only rapid-acting insulin to deliver basal and bolus with options of varying basal rates and customized bolus options, thereby closely mimicking physiological insulin secretion in those subjects who have mastered the techniques. Wireless integration of insulin pumps with next

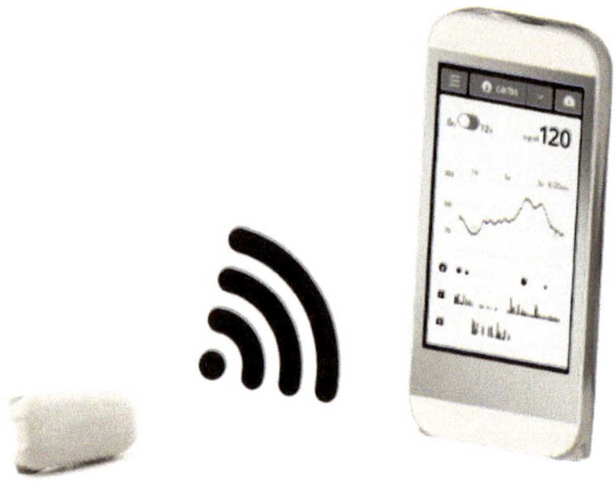

Fig. 5.2: iLET bihormonal pump.

generation continuous glucose sensors and control algorithms have opened the doors to fully closing the loop in the very near future. However, high cost and the necessity for aptitude and learning for the optimal usage of these devices will limit the benefits to a miniscule minority of the population, leaving behind the deserving majority.

REFERENCES

1. The effect of intensive treatment of diabetes on the development and progression of long-term complications in insulin-dependent diabetes mellitus. The Diabetes Control and Complications Trial Research Group. N Engl J Med. 1993;329:977-86.
2. Bode BW. Comparison of pharmacokinetic properties, physicochemical stability, and pump compatibility of 3 rapid-acting insulin analogues-aspart, lispro, and glulisine. Endocr Pract Off J Am Coll Endocrinol Am Assoc Clin Endocrinol. 2011;17:271-80.
3. Walsh J, Roberts R, Bailey T. Guidelines for optimal bolus calculator settings in adults. J Diabetes Sci Technol. 2011;5:129-35.
4. Lee SW, Cao M, Sajid S, et al. The dual-wave bolus feature in continuous subcutaneous insulin infusion pumps controls prolonged post-prandial hyperglycaemia better than standard bolus in Type 1 diabetes. Diabetes Nutr Metab. 2004;17:211-6.
5. Klupa T, Skupien J, Cyganek K, et al. The dual-wave bolus feature in type 1 diabetes adult users of insulin pumps. Acta Diabetol. 2011;48:11-4.
6. Bode BW. Insulin pump use in type 2 diabetes. Diabetes Technol Ther. 2010;12(Suppl 1):S17-21.
7. Raskin P, Bode BW, Marks JB, et al. Continuous subcutaneous insulin infusion and multiple daily injection therapy are equally effective in type 2 diabetes: a randomized, parallel-group, 24-week study. Diabetes Care. 2003;26:2598-603.
8. Herman WH, Ilag LL, Johnson SL, et al. A clinical trial of continuous subcutaneous insulin infusion versus multiple daily injections in older adults with type 2 diabetes. Diabetes Care. 2005;28:1568-73.
9. Wainstein J, Metzger M, Boaz M, et al. Insulin pump therapy vs. multiple daily injections in obese type 2 diabetic patients. Diabet Med J Br Diabet Assoc. 2005;22:1037-46.
10. Frias JP, Bode BW, Bailey TS, et al. A 16-week open-label, multicenter pilot study assessing insulin pump therapy in patients with type 2 diabetes suboptimally controlled with multiple daily injections. J Diabetes Sci Technol. 2011;5:887-93.
11. Edelman SV, Bode BW, Bailey TS, et al. Insulin pump therapy in patients with type 2 diabetes safely improved glycemic control using a simple insulin dosing regimen. Diabetes Technol Ther. 2010;12:627-33.

12. Reznik Y, Cohen O, Aronson R, et al. Insulin pump treatment compared with multiple daily injections for treatment of type 2 diabetes (OpT2mise): a randomised open-label controlled trial. Lancet. 2014;384:1265-72.
13. Kesavadev J, Balakrishnan S, Ahammed S, Jothydev S. Reduction of glycosylated hemoglobin following 6 months of continuous subcutaneous insulin infusion in an Indian population with type 2 diabetes. Diabetes Technol Ther. 2009;11:517-21.
14. Kesavadev J, Shankar A, Pillai PB, et al. CSII as an Alternative Therapeutic Strategy for Managing Type 2 diabetes: Adding the Indian Experience to a Global Perspective. Curr Diabetes Rev. 2016;12(4):314-14.
15. Sudhakaran C, Anjana RM, Rao K, et al. Role of continuous subcutaneous insulin infusion in patients with recalcitrant diabetes in South India. Diabetes Technol Ther. 2009;11:733-7.
16. Kesavadev J, Kumar A, Shankar A, et al. An Asian Indian woman with Wolfram syndrome on insulin pump: successful pregnancy and beyond. Diabetes Technol Ther. 2011;13:781-5.
17. Buse JB, Kudva YC, Battelino T, et al. Effects of sensor-augmented pump therapy on glycemic variability in well-controlled type 1 diabetes in the STAR 3 study. Diabetes Technol Ther. 2012;14:644-7.
18. Bergenstal RM, Tamborlane WV, Ahmann A, et al. Effectiveness of sensor-augmented insulin-pump therapy in type 1 diabetes. N Engl J Med. 2010;363:311-20.
19. Nørgaard K, Scaramuzza A, Bratina N, et al. Routine sensor-augmented pump therapy in type 1 diabetes: the INTERPRET study. Diabetes Technol Ther. 2013;15:273-80.
20. Kesavadev J, Jain SM, Muruganathan A, et al. Consensus evidence-based guidelines for use of insulin pump therapy in the management of diabetes as per Indian clinical practice. J Assoc Physicians India. 2014;62:34-41.
21. Kesavadev J, Das AK, Unnikrishnan R, et al. Use of insulin pumps in India: suggested guidelines based on experience and cultural differences. Diabetes Technol Ther. 2010;12:823-31.
22. Kesavadev J. Continuous insulin infusion systems in type 2 diabetes. J Assoc Physicians India. 2011;59(Suppl):41-3.
23. Kesavadev J. Fasting in Ramadan with an insulin pump. JPMA J Pak Med Assoc. 2015;65(5 Suppl 1):S47-50.
24. Saboo BD, Talaviya PA. Continuous subcutaneous insulin infusion: practical issues. Indian J Endocrinol Metab. 2012;16(Suppl 2):S259-62.
25. El-Khatib FH, Russell SJ, Nathan DM, et al. A bihormonal closed-loop artificial pancreas for type 1 diabetes. Sci Transl Med. 2010;2:27ra27.
26. Russell SJ, El-Khatib FH, Nathan DM, et al. Blood glucose control in type 1 diabetes with a bihormonal bionic endocrine pancreas. Diabetes Care. 2012;35:2148-55.
27. Russell SJ, El-Khatib FH, Sinha M, et al. Outpatient glycemic control with a bionic pancreas in type 1 diabetes. N Engl J Med. 2014;371:313-25.
28. El-Khatib FH, Russell SJ, Magyar KL, et al. Autonomous and continuous adaptation of a bihormonal bionic pancreas in adults and adolescents with type 1 diabetes. J Clin Endocrinol Metab. 2014;99:1701-11.
29. Russell SJ, Hillard MA, Balliro C, et al. Day and night glycaemic control with a bionic pancreas versus conventional insulin pump therapy in preadolescent children with type 1 diabetes: a randomised crossover trial. Lancet Diabetes Endocrinol. 2016;4:233-43.
30. Haidar A, Legault L, Dallaire M, et al. Glucose-responsive insulin and glucagon delivery (dual-hormone artificial pancreas) in adults with type 1 diabetes: a randomized crossover controlled trial. CMAJ. 2013;185:297-305.
31. Nimri R, Phillip M. Artificial pancreas: fuzzy logic and control of glycemia. Curr Opin Endocrinol Diabetes Obes. 2014;21:251-6.
32. Anderson SM, Raghinaru D, Pinsker JE, et al. Multinational home use of closed-loop control is safe and effective. Diabetes Care. 2016;dc152468.
33. Atlas E, Nimri R, Miller S, et al. MD-Logic Artificial Pancreas System. Diabetes Care. 2010;33(5):1072-6.

34. Nimri R, Danne T, Kordonouri O, et al. The "Glucositter" overnight automated closed loop system for type 1 diabetes: a randomized crossover trial. Pediatr Diabetes. 2013;14(3):159-67.
35. Miller S, Nimri R, Atlas E, et al. Automatic learning algorithm for the MD-logic artificial pancreas system. Diabetes Technol Ther. 2011;13(10):983-90.
36. Nimri R, Atlas E, Ajzensztejn M, et al. Feasibility study of automated overnight closed-loop glucose control under MD-logic artificial pancreas in patients with type 1 diabetes: the DREAM Project. Diabetes Technol Ther. 2012;14(8):728-35.
37. Nimri R, Muller I, Atlas E, et al. Night glucose control with MD-Logic artificial pancreas in home setting: a single blind, randomized crossover trial-interim analysis. Pediatr Diabetes. 2014;15(2):91-9.
38. Phillip M, Battelino T, Atlas E, et al. Nocturnal glucose control with an artificial pancreas at a diabetes camp. N Engl J Med. 2013;368(9):824-33.

CHAPTER 6

Diabetes in Older Adults

Medha N Munshi, Alan Sinclair

INTRODUCTION

Providing diabetes treatment to older adults requires consideration of issues that are typically not associated with the management of diabetes in younger adults. The pathophysiology of aging confers a multitude of comorbid conditions (such as vision and hearing loss, mobility issues, unstable balance and loss of dexterity) that have to be factored into the approach to treatment. Aging is also associated with a higher risk of developing conditions such as cognitive dysfunction, depression, chronic pain, and polypharmacy. Thus, in addition to macrovascular and microvascular complications associated with diabetes, it is important to recognize the subtle and not so subtle ways aging impacts on diabetes management. The best way to ensure successful diabetes management in older adults is to adapt our approaches to a patient's unique set of challenges and overall wellbeing and health status as well as personal preferences, and to aim for outcomes that are important for an individual's quality of life.

SCOPE OF THE PROBLEM

With increasing aging of the population and urbanization of lifestyle, the prevalence of diabetes has or is likely to reach epidemic levels in most countries. In the US, total diabetes prevalence is estimated to be 14% of the population and is highest in those aged ≥65 years; by the year 2050 diabetes prevalence could be as high as 33% of the whole population.[1] In the US National Health and Nutrition Examination Survey, the prevalence of diagnosed diabetes in those ≥75 years old was 14.9% and undiagnosed diabetes based on fasting plasma glucose and 2 hours oral glucose tolerance test was 13.4%.[2] This makes a total prevalence of diagnosed and undiagnosed diabetes of 28.3% with undiagnosed diabetes constituting a proportion of around 47%. The prevalence of "pre-diabetes" defined as either impaired fasting glycemia (IFG) or impaired glucose tolerance (IGT) was 46.7% in those aged ≥75 years old. Worldwide, the greatest proportional increase in the number of people with diabetes by age group is expected to occur in people between 60 and 79 years of age.[3] In 2014, approximately 387 million people around the world are believed to have diagnosed or undiagnosed diabetes. There will be a 69% increase in numbers of adults (aged 20–79 years) with diabetes in low- and middle-income countries compared to only 20% increase in higher income countries by the year 2030.[4] Over the next two decades, the number of people over 65 years of age is projected to increase markedly world-wide and will increase the number of older adults with diabetes further, making it an epidemic with significant personal and socioeconomic cost.

PATHOPHYSIOLOGY OF DIABETES IN OLDER ADULTS

Many of the differences between older patients compared to younger patients with diabetes stem from the pathophysiology of aging.[5] Inherent in the aging process is a progressive alteration in all aspects of glucose metabolism, including insulin secretion, insulin action, and hepatic glucose metabolism.[6,7] These changes are superimposed on a person's genetic background to magnify the incidence of type 2 diabetes as the aging process progresses. In some older people with diabetes, the loss of first phase insulin release occurs with the absence of the initial surge in postprandial insulin. Some evidence suggests that autoimmunity may play a role in the impairment of glucose-induced insulin secretion that occurs in lean, older people with diabetes.

PRESENTATION AND HETEROGENEITY IN OLDER ADULTS WITH DIABETES

It is not surprising that the clinical presentation of diabetes in the older patient can be different from that of younger adults (Table 6.1). It is important for clinicians to be aware of these differences so that they can adequately assess people as they age. Aging is associated with higher renal threshold for glucose, which leads to higher blood glucose levels in older patients before glycosuria occurs. Thus, one may not be able to detect glucose in the urine with dipsticks as expected. In addition, polyuria typically occurs following glycosuria. Thus, in older patients higher renal glucose threshold may prevent symptomatic polyuria. Further, polydipsia may be absent because of impaired thirst mechanisms in the older adults. The net result is that the classic symptoms of hyperglycemia—polyuria and polydipsia—are often not present (Box 6.1). In fact, dehydration is more common with aging because of altered thirst perception. As a result of all of these factors, infections, neuropathic pain, and failure to thrive may be the only clues for a diagnosis of diabetes among some older adults resulting in serious complication of nonketotic hyperosmolar state.

Table 6.1: Younger vs older adults with diabetes.

	Younger adults	***Older adults***
Presentation	Polyuria, polydipsia, polyphagia	Typical triad may be absent May present with neuroglycopenic or atypical symptoms
Comorbidities	Few	Comorbidities associated with longer duration of diabetes as well as those associated with aging
Polypharmacy (≥5 prescription medications/day)	Not typical	▪ Most elderly patients with diabetes have polypharmacy to control diabetes and other cardiovascular risk factors ▪ Pharmacokinetic change with aging affect metabolism and excretion of many antidiabetes medications as well as insulin

Box 6.1: Atypical clinical presentation of diabetes in the elderly.

- Atypical clinical presentation of diabetes in the elderly
- May not have typical symptoms such as polyuria, polydipsia
- Dehydration may result due to altered thirst perception and glycosuria
- May present with signs/symptoms of complications such as neuropathy, retinopathy at the time of diagnosis
- May not have typical symptoms of hypoglycemia such as tremors, palpitations, or sweating
- Hypoglycemia may present with neuroglycopenic symptoms like confusion, weakness, dizziness, etc.

Table 6.2: Traditional complications as comorbidities of diabetes.

Traditional complications of diabetes	***Comorbidities more likely to be seen in elderly with diabetes***
Cardiovascular disease Peripheral vascular disease Cerebrovascular disease Eye complications Renal complications Neurological complications	Cognitive dysfunction depression Physical disabilities Polypharmacy Chronic pain Urinary incontinence

Older adults with diabetes are a heterogeneous group with variable clinical, psychosocial and functional background. Some older individuals develop diabetes years earlier and may have significant complications with aging, while the others may present with newly diagnosed diabetes at an older age. In addition, some older adults are frail and have other underlying chronic conditions or limited physical or cognitive functioning while others have a few comorbidities and are very active. Older adults with diabetes can be highly functional community living individuals or they can be dependent on caregivers for their daily activities and may actually reside in assisted care facilities or nursing homes. The prevalence of diabetes in frail older adults living in nursing homes is certainly over 25%. Compared with community dwelling older individuals, nursing home patients with diabetes have a higher incidence of macrovascular complications, skin infections, and renal disease. The key point, therefore, is that these people need to be assessed as individuals in the context of their overall health and functional status, and with the recognition that adverse clinical, functional, and social circumstances often act as barriers to the older person's ability to perform diabetes self-management.

COMORBIDITIES AND COMPLICATIONS (TABLE 6.2)

As individuals age, they have a higher likelihood of developing multiple medical conditions, and with each of these conditions comes the probability that they will need to take multiple daily medications. In the past, the significant health burden in older people with diabetes was attributed primarily to higher risk of macrovascular and microvascular complications. However, many co-existing medical conditions (such as cognitive dysfunction, depression, functional disability, falls, polypharmacy, urinary incontinence, and chronic pain) not typically associated with diabetes occur at higher frequency in older adults with diabetes (Table 6.3). These conditions, often termed geriatric syndromes, may interfere with a patient's ability to

Table 6.3: Age-associated comorbidities in older adults with diabetes.

Comorbidities	***Impact on diabetes management***	***Strategies to improve care***
Cognitive dysfunction	▪ Behaviors affected include problem solving, planning, organization, insight, reasoning, and attention ▪ Difficulty with medical, nutritional, and exercise regimens adherence, e.g. omission of meals leading to hypoglycemia, incorrect dose or timing of insulin injections ▪ Difficulty in recognizing and reporting hypoglycemic episodes	▪ Red flags due to declining cognition include recent hypoglycemic episodes, deterioration of glycemic control after reasonable efforts, or feeling overwhelmed by self-care Actions: ▪ Simplify treatment plans to avoid hypoglycemia ▪ Liberalize glycemic goals ▪ Involve caregivers
Depression	Associated with poor glycemic control, decreased adherence to treatment strategies, increased functional disability, increased risk of coronary heart disease, higher mortality, and increased healthcare costs to society	Identify and treat depression
Physical disability	May require assistance from other caregivers or family members to implement tasks such as self-monitoring of blood glucose (SMBG), giving insulin injections, meal preparation and following a physical activity regimen	▪ Weigh benefits of improved glycemic control against need for caregiver support with intensive therapy ▪ Avoid factor that increase fall-risks such as use of complex insulin therapy ▪ Refer to an exercise physiologist and a supervised program for physical ▪ Use devices that facilitate self-care, e.g. talking meters, large font meters, insulin pens
Polypharmacy	▪ Increased probability of non-adherence and the potential for interactions between medications ▪ Some medications impair ability to recognize hypoglycemia ▪ Side effects of single or combination of drugs may exacerbate comorbidities ▪ Financial burden	▪ Keep the medication list current and review it at each medical visit ▪ Enlist others such as family members or caregivers ▪ Use of pill boxes and alarms

perform self-care tasks, including glucose monitoring, understanding the role of diet and exercise in glucose excursions, and coping with a complex insulin regimen. Difficulty with self-management may lead to increased risk of non-adherence or treatment errors, contributing to an increased risk of hypoglycemia and poor glycemic control, which in turn leads to further difficulty with self-management and ultimately increased risk of morbidity and mortality. Thus, before developing treatment and management plans for older adults, it is of key importance to conduct a careful and comprehensive assessment for all potential comorbidities, which will very possibly impact how you plan your therapeutic approach.

Cognitive Impairment

Cognitive dysfunction has been associated with both type 1 and type 2 diabetes, with a 1.5-fold greater risk of cognitive decline and 1.6-fold increase in risk of future dementia. In our study, 34% of highly functional older adults living in community screened positive for cognitive dysfunction.[8] Cognitive dysfunction in older adults affects many domains such as executive dysfunction, psychomotor efficiency, global cognition, episodic memory, semantic memory, and working memory. Many older patients with cognitive dysfunction remain undiagnosed; particularly in the early stages as subtle declines remain unrecognized by family as well as healthcare providers. In an everyday practice, short screening tools such as a clock drawing test and three word recall test (MiniCog) are useful.[9]

Depression

Depression is approximately twice as common in people with diabetes compared with the general population. Diabetes and depression have a bidirectional relationship of increased risk. Depression is frequently undiagnosed and remains untreated in this high-risk population. The risk of major depression is increased in people with diabetes who also have two or more co-existing chronic conditions, such as hypertension, coronary artery disease, or arthritis. Timely identification and treatment of depression is important.

Polypharmacy

Polypharmacy is commonly defined as use of 5 or more medications per day. Use of multiple drugs is a complex, challenging aspect of caring for older adults who often require multiple medications to manage their diabetes and associated conditions. Although, multiple medications are unavoidable in some patients to achieve glycemic control and to adequately control cardiovascular risk factors, a focus on appropriate prescribing, interventions to increase regimen adherence, and assessment of financial feasibility is important.

Physical Disability and Falls

Older adults with diabetes have a reduction in physical function and overall health status compared to age-matched controls living in the same community and is more likely to use a mobility aid such as a cane or a walker. They may have difficulty performing activities of daily living (bathing, toileting, eating, dressing, and grooming) as well as instrumental activities of daily living (travelling, shopping, using the telephone, managing finances, doing housework, and taking medications). Consulting with a social worker may help establish a support network for such people. Falls, especially the ones resulting in injury, are also more common in older adults. The increased risk of falls in older adults with diabetes is usually multifactorial. Presence of peripheral and/or autonomic neuropathy, cardiovascular disease, reduced renal function, muscle weakness, lower limb dysfunction, functional disability, loss of vision, polypharmacy, and comorbidities like osteoarthritis or even hypoglycemia may contribute to, and worsen the impact of, falls in frail older adults. People who develop a fear of falling are usually reluctant to follow physical activity recommendations.

Urinary Incontinence

Diabetes increases a woman's risk of developing urinary incontinence. This condition in older patients with diabetes, especially women, is also multifactorial in etiology. Risk factors include urinary tract infection, vaginal infection, autonomic neuropathy (resulting in either neurogenic bladder or fecal impaction) and polyuria due to hyperglycemia. Although there is no direct evidence to suggest a deleterious effect of incontinence on diabetes control, identification and treatment are recommended to improve quality of life.

Chronic Pain

Pain is considered the 5th vital sign with huge impact on patients' quality of life, and should be evaluated at each visit. Many older adults are reluctant to complain about pain. However, pain can increase depression, distract people from diabetes self-care, reduce the likelihood that they are active, and increase adrenalin levels, which can impact glucose levels. Management of pain improves overall quality of life in this vulnerable population in addition to increasing the efficacy and outcomes of diabetes treatments.

HYPOGLYCEMIA

Hypoglycemia is usually the limiting factor in achieving recommended levels of glycemic control at any age. In an aging population specifically, hypoglycemia can lead to poor outcomes such as, precipitation of cardiovascular or cerebrovascular events, and exacerbation of cognitive dysfunction. Thus, avoidance of hypoglycemia is an important consideration while establishing goals for glycemic control and choosing medical regimen. The risks of hypoglycemia are multifactorial (Box 6.2) and should be carefully looked for at each visit in these patients.

However, simply moderating the A1c goal to a higher level may not actually prevent hypoglycemia. A small study using continuous glucose monitoring (CGM) in older people with poorly controlled diabetes [A1c>8% (>64 mmol/mol)], showed frequent and often unrecognized hypoglycemic episodes. Thus, merely chasing high glucose levels with more insulin may not always be successful in improving glucose control; for example, in the context of an older person who does not recognize hypoglycemic symptoms can foster increased episodes of unrecognized hypoglycemia and rebound hyperglycemia, further prompting patients and providers to chase with more insulin. In such instances, simplification of treatment regimen to match an older patient's coping skills may help achieve the best glycemic control balanced with a more significantly reduced risk of hypoglycemia.[10] This was shown in a recent study of older adults on complex insulin regimen. Simplification of regimen with once day long-acting insulin in combination with other noninsulin agents decreases the risk of hypoglycemia without compromising glycemic control.

Glycemic Goals and Goal Setting

The goals for glycemic control as well as risk factor management in older adults should be individualized, reflecting the individual's overall health status and self-care, or assisted-care, limitations (Table 6.4). Acute complications of hyperglycemia in older adults include

Box 6.2: Hypoglycemia in older adults.

- Atypical clinical presentation with neuroglycopenic manifestations of hypoglycemia (e.g. cognitive changes, delirium, weakness, dizziness) as compared to the adrenergic manifestations (e.g. tremors, sweating, palpitations) is common
- Neuroglycopenic symptoms may be misconstrued as primary neurological disease (such as a transient ischemic attack) by patients or caregivers, leading to difficulty in diagnosis
- Diminished glucose counter-regulation involving glucagon, epinephrine, and growth hormone responses to hypoglycemia increase the risk
- Reduction in autonomic warning symptoms interferes with recognition and timely treatment
- Gastroparesis increase the risk of hypoglycemia immediately after meals, if medications are not adjusted for the delay in food absorption
- Forgetting to eat meals on time, difficulty with meal preparations, anorexia and weight-loss after acute illness add to the risk of hypoglycemia
- Even a mild episode of hypoglycemia in combination with other comorbidities may lead to increased risk of falls and fracture leading to severe compromise in quality of life
- Carefully monitor for hypoglycemia in people who exercise periodically, miss meals, abuse alcohol, have impaired renal, cardiac, or gastrointestinal disease, and after recent hospitalization
- Avoid glucose-lowering medication with high risk of hypoglycemia such as sulfonylureas and insulin in older patients if possible.

Table 6.4: Glycemic goals based on expert opinions and guidelines.

	Healthy ▪ Few comorbidities ▪ No cognitive dysfunction ▪ Intact functionality	Intermediate ▪ Multiple comorbidities ▪ Mild-moderate cognitive dysfunction ▪ 2+IADL dependency	Complex ▪ Multiple and severe comorbidities ▪ Severe cognitive dysfunction ▪ 2+ADL dependency	Limited life expectancy ▪ End-stage comorbidities ▪ On hospice or palliative care
Glycemic control	<7.5%	<8%	<8.5%	Not reliable or important
Fasting and pre-meal glucose	80–130	90–150	100–200	Avoid symptomatic hyperglycemia
Blood pressure	<140/90	<150/90	<150/90	<160/95
Cholesterol	Statin unless not tolerated	Statin unless not tolerated	Statin unless not tolerated or high treatment burden	Consider stopping statin if low life expectancy

Contd...

Contd...

Diet	▪ Minimize complexity of diet planning ▪ Stress consistency in carbohydrate intake and timing	Avoid large carbohydrate peaks	Liberalize diet and encourage what patient enjoys	Avoid any dietary restrictions
Exercise	Encourage all types of exercise: aerobic, resistance training, and those of range or movement and flexibility	Provide safe environment to exercise to avoid falls	Encourage as much as activity as possible to improve conditioning	Focus activities to improve quality of life

(IADL: Instrumental activities of daily living [e.g. medication management, shopping, house-keeping, transportation, etc.]; ADL: Activities of daily living [e.g. transferring, bathing, dressing, toileting, eating])

Box 6.3: General principles in developing treatment plans and goals.

- Overall health status versus chronological health
- Comorbidities, complications, and overall treatment burden
- Social and financial resources
- Life expectancy
- Patient's own preferences and quality of life

dehydration, impaired vision, and cognition; all of which contribute to functional decline and an increased risk of falling. Conversely, the adverse effects of too aggressive diabetes treatment, most notably hypoglycemia, can also result in poor outcomes, such as traumatic falls and exacerbation of comorbid conditions. Thus, a careful balance must be sought and clinicians need to differentiate between older people's chronological age verses actual health status, duration of disease and age of onset, presence of complications and comorbidities, variable life expectancy, social support systems and their financial status (Box 6.3). It is often these latter factors that are more important in setting therapeutic goals. Recently several organizations have published guidelines to help clinicians care for their older patients with diabetes.[11-14]

Hemoglobin A1C (A1c)

It is the most commonly used test to assess average glycemic control and monitor treatment efficacy in people with diabetes. The A1c test is now also recommended for the diagnosis of diabetes excluding some circumstances.[15] There is some concern that the interpretation of A1c and its translation to estimated average glucose may not be consistent in different population of different age and ethnicity. In older adults with diabetes usually have multiple co-existing medical conditions, many of which (such as anemia, renal insufficiency, uremia, acidosis, hemodialysis, erythropoietin therapy) falsely increase or decrease A1c levels.[16] Aging itself is associated with elevation of A1c. A large cross-sectional study showed that in the nondiabetic population, A1c was positively associated with age.[17] The prevalence of all these conditions affecting A1c levels is even higher in the nursing home population. At present, there are no studies evaluating how much effect each condition exerts on A1c. Recently, a small study have raised caution in interpreting A1c and estimated average glucose levels in older people using the same formula as for younger adults.[18] In recent years, A1c has been used as the quality indicator for diabetes management in surveys assessing the number of patients achieving treatment goals, and by insurance companies assessing medical care provided by physicians. Consequently, lowering A1c to a certain number becomes a goal for clinicians striving to provide quality care to patients with diabetes. The biggest problem with this scenario is that overtreatment due to falsely elevated A1c can have deleterious effects on patients, especially due to hypoglycemia. The older population has worse outcomes due to hypoglycemia, which can lead to falls, fractures, and exacerbation of chronic conditions like cognitive dysfunction. On the other hand, undertreatment due to falsely low A1c levels can lead to false reassurance and complications of hyperglycemia. In addition, diabetes management guidelines and treatment algorithms use only A1c levels to define glycemic goals. A1c continues to be an excellent marker for moderate to long-term glycemic control, as long as its short comings are well understood, and watched for.

PHARMACOTHERAPY

All types of glucose-lowering medications and insulins can be used successfully in older patients when used carefully. Most people with diabetes and their medical providers prefer to use the oral medications as the first-line therapy. However, patients with significant hyperglycemia and glucose toxicity with very high glucose values at presentation are now available to target hyperglycemia. The Table 6.5 shows mechanisms of action, advantages, disadvantages, and caveats of these classes of medications in the older population. Metformin remains an attractive agent to use due to a low risk of hypoglycemia in older adults with diabetes. It is important to remember that in frail older adults with reduced muscle may need insulin initially to establish control. It is usually possible to change the regimen to an oral medication once the glucose levels are controlled and the effects of glucose toxicity have resolved. "Start low and go slow" is a good principle to follow when starting new medications or adjusting insulin in an older patient.

Many different classes of glucose-lowering agents mass, serum creatinine may not reflect true renal function. Calculated creatinine clearance or glomerular filtration rate (GFR) are used for dosing and monitoring the treatment. If the GFR is below 60 mL/min/1.73 m^2, careful and frequent monitoring should be conducted. If the GFR is below 45 mL/min/1.73 m^2, metformin half maximum dose should be used. It is best to avoid metformin if the GFR is below 30 mL/min/1.73 m^2.[19] Any older patient treated with metformin should stop taking the drug immediately if they become ill for any reason, or if they are to undergo a procedure requiring the use of iodinated contrast material. The longer-acting insulin secretagogues, the sulfonylureas are usually well tolerated in younger population but should be avoided in older people due to risk of hypoglycemia.[20] However, lower cost of these drugs still makes them attractive agents in areas where patients pay out of pocket for medications. Thiazolidinediones do not pose risk of hypoglycemia, making them an excellent choice for some older people. Possibility of increased bladder cancer risk with pioglitazone has dampened enthusiasm to some extent for

Table 6.5: Oral and injectable antidiabetic medications for older patients.

Oral glucose-lowering medications				
Class	***Mechanism of action***	***Advantages in older population***	***Disadvantages in older population***	***Caveats for use in older population***
Biguanides Metformin	Decrease hepatic glucose production, increase GLP-1 secretion	▪ Low risk for hypoglycemia ▪ Low cost ▪ Well understood side effects	▪ Not useful in decompensated ▪ CHF, GFR < 45, acute illnesses, and dehydration–frequently seen in elderly ▪ Side effects include gas, diarrhea, B_{12} deficiency, lactic acidosis ▪ Weight loss can be problematic in frail elderly	▪ Use as initial therapy unless contraindicated ▪ Initiate at low dose, increase dose slowly and take with food to decrease gas, diarrhea ▪ Extended release formulation may decrease GI symptoms ▪ May cause weight loss ▪ GI symptoms may develop after prolonged use ▪ Measure liver functions, serum creatinine and eGFR initially, then periodically and with any increase in dose ▪ Avoid initiating and stop use if eGFR <45
Insulin secretagogues Sulfonylureas	Stimulate beta cell insulin secretion	Low cost	Risk of hypoglycemia especially with longer acting sulfonylureas such as chlorpropamide (first generation sulfonylurea) and glyburide	▪ Avoid use if possible due to risk of hypoglycemia ▪ Consider use of short acting sulfonylurea in the setting of renal disease to reduce the risk for hypoglycemia

Contd...

Contd...

Class	***Mechanism of action***	***Advantages in older population***	***Disadvantages in older population***	***Caveats for use in older population***
Meglitinides ▪ Repaglinide ▪ Nateglinide				▪ Repaglinide or nateglinide may be useful for those with postprandial hyperglycemia or with hypo-glycemia on sulfonylurea ▪ Watch for increased risk of hypoglycemia with acute illness, hospitalization, weight loss, lack of appetite, skipped meals and those with memory issues
Thiazolidinedi-ones (TZDs) ▪ Pioglitazone ▪ Rosiglitazone	Improve glucose transport, and decrease hepatic glucose production	▪ Low risk of hypoglycemia ▪ May increase fluid retention	▪ Fluid retention and CHF are common co-morbidities in older people preventing use ▪ Increases bone loss and risk for bone fracture ▪ May increase risk for macular edema	▪ Side effects of fluid retention- can be limiting factors in using this class of medications ▪ Concerns regarding potential small increase in bladder cancer are less in those with limited life expectancy
Alpha-glucosidase inhibitors ▪ Acarbose ▪ Miglitol	Delay absorption and breakdown of carbohydrates	▪ Low cost ▪ Low risk of hypoglycemia ▪ Use if postprandial hyperglycemia predominates	▪ May cause gas, diarrhea and aggravate chronic intestinal disorders ▪ Do not use in renal impairment (creatinine > 2.0)	▪ Modest glucose lowering affect ▪ Initiate at low dose and increase slowly to lower GI side effects

Contd...

Contd...

Class	Mechanism of action	Advantages in older population	Disadvantages in older population	Caveats for use in older population
DPP-4 Inhibitors ▪ Sitagliptin ▪ Saxagliptin ▪ Linagliptin ▪ Alogliptin	In a glucose dependent manner, these medications slow the inactivation of incretin hormones, resulting in increased insulin secretion and decreased glucagon levels	▪ Low risk of hypoglycemia ▪ Better for controlling postprandial glucose elevations	▪ Occasional diarrhea and stomach discomfort ▪ Safety of use in the setting of prior pancreatitis is unknown ▪ Lower glucose lowering efficacy may result in the need for a multidrug program ▪ Increased risk for CHF with saxagliptin	▪ Good drug for frail older people, with newly diagnosed DM ▪ Reduce dose in renal disease with some members of the class ▪ Postmarketing reports of hepatic failure with alogliptin
SGLT-2 ▪ Canagliflozin ▪ Dapagliflozin ▪ Empagliflozin	Blocks the reabsorption of glucose by the proximal tubule of the kidney thereby increasing excretion of glucose in the urine	Low risk of hypoglycemia	▪ Not for use with moderate-severe renal dysfunction ▪ May reduce blood pressure ▪ Increased risk for genital mycotic infections and UTI ▪ Risk of dehydration, weight loss, hyperkalemia, increased LDL cholesterol ▪ Little data available for safety in the older population	▪ Adjust dose in mild kidney disease ▪ To decrease the risk of hypotension and dehydration, consider antihypertensive medication adjustment especially diuretics when starting this class of medications ▪ Do not use dapagliflozin in setting of bladder cancer, use with caution with a history of bladder cancer

Contd...

Contd...

Injectable antidiabetic medications				
Class	***Mechanism of action***	***Advantages in older population***	***Disadvantages in older population***	***Caveats for use in older population***
Incretin mimetics ▪ Exenatide ▪ Liraglutide ▪ Extended release exenatide ▪ Albiglitude ▪ Dulaglutide	In a glucose dependent manner increase insulin secretion, decrease glucagon secretion, slow gastric emptying, and increase satiety	▪ Use may be associated with weight loss, this is helpful in the overweight/ obese person ▪ Low risk of hypoglycemia	▪ These are injectable medications ▪ Dosing frequency is dependent on the medication and can range from twice a day to once weekly ▪ Side effects include nausea, diarrhea and increased satiety, which can affect nutritional status in the older adult ▪ Increased risk for pancreatitis ▪ Risk for acute renal impairment ▪ High cost ▪ Limited data on safety in the older population	▪ Low risk of hypoglycemia and formulation that can be used once weekly makes this an attractive agent to use in older people ▪ Consider the person's cognitive abilities, dexterity and visual acuity before considering use of any injectable medication ▪ To decrease risk of hypoglycemia if using with a sulfonylurea or basal insulin, consider initially decreasing sulfonylurea or insulin dose

its use. Alpha-glucosidase inhibitors have relatively lower efficacy but are safe in older adults. The main side effects that limit their use are flatulence and diarrhea, which are very common. The incretin-mimetic agents and DPP-4 inhibitors are well-tolerated by older individuals.

Designing Treatment Strategies for Older Adults with Diabetes

Beyond the considerations of degree of β-cell dysfunction and insulin resistance, the treatment strategies in older adults also require consideration of comorbidities, ability to perform self-care, caregiver support system, and finances. In addition, if the glycemic goals are not met after reasonable efforts, the patient should be evaluated for contributing causes, such as difficulty adhering to the medication, side effects, or poor understanding of the nutrition plan. Recently, there is an increased focus on patient-centered approach to diabetes management. An update to a position statement of the American Diabetes Association (ADA) and the European Association for the Study of Diabetes (EASD) have identified practical algorithms to guide clinicians on how to start and intensify both antidiabetic medications as well as insulin therapy in adults with diabetes.[21] In addition, the International Diabetes Federation (IDF) has published global guidelines for managing older people with type 2 diabetes.[22] The stepwise approach starts with the lifestyle modifications and metformin as the drug of first choice and then choosing next class of medications based on cost, risk of hypoglycemia, efficacy, side-effect profile, and impact on weight. These guidelines and algorithms can be useful tools in developing individualized approaches for goal setting and for the use of glucose-lowering medication in older adults.

Insulin

When other glucose-lowering medications are not able to adequately control hyperglycemia, insulin can be used carefully in older adults. The risk of hypoglycemia is higher with insulin compared with other glucose-lowering medications. A higher complexity insulin regimen can be worse for increasing risk of hypoglycemia than once day basal insulin. It is common to see an older adult's ability to manage a complicated insulin regimen change with increasing age or worsening overall health. Before beginning insulin therapy, it is important to evaluate whether or not the patient is physically and cognitively capable of drawing up and giving the appropriate dose of insulin using syringes and vials or using an insulin pen, monitoring blood glucose, and recognizing and treating hypoglycemia. Errors in insulin technique are frequently seen in older adults even after many years of previously successful self-managed insulin treatment. Thus, periodical assessment and education about the correct injection technique is important in this population.

Currently, there are various types of insulins available with different time-action curves making it easier to target hyperglycemia and avoid hypoglycemia. The algorithm for using different types of insulin, their initiation, and intensification are well described in the guidelines from the ADA, EASD, and IDF.[21,22] The algorithm underscores the point that as the number of insulin injections increases during the day, the flexibility in meals and activity increases along with complexity of the regimen. However, avoiding complex regimens is prudent for older populations of patients. In a recent prospective study, simplification of the insulin regimen was performed by replacing multiple insulin injections/day with once day basal insulin combined with non-insulin agents (Munshi et al, in press JAMA Int Med 2016). This simplification resulted in a lower risk of hypoglycemia as shown by duration of glucose<70 mg/dL (<3.9 mmol/L) on continuous glucose monitoring (CGM) without worsening glycemic control (A1c). Diabetes-related distress was also improved after simplification in this study.

EDUCATIONAL STRATEGIES IN OLDER ADULTS WITH DIABETES

In the light of the unique needs of older patients, effective geriatric diabetes education programs are increasingly important. To positively impact self-care and quality of life in older people with diabetes, education programs must be tailored to patients' individual needs.[23] However, education programs developed especially for older populations with diabetes are rare. The American Association of Diabetes Educators (AADE)[https://www.diabeteseducator.org/docs/default-source/default-document-library/special-considerations-in-the-management-of-older-persons-with-diabetes.pdf?sfursn=0] and the ADA along with American Geriatrics Society (AGS)[11] have formulated guidelines for diabetes education in older patients largely based on expert consensus. These guidelines take in to consideration the clinical and functional heterogeneity seen in older population. These factors need to be assessed in all elders presenting for diabetic education and reassessed on a regular basis, since patient's ability to learn and retain information can change with aging and progression of medical comorbidities.

SELF-MONITORING PROGRAMS

Self-monitoring of blood glucose (SMBG) is a central component of self-care for all people with diabetes. It allows people to visualize their glycemic patterns, and consider them in the context of the other factors that impact glucose control such as food intake, activity, timing of various daily activities, stress. The ability to perform SMBG, as well as assess the implications of its results on a daily basis, is often a key factor in determining what type of diabetes treatment program is appropriate for any given individual. The monitoring numbers are important for the healthcare provider to assess the effectiveness of treatment and risk of hypoglycemia. Devices such as talking meters for the visually impaired and large meters for patients with arthritis should be considered when appropriate. The frequency of monitoring is usually influenced by the stability of blood glucose excursions, the nature of the treatment strategy, the patients' cognitive and physical abilities, caregiver support, and availability of resources. The questions that can be answered by self-monitoring are:

- Are there unrecognized hypoglycemic events occurring at different times of the day?
- When are the hyperglycemic excursions more predominant? Fasting? Before meals? Which meal?
- How are the glycemic patterns trending over time? Stable? Changing?
- Which insulin/medication doses need change?

Take Home Points in the care of older adults with diabetes

- The decision process to manage diabetes older adults often requires a more complex combination of data, clinical skills, and formal evaluation for multiple diseases and conditions to determine the best approach.
- When evaluating an older patient with diabetes, goal setting for both hyper- and hypoglycemia is equally important.
- The unique presentations of hypoglycemia and hypoglycemic unawareness require the need to keep a high degree of suspicion even when the patient denies having hypoglycemia.
- It is good practice to repeat conversations about important issues in self-management such as recognition and treatment of hypoglycemia at every visit.
- Medications have potentially higher side effects in older adults. Thus, choosing an agent that is least harmful to the patient with his/her comorbidities is appropriate.
- When patients on complex insulin regimen are unable to cope with self-care, simplification of the regimen can achieve lower risk of hypoglycemia without compromising glycemic control.
- Health is dynamic in older adults. Hospitalization, delirium, anorexia, weight loss and deconditioning are seen frequently in elderly who become unwell. Increased or decreased needs for medications/ insulin should be carefully assessed.
- Role of caregivers is critical. Spouse, family or other caregivers such as visiting nurses should be educated along with the patients.

REFERENCES

1. Boyle JP, Thompson TJ, Gregg EW, et al. Projection of the year 2050 burden of diabetes in the US adult population: dynamic modeling of incidence, mortality, and prediabetes prevalence. Popul Health Metr. 2010;8:29.
2. Cowie CC, Rust KF, Ford ES, et al. Full accounting of diabetes and pre-diabetes in the US population in 1988-1994 and 2005-2006. Diabetes Care. 2009;32(2):287-94.
3. Whiting DR, Gauriguata L, Weil C, et al. IDF diabetes atlas: global estimates of the prevalence of diabetes for 2011 and 2030. Diabetes Res Clin Pract. 2011;94(3):311-21.
4. Shaw JE, Sicree RA, Zimmet PZ. Global estimates of the prevalence of diabetes for 2010 and 2030. Diabetes Res Clin Pract. 2010;87(1):4-14.
5. Meneilly GS. The pathophysiology of diabetes in the elderly. In: Lipsitz LA, Munshi MN (Eds). Geriatric Diabetes, Informa Healthcare: New York, NY. 2007. pp. 29-36.
6. Meneilly GS, Elahi D. Metabolic alterations in middle-aged and elderly lean patients with type 2 diabetes. Diabetes Care. 2005;28(6):1498-9.
7. Meneilly GS, Elliott T. Metabolic alterations in middle-aged and elderly obese patients with type 2 diabetes. Diabetes Care. 1999;22(1):112-8.
8. Munshi M, Grande L, Hayes M, et al. Cognitive dysfunction is associated with poor diabetes control in older adults. Diabetes Care. 2006;29(8):1794-9.
9. Sinclair AJ, Gadsby R, Hillson R, et al. Brief report: Use of the Mini-Cog as a screening tool for cognitive impairment in diabetes in primary care. Diabetes Res Clin Pract. 2013;100(1):e23-5.
10. Munshi MN, Hayes M, Sternthal A, et al. Use of serum c-peptide level to simplify diabetes treatment regimens in older adults. Am J Med. 2009;122(4):395-7.
11. Kirkman MS, Briscoe VJ, Clark N, et al. Diabetes in older adults. Diabetes Care. 2012;35(12):2650-64.
12. Sinclair AJ, Paolisso G, Gastro M, et al. European Diabetes Working Party for Older People 2011 clinical guidelines for type 2 diabetes mellitus. Executive summary. Diabetes Metab. 2011; 37(Suppl 3):S27-38.
13. Munshi MN, Florez H, Huang ES, et al. Management of diabetes in long-term care and skilled nursing facilities: a position statement of the American Diabetes Association. Diabetes Care. 2016;39(2):308-18.
14. Cho NH, CS, Distiller L, Dong B, Dunning T, Gadsby R, Goel A, Munshi MN, Sinclair A, Sinay I. IDF Global Guideline for Managing older people with Type 2 Diabetes, 2013.
15. Standards of medical care in diabetes—2012. Diabetes Care, 2012;35(Suppl 1): S11-63.
16. Inzucchi SE. Clinical practice. Diagnosis of diabetes. N Engl J Med. 2012;367(6):542-50.
17. Pani LN, Korenda L, Meigs JB, et al. Effect of aging on A1C levels in individuals without diabetes: evidence from the Framingham Offspring Study and the National Health and Nutrition Examination Survey 2001-2004. Diabetes Care. 2008;31(10):1991-6.
18. Munshi MN, Segal AR, Suhl E, et al. Shortfalls of the use of HbA1C-derived eAG in older adults with diabetes. Diabetes Res Clin Pract. 2015;110(1):60-5.
19. Lipska KJ, Bailey CJ, Inzucchi SE. Use of metformin in the setting of mild-to-moderate renal insufficiency. Diabetes Care. 2011;34(6):1431-7.
20. Shorr RI, Ray WA, Daugherty JR, et al. Incidence and risk factors for serious hypoglycemia in older persons using insulin or sulfonylureas. Arch Intern Med. 1997;157(15):1681-6.
21. Inzucchi SE, Bergenstal RM, Buse JB, et al. Management of hyperglycemia in type 2 diabetes, 2015: a patient-centered approach: update to a position statement of the American Diabetes Association and the European Association for the Study of Diabetes. Diabetes Care. 2015;38(1):140-9.
22. Global Guidelines for Managing Older People with Type 2 Diabetes, 2014.
23. Suhl E, Bonsignore P. Diabetes: Self-management education for older adults. Diabetes Spectrum. 2006;19:234-40.

CHAPTER 7

Diabetic Retinopathy

Paolo S Silva, Jerry D Cavallerano

INTRODUCTION

Diabetic retinopathy is a common microvascular complication of diabetes mellitus (DM), affecting virtually all individuals with type 1 or type 2 DM duration of 15–20 years or more. The World Health Organization estimates that in 2002 diabetic retinopathy accounted for approximately 5% of blindness worldwide, accounting for approximately 5 million blind persons. This blindness generally results from nonresolving vitreous hemorrhage, traction retinal detachment, or diabetic macular edema. Currently, there are no means of preventing diabetic retinopathy and there is no cure for the condition. It is not surprising, therefore, that loss of vision is consistently reported to be the most feared complication of DM. Nevertheless, beginning in the late 1960s with the advent of laser photocoagulation and other effective therapies, the advent of intravitreous injections of corticosteroids and a variety of agents targeting antivascular endothelial growth factor (anti-VEGF), greater understanding of diabetic retinopathy, and recognition of the impact of glycemic control and other comorbidities such as hypertension, dyslipidemia, hypercholesterolemia, renal disease, and anemia, the risk of moderate and severe vision loss from diabetic retinopathy can be virtually eliminated with appropriate care.

While diabetic retinopathy remains a leading cause of new-onset blindness worldwide, the 5-year risk of severe visual loss can be reduced to less than 5% if a person with diabetic retinopathy approaching or just reaching high-risk proliferative retinopathy undergoes scatter (panretinal) laser photocoagulation surgery or has intravitreous injection of an anti-VEGF agent. Furthermore, people with diabetic macular edema can have the risk of moderate visual loss reduced through intravitreous injection of anti-VEGF agents and appropriate focal laser photocoagulation when indicated. Since diabetic retinopathy is often asymptomatic in its most treatable stages, early detection of diabetic retinopathy through regularly scheduled ocular examinations becomes critical.

EPIDEMIOLOGY

For the past 50 years, diabetic retinopathy has remained the most common cause of blindness in the working age adult population in the United States and other developed countries. Nearly all persons with 15 or more years of diabetes develop some form of clinically evident diabetic retinopathy, making it one of the most frequently occurring microvascular complications of diabetes. Diabetic macular edema is a manifestation of diabetic retinopathy that may occur in any stage of the retinopathy, but increases in prevalence with advancing diabetic retinopathy severity and often leads to loss of central vision. Pooled data from eight population-based studies estimate that among persons 40 years of age and older, the prevalence of diabetic retinopathy was 40% and the prevalence of severe retinopathy (severe-very severe nonproliferative diabetic retinopathy and proliferative diabetic retinopathy or diabetic macular edema) was 8%. Based on these estimates, it is projected that the diabetic population having 40 years of age or older in the United States is over 4 million persons with diabetic retinopathy and 900,000 persons with vision-threatening diabetic retinopathy. These epidemiologic estimates provide us with the magnitude of the public health program of the diabetic retinal disease and allow us to develop public health strategies to prevent or reduce the occurrence or progression of this complication.

PATHOPHYSIOLOGY

The pathogenesis of diabetic retinopathy is not fully understood but represents an end-organ response to a systemic condition. The chronic state of hyperglycemia leads to interconnected biochemical, hemodynamic, and cellular changes within the retina. The development and progression of diabetic retinopathy result from a complex interplay of multiple factors that may differ between individuals. The relative contributions of different mechanisms vary in importance at different stages of diabetic retinopathy. Advanced glycation end products (AGEs), protein kinase C and polyol pathways, and changes in retinal blood flow are particularly important early in the course of the disease when no clinically evident changes are seen. Retinal ischemia and angiogenic factors such as VEGF and insulin-like growth factor are particularly important in the more advanced stages of the disease and play a role in the development of proliferative diabetic retinopathy and diabetic macular edema. Genetic differences and observed variability in susceptibility among individuals at different stages of the disease are likely brought about by inter- and intra-individual variations in biochemical or physiologic responses to hyperglycemia. This variability may in part explain why some diabetic persons have minimal diabetic retinopathy despite years of severe hyperglycemia, whereas in others severe diabetic retinopathy develops in a short period despite relatively good glycemic control. The precise pathophysiology of diabetic retinal disease, although extensively studied, has remained elusive due to the multiple pathways involved and the variability in the clinical outcomes observed, making direct casual relationships relatively difficult to establish.

LESIONS OF DIABETIC RETINOPATHY

Biochemical, vascular, inflammatory, and neuroretinal changes result in the commonly observed clinical lesions of diabetic retinopathy. The presence and extent of these lesions are related to the risk of progression of diabetic retinopathy and the risk of vision loss.

Hemorrhages and Microaneurysms

Microaneurysms are generally the first clinically observable sign of diabetic retinopathy (Fig. 7.1A). Microaneurysms are circular, generally 125 μ in diameter, and have sharp edges. Microaneurysms result from loss of functional pericytes, which are critical for supporting retinal capillaries, and their loss of function or decreased number leads to outpouchings of the capillary walls. These microaneurysms can leak fluid, protein, and other molecules into the retina.

Ruptured microaneurysms, decompensated retinal capillaries, and intraretinal microvascular abnormalities can result in intraretinal hemorrhages. Circular lesions larger than 125 μ in diameter are generally dot or punctate hemorrhages, which are usually larger than microaneurysms, have irregular borders, and may be of variable density. Dot hemorrhages and microaneurysms lie within the retinal tissue itself. The clinical appearance of these hemorrhages reflects the retinal architecture at the level at which the hemorrhages occur, so hemorrhages deeper in the retina, at which point the arrangement of cells is more or less perpendicular to the surface of the retina, assume a pinpoint or dot shape. Since the clinical distinction between microaneurysms and dot hemorrhages may be difficult, clinically it is common to combine the description as hemorrhages and/or microaneurysms. Hemorrhages can also have a blot or linear appearance, particularly when present in the nerve fiber layer of the retina (Fig. 7.1A).

Hemorrhages that are anterior to the retinal surface and posterior to the vitreous face are classified as preretinal hemorrhages. Hemorrhages that have broken into the vitreous cavity are classified as vitreous hemorrhages, which are usually associated with fibrovascular proliferation or retinal tears.

Venous Caliber Abnormalities

Venous caliber abnormalities include venous dilatation, venous narrowing, venous beading, venous loop formation, or venous reduplication. Venous caliber abnormalities develop in the presence of severe retinal hypoxia and there are often large areas of nonperfusion adjacent to these veins. Scatter (panretinal) photocoagulation may cause these abnormal veins to become less dilated and more regular (Fig. 7.1B).

Intraretinal Microvascular Abnormalities

Intraretinal microvascular abnormalities, unlike retinal neovascularization described here, are visible within the retinal layers. Intraretinal microvascular abnormalities are most likely preexisting vessels with endothelial cell proliferations that become “shunts” through areas of no perfusion. Cotton wool spots, sometime referred to as soft exudates, may be present adjacent to intraretinal microvascular abnormalities (Fig. 7.1C).

Cotton Wool Spots (Soft Exudates)

Cotton wool spots, sometime referred to as soft exudates, develop in response to multiple retinal and systemic disease. Although cotton wool spots are relatively easy to identify clinically, they are not generally used to determine the clinical level of diabetic retinopathy. Cotton wool spots are superficial swellings in the nerve fiber layer of the retina. They are round or oval in shape, white or pale yellow-white in color, and have feathery edges, representing the orientation of the retinal nerve fiber layer, which runs longitudinally along the retinal surface.

Hard Exudates

Unlike cotton wool spots, hard exudates are located in the outer layers of the retina. Hard exudates are also white or yellow-white in color but hard exudates are small and generally have sharp borders, representing the layers of the retinal that run perpendicular to the surface of the retina. Hard exudates result from leakage of fluids and proteins from diseased retinal capillary bed. The hard exudates may be isolated or arranged in a full or partial ring. Hard exudates are generally not predictive of the risk of progression of retinopathy, but hard exudates in the macular area are signs of macular edema and a risk for vision loss if they occur within 1,500 μ from the center of the macula.

Neovascularization

Retinal neovascularization is the hallmark of proliferative disease. Neovascularization marks the development of new vessels on the retinal surface or extending forward above the retinal surface. Neovascularization results from proliferating endothelial cell tubules and the rate of growth of these new vessels is variable. The vessels can grow on or near (within one disc diameter) the optic disc (neovascularization of the disc) or elsewhere in the retina (neovascularization elsewhere) (Figs. 7.1D and E).

Fibrous Proliferation

Translucent fibrous tissue often appears adjacent to the new vessels, although fibrous tissue may appear with no apparent accompanying new vessels. This tissue appears white or opaque and may adhere to the adjacent vitreous. As with retinal neovascularization, fibrous proliferations are categorized as fibrous proliferations on the optic disc or fibrous proliferations elsewhere (i.e., not on or near the optic disc).

CLASSIFICATION OF DIABETIC RETINOPATHY AND SEVERITY LEVELS

Diabetic retinopathy is marked by gradually progressive stages, which result from alterations in the retinal microvasculature, leading to areas of retinal nonperfusion, increased vascular permeability, and pathologic intraocular proliferation of retinal vessels. The presence and degree of the various retinal lesions, predominantly hemorrhages and/or microaneurysms, venous beading or venous caliber abnormalities, and intraretinal microvascular abnormalities, determine the level of nonproliferative diabetic retinopathy and the risk of progression to sight-threatening proliferative diabetic retinopathy. Diabetic retinopathy is generally broadly classified into two main categories: (1) Nonproliferative diabetic retinopathy, and (2) Proliferative diabetic retinopathy. Diabetic macular edema is a separate retinal complication associated with increased vascular permeability in the macular area, and is usually designated in addition to the level of nonproliferative diabetic retinopathy and proliferative diabetic retinopathy.

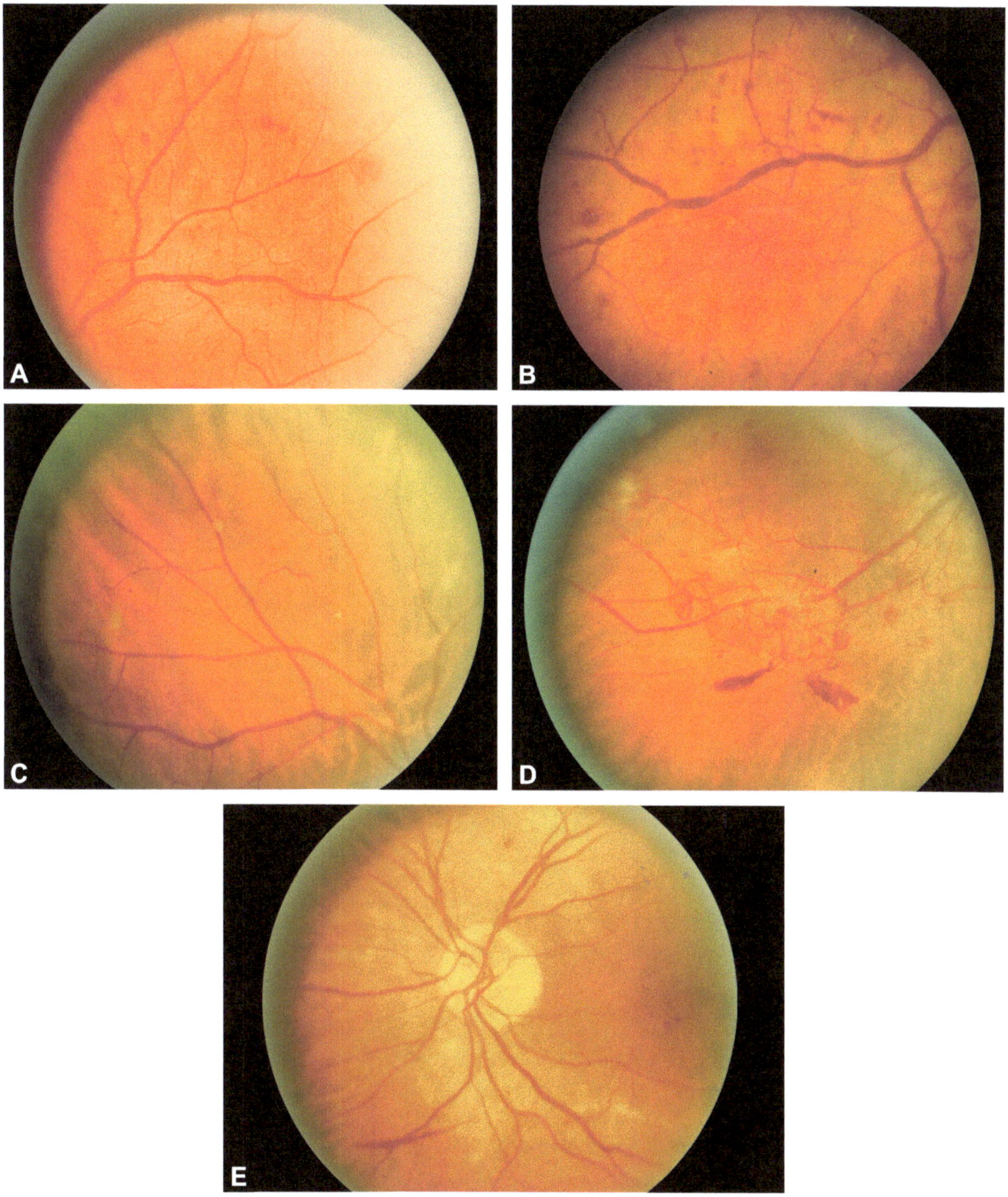

Figs. 7.1A to E: Selected Early Treatment Diabetic Retinopathy Study (ETDRS) standard photographs. Figures 7.1A to C show standards for nonproliferative diabetic retinopathy lesions. Figures 7.1D and E show standards for proliferative diabetic retinopathy lesions. (A) Standard photograph 2A showing severe hemorrhages and/or microaneurysms; (B) Standard photograph 6B showing severe venous beading; (C) Standard photograph 8A showing severe intraretinal microvascular abnormalities; (D) Standard photograph 7 showing new vessels on the retina; and (E) Standard photograph 10A showing new vessels on the disc.

Proliferative diabetic retinopathy is a risk for severe vision loss (best correct visual acuity of 5/200 or worse) and diabetic macular edema is a risk for moderate vision loss [doubling of the visual angle (e.g., 20/20 reduced to 20/40 or 20/50 reduced to 20/100)]. These risks are dramatically reduced with appropriate medical and ophthalmologic care and more than 90% of vision loss resulting from proliferative diabetic retinopathy can be prevented. Accurate diagnosis of a person's level of diabetic retinopathy is critical because there is a varying risk of progression to proliferative diabetic retinopathy and high-risk proliferative diabetic retinopathy depending on the specific nonproliferative diabetic retinopathy. There are various classification systems for diabetic retinopathy, some more useful in a clinical arena and some more useful for research. The classification systems used in this chapter will highlight the International Classification of Diabetic Retinopathy and Diabetic Macular Edema, which is usual in clinical arenas, and the Early Treatment Diabetic Retinopathy Study (ETDRS) classification, which is useful in research arenas (Tables 7.1 to 7.3).

Table 7.1: Early Treatment Diabetic Retinopathy Study (ETDRS) severity levels.

ETDRS level	***Retinopathy severity***
10	DR absent
14/15	DR questionable
20	Microaneurysms only
35	Mild NPDR
43	Moderate NPDR
47	Moderately severe NPDR
53	Severe NPDR
61	Mild PDR
65	Moderate PDR
71/75	High-risk PDR
90	Cannot determine

(DR: Diabetic retinopathy; NPDR: Nonproliferative diabetic retinopathy; PDR: Proliferative diabetic retinopathy)

Table 7.2: International Clinical Diabetic Retinopathy and Diabetic Macular Edema Scale.

Level of diabetic retinopathy	***Findings***
No apparent retinopathy	No abnormalities
Mild NPDR	Microaneurysms only
Moderate NPDR	More than microaneurysms, but less than severe NPDR
Severe NPDR	Any of the following: >20 intraretinal hemorrhages in each four retinal quadrants; definite VB in two or more retinal quadrants; prominent IRMA in one or more retinal quadrants; and no PDR
PDR	One or more of the following: ▪ Neovascularization, vitreous/preretinal ▪ Hemorrhage.

Contd...

Contd...

Level of DME	***Findings***
DME apparently absent	No apparent retinal thickening or HE in the posterior pole
DME apparently present	▪ *Mild DME:* Some retinal thickening or HE in the posterior pole, but distant from center of the macula ▪ *Moderate DME:* Retinal thickening or HE approaching the center, but not involving the center ▪ *Severe DME:* Retinal thickening or HE involving the center of the macula.

(DME: Diabetic macular edema; IRMA: Intraretinal microvascular abnormality; NPDR: Nonproliferative diabetic retinopathy; PDR: Proliferative diabetic retinopathy; HE: Hard exudates)

Table 7.3: Comparison of International and ETDRS levels of retinopathy.

International classification	***ETDRS levels***
No apparent retinopathy	Level 10: DR absent
Mild NPDR	Level 20: Mild NPDR
Moderate NPDR	Levels 35, 43, and 47: Moderate NPDR
Severe NPDR	Levels 53A–E: Severe-very severe NPDR
Proliferative DR	Levels 61, 65, 71, 75, 81, and 85
PDR, high-risk PDR, and very severe PDR	

(DR: Diabetic retinopathy; ETDRS: Early Treatment Diabetic Retinopathy Study; NPDR: Nonproliferative diabetic retinopathy; PDR: Proliferative diabetic retinopathy)

Nonproliferative Diabetic Retinopathy

In the ETDRS classification, mild nonproliferative diabetic retinopathy is marked by at least one retinal microaneurysm, but hemorrhages and microaneurysms are less than those in ETDRS standard photograph 2A (Fig. 7.1A). No other retinal lesion or abnormality associated with diabetes is present. Those with mild nonproliferative diabetic retinopathy have approximately a 5% risk of progression to proliferative diabetic retinopathy within 1 year and a 15% risk of progression to high-risk proliferative diabetic retinopathy within 5 years. In the International Classification of Diabetic Retinopathy, mild nonproliferative diabetic retinopathy is marked by microaneurysms only.

In the ETDRS classification, moderate nonproliferative diabetic retinopathy is characterized by hemorrhage and/or microaneurysm (H/Ma) greater than those pictured in ETDRS standard photograph 2A in 1–3 retinal quadrants. Soft exudates, venous beading, and intraretinal microvascular abnormalities may be present to a mild degree. The risk of progression to proliferative diabetic retinopathy within 1 year is 12–27%, and the risk of progression to high-risk proliferative diabetic retinopathy within 5 years is 33%. In the International Classification of Diabetic Retinopathy, moderate nonproliferative diabetic retinopathy is marked by more than microaneurysms but does not reach the description of severe nonproliferative diabetic retinopathy.

Treatment for mild or moderate nonproliferative diabetic retinopathy generally includes careful observation every 6–12 months and efforts to control glucose levels and comorbidities such as hypertension, renal disease, anemia, cholesterol, and lipids. Shorter follow-up periods are necessary in the presence of diabetic macular edema, even with mild or moderate degrees of nonproliferative diabetic retinopathy. The presence of uncontrolled coincident medical problems or pregnancy will influence the period of reevaluation.

In the ETDRS classification, severe nonproliferative diabetic retinopathy, based on the severity of H/Ma, intraretinal microvascular abnormalities, and venous beading, is characterized by any one of the following lesions:

- Hemorrhages and/or microaneurysms greater than or equal to standard photograph 2A (Fig. 7.1A) in four quadrants or
- Venous beading (Fig. 7.1B) in two or more quadrants or
- Intraretinal microvascular abnormalities greater than or equal to standard photograph 8A (Fig. 7.1C) in at least one quadrant.

In the International Classification of Diabetic Retinopathy, severe nonproliferative diabetic retinopathy is marked by any of the following: more than 20 intraretinal hemorrhages in each of the four retinal quadrants, definite venous beading in two or more retinal quadrants, or prominent intraretinal microvascular abnormalities in one or more retinal quadrants and no proliferative diabetic retinopathy (Figs. 7.2A and B).

In the ETDRS, eyes with severe nonproliferative diabetic retinopathy had a 52% risk of developing proliferative diabetic retinopathy within 1 year and a 60% risk of developing high-risk proliferative diabetic retinopathy within 5 years. These patients require follow-up evaluation in 3–4 months. Treatment of diabetic macular edema is strongly indicated because of the risk of the development of proliferative diabetic retinopathy and high-risk proliferative diabetic

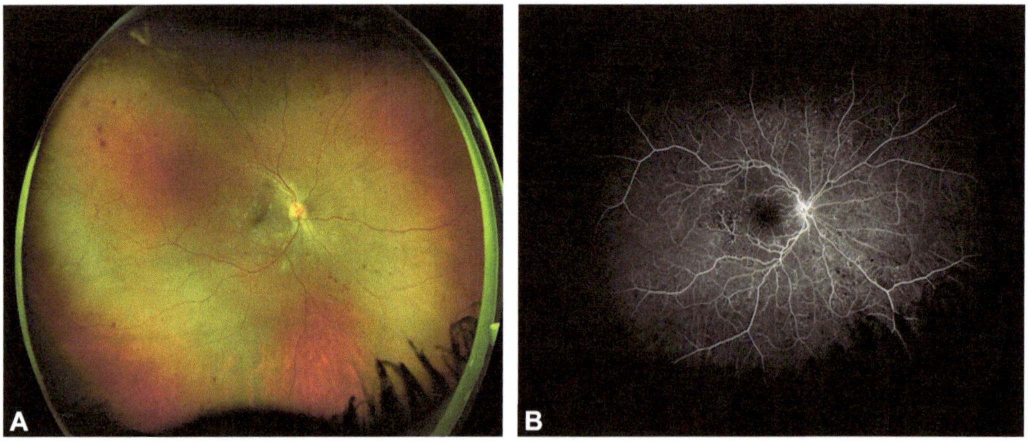

Figs. 7.2A and B: Ultrawide field retinal images of an eye with very severe nonproliferative diabetic retinopathy. (A) Color composite image showing hemorrhages and/or microaneurysms greater than standard 2A in four fields, intraretinal microvascular abnormalities greater than standard 8A; and (B) Corresponding fluorescein angiogram showing areas of hyper- and hypofluorescence corresponding to the lesions seen on color image.

retinopathy. In addition, some eyes with macular edema, even if not clinically significant, may require intervention in preparation for impending scatter (panretinal) laser surgery.

In the ETDRS classification, eyes with very severe nonproliferative diabetic retinopathy have two or more lesions of severe nonproliferative diabetic retinopathy but no frank neovascularization. There is a 75% risk of developing proliferative diabetic retinopathy within 1 year. There is no corresponding classification of very severe nonproliferative diabetic retinopathy in the International Classification of Diabetic Retinopathy and this category is not separately designated in the International Classification of Diabetic Retinopathy.

Patients with very severe nonproliferative diabetic retinopathy may be candidates for scatter (panretinal) laser surgery, and macular edema, if present, may require treatment. Very close follow-up evaluation at 2–3 months interval is important. For individuals with type 2 diabetes, early scatter laser photocoagulation may be considered for patients with severe or very severe nonproliferative diabetic retinopathy.

Proliferative Diabetic Retinopathy

Proliferative diabetic retinopathy is marked by new vessel growth on the optic disc or elsewhere on the retina or by fibrous tissue proliferation on the optic disc or elsewhere (Fig. 7.3). Eyes with early proliferative diabetic retinopathy have a 75% risk of developing high-risk proliferative diabetic retinopathy within a 5-year period. These eyes may require scatter (panretinal) laser surgery, and macular edema, even if not clinically significant, may benefit from treatments before scatter treatment is initiated. In the international classification, proliferative diabetic

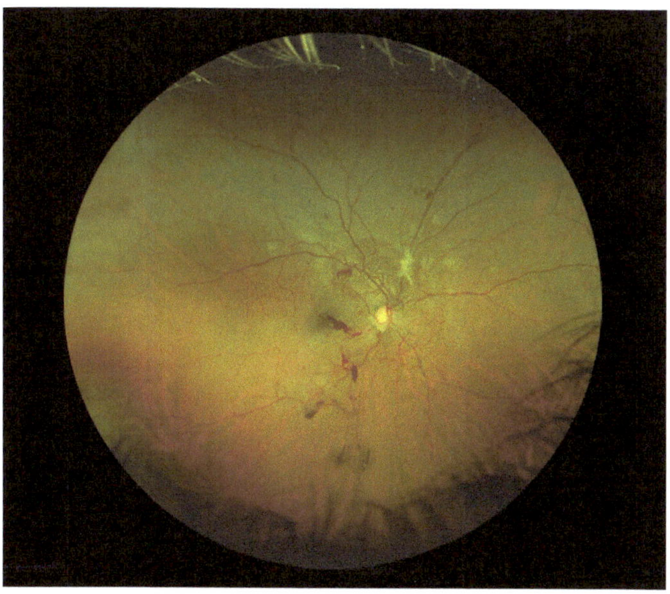

Fig. 7.3: Ultrawide field retinal images of an eye with proliferative diabetic retinopathy with high-risk characteristics showing extensive preretinal hemorrhages and new vessels on the disc greater than standard photograph 10A.

retinopathy is characterized by any one of the following: any retinal neovascularization, vitreous hemorrhage, or preretinal hemorrhage.

Individuals with severe and very severe nonproliferative diabetic retinopathy and early proliferative diabetic retinopathy (less than high-risk proliferative diabetic retinopathy) may be considered for early scatter (panretinal) laser surgery, particularly with type 2 diabetes or if there are new vessels in the presence of severe or very severe nonproliferative diabetic retinopathy, elevated new vessels, or new vessels on the disc.

Eyes that have new vessels on the disc that cover one-third to one-fourth of the optic disc or that have new vessels on the disc less than one-fourth to one-third of disc area with fresh preretinal or vitreous hemorrhage present, or that have new vessels elsewhere greater than half of disc area with fresh preretinal or vitreous hemorrhage present, are classified as having high-risk proliferative diabetic retinopathy. An eye with high-risk proliferative diabetic retinopathy has a 50–75% risk of developing severe vision loss within 5 years; timely and appropriate laser photocoagulation can reduce the risk to less than 5%.

Diabetic Macular Edema

Structural Changes

Diabetic macular edema can be present with any level of nonproliferative or proliferative diabetic retinopathy. Diabetes affects macular function and structure in any of the following ways:

- Macular edema (a collection of intraretinal fluid in the macula with or without lipid exudates and with or without cystoid changes)
- Nonperfusion of parafoveal capillaries with or without intraretinal fluid
- Traction in the macula by fibrous tissue proliferation causing dragging of the retinal tissue, surface wrinkling, or detachment of the macula
- Intraretinal or preretinal hemorrhage in the macula
- Lamellar or full-thickness retinal hole formation
- Any combination of the preceding.

Clinical Classification

Clinically, macular edema is retinal thickening within 1.5-2 disc diameters (1,500-2,000 μ) of the center of the macula. The ETDRS considered diabetic macular edema that involved or threatened the center of the macula as clinically significant macular edema. In the ETDRS, any one of the following conditions was considered clinically significant macular edema:

- Retinal thickening at or within 500 μ of the center of the macula
- Hard exudates at or within 500 μ of the center of the macula if there is thickening of the adjacent retina
- An area or areas of retinal thickening at least 1 disc area in size, at least part of which is within 1 disc diameter of the center of the macula.

The International Classification of Diabetic Macular Edema classified diabetic macular edema as mild, moderate, or severe as follows:

- *Mild diabetic macular edema:* Some retinal thickening or hard exudates in posterior pole but distant from the center of the macula

- *Moderate diabetic macular edema:* Retinal thickening or hard exudates approaching the center but not involving the center
- *Severe diabetic macular edema:* Retinal thickening or hard exudates involving the center of the macula.

The Diabetic Retinopathy Clinical Research Network (DRCR.net) modified these descriptions to match the change in treatment paradigm demonstrated by the DRCR.net. The DRCR.net considers diabetic macular edema as central-involved diabetic macular edema or not central-involved diabetic macular edema, with central-involved diabetic macular edema amenable to treatment with an intravitreous anti-VEGF agent, as described here.

CURRENT TREATMENT FOR DIABETIC RETINOPATHY

Current treatment strategies for diabetic retinopathy are based on high levels of clinical evidence derived from multicentered, randomized clinical trials. These strategies include direct ocular intervention with laser photocoagulation and intravitreous injections of anti-VEGF agents and steroids and optimization of medical management of diabetes and comorbidities.

Nonproliferative and Proliferative Diabetic Retinopathy

The Diabetic Retinopathy Study, sponsored in the United States by the National Eye Institute and conducted from 1971 to 1975, demonstrated that scatter (panretinal) retinal laser photocoagulation versus no photocoagulation reduced the risk of severe vision loss from proliferative diabetic retinopathy by 60%. The ETDRS, again sponsored by the National Eye Institute and conducted from 1979 to 1991, elucidated optimal timing for scatter laser, demonstrating that both early photocoagulation and deferral of photocoagulation until an eye reaches the high-risk stage of proliferative diabetic retinopathy are effective in preventing severe vision loss. Subsequent analysis of the ETDRS data showed that early scatter laser photocoagulation is particularly beneficial for patients with type 2 diabetes. As a result, early scatter photocoagulation may be indicated for persons with severe or very severe nonproliferative diabetic retinopathy or with proliferative diabetic retinopathy less than high risk, particularly if there is likelihood that follow-up evaluations and/or the opportunity for timely treatment may be delayed.

Scatter laser photocoagulation consists of applying approximately 1,200–1,800 individuals laser scars to the retina, avoiding the macula area, large vessels, and areas of hemorrhage. More recent lasers such as the PAtterned SCAnning Laser (PASCAL) apply up to 25 burns at a time in a grid-like pattern, reducing the time for laser treatments (Fig. 7.4).

Vitrectomy surgery for proliferative diabetic retinopathy that results in nonresolving vitreous hemorrhage or traction retinal detachment is effective in preventing severe vision loss if the traction retinal detachment threatens central vision and is frequently effective in restoring vision. During vitrectomy surgery, vitreous hemorrhage, retinal membranes, and scar tissue causing traction on the retina are surgically removed, and laser photocoagulation may be performed during the surgical procedure (endolaser).

Scatter laser photocoagulation according to ETDRS protocol is effective in reducing the risk of severe vision loss from proliferative diabetic retinopathy to less than 4%. While laser photocoagulation and vitrectomy surgery when indicated are the current standards for treating

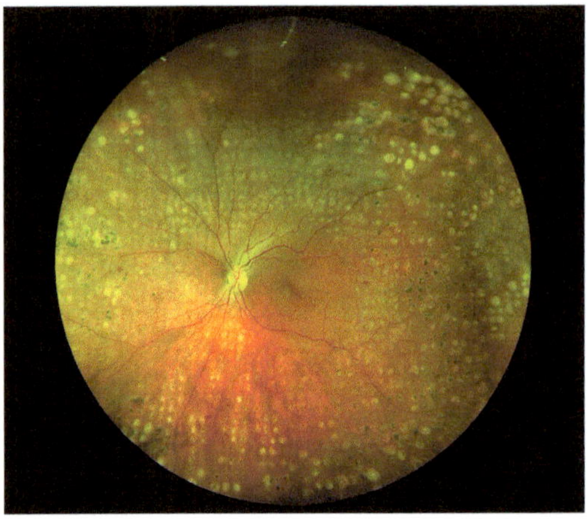

Fig. 7.4: Ultrawide field retinal images of an eye with quiescent proliferative diabetic retinopathy after panretinal laser photocoagulation. The grayish spots on the retina correspond to prior laser treatment.

proliferative diabetic retinopathy, intravitreous injection of anti-VEGF agents is currently under investigation in the DRCR.net in an attempt to make treatments more effective and less destructive than laser photocoagulation and the DRCR.net has demonstrated that intravitreal anti-VEGF agents are as effective as scatter laser photocoagulation in preserving vision.

Diabetic Macular Edema

The ETDRS conclusively demonstrated that focal laser photocoagulation for clinically significant macular edema reduces the risk of moderate vision loss by 50% compared to no treatment. Focal laser photocoagulation consists of either direct laser treatment, grid laser treatment, or a combination of direct laser to focal leaks and grid laser treatment to diffuse leakage or thickened avascular zones. Laser burns for macular edema are of smaller, less intense, and shorter duration than the burns for scatter laser photocoagulation.

Although laser photocoagulation is effective in preserving vision, the procedure is inherently destructive; consequently, efforts continue to be made to develop more effective treatments. Intravitreal injections of steroids, predominantly triamcinolone, and anti-VEGF agents were used extensively to treat diabetic macular edema. In 2010, the DRCR.net demonstrated that in a multicentered, controlled clinical trial, intravitreous injection of the anti-VEGF agent ranibizumab was superior to focal laser photocoagulation and combination focal laser photocoagulation and intravitreous injection of triamcinolone both in preventing vision loss and in restoring loss vision in eyes with center-involved diabetic macular edema. Subsequent DRCR.net clinical trials have shown the effectiveness of other intravitreous anti-VEGF agents in preserving vision and increasing the odds of recurring lost vision from diabetic macular edema. Studies of additional intravitreous agents are ongoing.

Medical Interventions

The Diabetic Retinopathy Study, ETDRS, and completed and ongoing DRCR.net trials provide solid evidence-based protocols for caring for diabetic retinopathy and diabetic macular edema.

Two major clinical studies have demonstrated the benefits of intensive glucose control for both type 1 and type 2 diabetes. The United Kingdom Prospective Diabetes Study enrolled 3,867 patients with newly diagnosed type 2 DM and randomized subjects to either intensive glucose control or conventional control with either sulfonylureas or insulin. Intensive glucose control resulted in a 17% risk reduction for progression of diabetic retinopathy, a 29% risk reduction in the need for laser photocoagulation surgery, a 23% risk reduction for the development of vitreous hemorrhage, and a 16% risk reduction in legal blindness. The United Kingdom Prospective Diabetes Study also identified elevated blood pressure to be an independent risk factor for the onset and progression of diabetic retinopathy. While monitoring subjects after the completion of the study, subjects in the intensive treatment group continued to have slower progression of diabetic retinopathy than the conventional treatment group despite convergence of hemoglobin A1c (HbA1c) levels. This "legacy effect" demonstrates the importance of early intervention to reduce the risk of onset and progression of diabetic retinopathy. Studies in Japan with type 2 diabetes subjects had similar findings.

The Diabetes Control and Complications Trial (DCCT) and the continued monitoring of participants in the trial through the Epidemiology of Diabetes Interventions and Complications (EDIC) study similarly tested intensive glucose control versus conventional control in patients with recent-onset type 1 diabetes. The DCCT found that regardless of the baseline level of glycemic control, a 10% reduction of glycosylated hemoglobin level significantly reduced the risk of onset of diabetic retinopathy, retarded the progression of diabetic retinopathy, and reduced the need for laser treatment. Intensive therapy reduced the risk of onset of retinopathy by 76% and resulted in a 63% reduction in the risk of progression of retinopathy. The risk of developing severe nonproliferative diabetic retinopathy or proliferative diabetic retinopathy was reduced by 47%, the risk of developing clinically significant macular edema was reduced by 23%, and there was a 56% reduction in the risk of requiring laser surgery for those on intensive therapy was reduced by 56%. Once again, ongoing follow-up evaluation in the EDIC study demonstrated a legacy effect with the benefits of intensive control persisting for more than 10 years following the completion of the study, despite convergence of glycemic control for both groups after 4–7 years. Similar reduction of risks was identified for other microvascular complications of DM, such as renal disease and neuropathy.

RISK FACTORS FOR ONSET AND PROGRESSION OF DIABETIC RETINOPATHY

While baseline level of diabetic retinopathy is an important factor in determining the risk of progression of diabetic retinopathy and subsequent vision loss, there are significant systemic conditions that influence the risk of onset and progression of diabetic retinopathy in addition to diabetes control.

Well-designed prospective and retrospective studies have demonstrated that hypertension, dyslipidemia, elevated cholesterol, renal disease, and anemia are independent or associated risk factors for the onset and progression of diabetic retinopathy. Pregnancy in the presence of established diabetes, particularly when accompanied by hypertension or sudden and rapid lower of HbA1c, may also accelerate the progression of diabetic retinopathy. Optimized control of glucose levels and comorbidities is essential to reducing the burden of vision loss from diabetes.

NONRETINAL COMPLICATIONS OF DIABETES

While diabetic retinopathy is the most often mentioned complication of diabetes, all structures of the eye and many aspects of visual function are susceptible to the deleterious effects of diabetes.

Glaucoma

Type 2 diabetes is a known risk factor for primary open-angle glaucoma and there are reports that open-angle glaucoma is 1.4 times more common in the diabetic population than in the nondiabetic population. Additionally, the prevalence of glaucoma increase with age and duration of diabetes, but medical therapy for open-angle glaucoma is generally effective.

Nerve Palsy

Diabetes may be the underlying etiology of mononeuropathies of the third, fourth, or sixth cranial nerves. The percentage of all extraocular muscle palsies attributable to DM is estimated at 4.5–6%. These palsies are considered to be secondary to ischemic infarction of the affected nerve. The third and sixth cranial nerves are the most frequently affected, although the fourth nerve can also be affected. Mononeuropathies also may be the initial presenting sign of new-onset diabetes. The presenting symptom is usually diplopia, and treatment includes ruling out nondiabetic causes of the condition and possible patching to eliminate diplopia.

Cornea

Diabetes may cause a cornea to injure more easily and heal more slowly. Reduced corneal sensitivity may result in reduced reflex tearing and unawareness of ocular foreign bodies. The reduction of corneal sensitivity may predispose a person to the development of neurotrophic corneal ulcerations. Alterations in the basement membrane layer of the corneal epithelium may retard corneal healing.

Decreased corneal sensitivity may affect contact lens wear and all diabetic contact lens users should be properly educated to be aware of potential problems, early signs of lens rejection and infection, or corneal abrasion. While diabetes is not a contraindication for photorefractive surgery to reduce myopia or hyperopia, diabetic persons should be evaluated carefully prior to undergoing LASIK or other photorefractive surgical techniques.

Iris

The most serious diabetic complication affecting the iris is neovascularization of the iris or rubeosis iridis, a growth of new blood vessels on the iris. These vessels generally are first observed at the pupillary border and may resemble grape clusters in appearance. If the vessels progress, a fine network of vessels may grow over the iris tissue and into the filtration angle of the eye. Fibrovascular growth in the filtration angle may result in closure of the angle, resulting in neovascular glaucoma, although intraocular pressure may be elevated prior to angle involvement because of protein and cellular leakage from the proliferating vessels. Diabetes is a leading cause of neovascular glaucoma, accounting for 32.2% of cases, as opposed to 36.1% of cases resulting from retinal venous obstructive disease. Treatment for neovascularization of the iris and neovascular glaucoma includes scatter (panretinal) laser photocoagulation, topical antiglaucoma medications, systemic antiglaucoma medications, anti-VEGF agents, antiglaucoma filtration surgery, including Molteno valve implants, or a combination of one or more of these therapies.

Lens

Diabetes affects the crystalline lens in a variety of ways, resulting in structural and functional changes.

Refractive Change

Refractive changes related to fluctuation of blood glucose levels are frequent. Elevated blood glucose levels may result in blurred vision that is frequently the presenting symptom for new-onset diabetes. Stabilization of refractive changes, due to either new-onset or poorly controlled diabetes, may take 4–6 weeks to occur.

Cataract

Cataracts tend to developer at a younger age and progress more rapidly in the presence of diabetes. This increased risk of cataract development occurs in both type 1 and type 2 diabetes. Multiple factors influence cataract development, including duration of diabetes, retinopathy status, the use of diuretics, and diabetes control. In individuals with type 2 diabetes, additional risk factors may include smoking and lower diastolic blood pressure. Current surgical procedures are 90–95% successful in restoring useful vision, but there are potential complications unique to diabetes, such as delayed wound healing, acceleration of diabetic retinopathy, iris or retinal neovascularization, and macular edema.

Reversible "diabetic" cataracts can occur and are most frequently related to poor metabolic control of diabetes. These cataracts are usually bilateral and are characterized by dense bands of white, subcapsular spots that are snowflake in appearance, or fine, needle-shaped opacities. Since these diabetic cataracts are related to prolonged periods of severe hyperglycemia and untreated DM, they are only rarely now seen in the United States and other industrialized countries.

RECOMMENDED EYE EXAMINATION FREQUENCY

In the absence of any preventive or curative measures, the mainstay of diabetic retinopathy care relies on periodic, lifelong retinal evaluation. In general, annual retinal examination is advisable, since current treatments are most effective before vision has been loss and diabetic retinopathy and diabetic macular edema frequently cause no symptoms when the conditions are most amenable to treatment. Table 7.4 summarizes recommended examination frequency.

Table 7.4: Schedule for initial ophthalmologic examination.

Diabetes type	*Recommended first examination*	*Minimum routine follow-up**
Type 1	Within 3–5 years after diagnosis of diabetes or once patient is 10 years of age or older	Yearly
Type 2	At time of diagnosis of diabetes	Yearly
Pregnancy	Prior to conception and during the 1st trimester	Physician discretion

*Abnormal findings necessitate more frequent follow-up.

FUTURE DIRECTIONS

Although significant strides have been made in diagnosing and treating diabetic retinopathy, there currently is no means to prevent or cure diabetic retinopathy. Current diagnostic tools are now probing down to the cellular level to enhance our understanding of the disease in an attempt to understand possible preventive or curative measures or make treatments more effective by tailoring treatments to specific characteristics of an individual's diabetic retinopathy.

Intravitreous injections of anti-VEGF agents and other agents hold promise of more personalized treatment regimens. Laser photocoagulation for diabetic macular edema, which was the mainstay of treatment since the mid-1980s, has now been supplanted in most cases with intravitreous anti-VEGF. New treatments are likely to improve outcomes, perhaps with the use of multiple agents. Understanding the underlying neuronal, vascular, and inflammatory components of diabetic retinopathy and diabetic macular edema may lead to breakthroughs in preventing or curing diabetic retinopathy.

CONCLUSION

The current management of diabetic requires optimal control of systemic risk factors to prevent the development or progression of vision-threatening complications. It is only with the coordinated care between eye care providers and the many other members of the diabetic patient's medical care team can optimal ophthalmic outcomes be achieved.

Conflict of interest: All authors report no conflicting relationship.

BIBLIOGRAPHY

1. Aiello LP, Cahill MT, Wong JS. Systemic considerations in the management of diabetic retinopathy. Am J Ophthalmol. 2001;132:760-6.
2. Diabetes Control and Complications Trial/Epidemiology of Diabetes Intervention and Complications Research Group, Lachin JM, Genuth S, et al. Retinopathy and nephropathy in patients with type 1 diabetes four years after a trial of intensive therapy. N Engl J Med. 2000;342:381-9.
3. Diabetic Retinopathy Clinical Research Network, Elman MJ, Aiello LP, et al. Randomized trial evaluating ranibizumab plus prompt or deferred laser or triamcinolone plus prompt laser for diabetic macular edema. Ophthalmology. 2010;117:1064-77.e35.
4. Diabetic Retinopathy Clinical Research Network, Elman MJ, Qin H, et al. Intravitreal ranibizumab for diabetic macular edema with prompt versus deferred laser treatment: three-year randomized trial results. Ophthalmology. 2012;119:2312-8.

5. Diabetic Retinopathy Clinical Research Network, Wells JA, Glassman AR, et al. Aflibercept, bevacizumab, or ranibizumab for diabetic macular edema. N Engl J Med. 2015;372:1193-203.
6. Effects of aspirin treatment on diabetic retinopathy. ETDRS report number 8. Early Treatment Diabetic Retinopathy Study Research Group. Ophthalmology. 1991;98:757-65.
7. Fluorescein angiographic risk factors for progression of diabetic retinopathy. ETDRS report number 13. Early Treatment Diabetic Retinopathy Study Research Group. Ophthalmology. 1991;98:834-40.
8. Fundus photographic risk factors for progression of diabetic retinopathy. ETDRS report number 12. Early Treatment Diabetic Retinopathy Study Research Group. Ophthalmology. 1991;98:823-33.
9. Grading diabetic retinopathy from stereoscopic color fundus photographs—an extension of the modified Airlie House classification. ETDRS report number 10. Early Treatment Diabetic Retinopathy Study Research Group. Ophthalmology. 1991;98:786-806.
10. Holman RR, Paul SK, Bethel MA, et al. 10-year follow-up of intensive glucose control in type 2 diabetes. N Engl J Med. 2008;359:1577-89.
11. Intensive blood-glucose control with sulphonylureas or insulin compared with conventional treatment and risk of complications in patients with type 2 diabetes (UKPDS 33). UK Prospective Diabetes Study (UKPDS) Group. Lancet. 1998;352:837-53.
12. Klein R, Klein BE, Moss SE, et al. The Wisconsin Epidemiologic Study of Diabetic Retinopathy: XVII. The 14-year incidence and progression of diabetic retinopathy and associated risk factors in type 1 diabetes. Ophthalmology. 1998;105:1801-15.
13. Klein R, Klein BE, Moss SE, et al. The Wisconsin Epidemiologic Study of Diabetic Retinopathy. XV. The long-term incidence of macular edema. Ophthalmology. 1995;102:7-16.
14. Klein R, Klein BE, Moss SE, et al. The Wisconsin Epidemiologic Study of Diabetic Retinopathy. II. Prevalence and risk of diabetic retinopathy when age at diagnosis is less than 30 years. Arch Ophthalmol. 1984;102:520-6.
15. Klein R, Klein BE, Moss SE, et al. The Wisconsin Epidemiologic Study of Diabetic Retinopathy. III. Prevalence and risk of diabetic retinopathy when age at diagnosis is 30 or more years. Arch Ophthalmol. 1984;102:527-32.
16. Klein R, Klein BE, Moss SE, et al. The Wisconsin Epidemiologic Study of Diabetic Retinopathy. IX. Four-year incidence and progression of diabetic retinopathy when age at diagnosis is less than 30 years. Arch Ophthalmol. 1989;107:237-43.
17. Klein R, Klein BE, Moss SE, et al. The Wisconsin Epidemiologic Study of Diabetic Retinopathy. X. Four-year incidence and progression of diabetic retinopathy when age at diagnosis is 30 years or more. Arch Ophthalmol. 1989;107:244-9.
18. Klein R, Knudtson MD, Lee KE, et al. The Wisconsin Epidemiologic Study of Diabetic Retinopathy XXIII: the twenty-five-year incidence of macular edema in persons with type 1 diabetes. Ophthalmology. 2009;116:497-503.
19. Klein R, Knudtson MD, Lee KE, et al. The Wisconsin Epidemiologic Study of Diabetic Retinopathy: XXII. The twenty-five-year progression of retinopathy in persons with type 1 diabetes. Ophthalmology. 2008;115:1859-68.
20. Kohner EM, Aldington SJ, Stratton IM, et al. United Kingdom Prospective Diabetes Study, 30: diabetic retinopathy at diagnosis of non-insulin-dependent diabetes mellitus and associated risk factors. Arch Ophthalmol. 1998;116:297-303.
21. Ohkubo Y, Kishikawa H, Araki E, et al. Intensive insulin therapy prevents the progression of diabetic microvascular complications in Japanese patients with non-insulin-dependent diabetes mellitus: a randomized prospective 6-year study. Diabetes Res Clin Pract. 1995;28:103-17.
22. Photocoagulation for diabetic macular edema. Early Treatment Diabetic Retinopathy Study report number 1. Early Treatment Diabetic Retinopathy Study research group. Arch Ophthalmol. 1985;103:1796-806.

23. Rask-Madsen C, King GL. Vascular complications of diabetes: mechanisms of injury and protective factors. Cell Metab. 2013;17:20-33.
24. Shichiri M. Intensive insulin therapy prevents the progression of diabetic microvascular complications in Japanese patients with non-insulin-dependent diabetes mellitus: a randomized prospective 6-year study. Diabetes Res Clin Pract. 1995;28:103-17.
25. Silva PS, Cavallerano JD, Aiello LM. Ocular telehealth initiatives in diabetic retinopathy. Curr Diab Rep. 2009;9:265-71.
26. Silva PS, Cavallerano JD, Sun JK, et al. Effect of systemic medications on onset and progression of diabetic retinopathy. Nat Rev Endocrinol. 2010;6:494-508.
27. The Diabetes Control and Complications Trial Research Group. The effect of intensive treatment of diabetes on the development and progression of long-term complications in insulin-dependent diabetes mellitus. N Engl J Med. 1993;329:977-86.
28. Writing Committee for the Diabetic Retinopathy Clinical Research Network, Gross JG, Glassman AR, et al. Panretinal photocoagulation vs intravitreous ranibizumab for proliferative diabetic retinopathy: a randomized trial. JAMA. 2015;314:2137-46.
29. Writing Team for the Diabetes Control and Complications Trial/Epidemiology of Diabetes Interventions and Complications Research Group. Effect of intensive therapy on the microvascular complications of type 1 diabetes mellitus. JAMA. 2002;287:2563-9.
30. Writing Team for the Diabetes Control and Complications Trial/Epidemiology of Diabetes Interventions and Complications Research Group. Sustained effect of intensive treatment of type 1 diabetes mellitus on development and progression of diabetic nephropathy: the Epidemiology of Diabetes Interventions and Complications (EDIC) study. JAMA. 2003;290:2159-67.

CHAPTER 8

Diabetic Kidney Disease

Robert C Stanton

INTRODUCTION

Diabetic kidney disease is the major cause of kidney disease worldwide. This is primarily driven by the epidemic rise in the numbers of people with type 2 diabetes mellitus. The development of diabetic kidney disease has major consequences as either an increase in urine albumin level or a decrease in estimated glomerular filtration rate will lead to a significantly higher risk of cardiovascular disease. This increased risk leads to greater morbidity and mortality in people with diabetic kidney disease. This it is very important for the clinician to be aware of these issues in order to provide optimal care to the patient with diabetic kidney disease. In this chapter the epidemiology, diagnosis, prevention, and treatment of diabetic kidney disease will be reviewed.

EPIDEMIOLOGY

Diabetic kidney disease (DKD) is growing at an epidemic rate throughout the world.[1] One of the best ways to see the growth of this disease is to examine the rise in the numbers of patients with end stage kidney disease (ESKD). This is because one could debate how many people actually have chronic kidney disease (CKD) (as the clinical criteria are not definitive as discussed here) but there is no debate as to the number of people with ESKD (defined as those either on dialysis or with a kidney transplant). As of the most recent data (2013) in the United States, about 661,000 people have ESKD. In 1978, there were about 41,000 ESKD patients (35,000 dialysis patients and about 6,000 transplant recipients). The number of patients with ESKD in 1996 was about 307,000. Diabetes mellitus is the main cause of ESKD comprising 248,000 of the cases in 2013 (increased from 99,000 in 1996). Indeed type 2 diabetes mellitus has been the major reason for the increase in ESKD with hypertension as the second most common cause. In 1996, there were about 1.3 cases of ESKD due to diabetes mellitus as compared to hypertension and in 2013 there was about 1.5 cases of ESKD as compared to hypertension. Of new cases in 2013, 44% were due to diabetes mellitus and 29% were due to hypertension. The other causes include glomerulonephritis, cystic diseases, and less common diseases. The development of ESKD leads to significant increase in morbidity, mortality, and increased financial costs. In 2013, the United States Government spent a very large amount of money (about 31 billion dollars that is about 6% of the

Box 8.1: Epidemiology statistics.

- About 14.8% of the US population has chronic kidney disease (CKD) as defined as glomerular filtration rate (GFR) of less than 60 mL/min or elevated urine albumin level
- Most of the CKD is caused by diabetes
- Most CKD patients die of heart disease before reaching end stage kidney disease (ESKD)
- About 700,000 people have ESKD. Diabetes is responsible for 44% of the ESKD patients
- Death rates are 15–20% per year for dialysis patients in the USA
- Medicare spent $37 billion in 2015 on ESKD, which is about 7.3% of the Medicare budget. And at least $50 billion more was spent on CKD patients.

United States healthcare budget—this cost has approximately doubled in 10 years) on just 0.2% of the population. The overall personal and financial costs to society are much greater though when considering all patients with CKD, which numbers in the millions in the USA (Box 8.1).

Chronic kidney disease is estimated to affect 13.6% of the United States population in 2013. CKD is defined as an estimated glomerular filtration rate (eGFR) of less than 60 mL/min or a urine albumin/creatinine ratio more than 30 mg/g. This may be an overestimate of the number of people with CKD as eGFR declines normally from about 0.5–1.0 mL/min/year. As we are born with an eGFR of 110–130 mL/min (women are born with lower GFRs than men), many people over the age of 70 years old may well have an eGFR of less than 60 mL/min just by normal aging. But the exact number of people has to be in the millions due to the following well-documented facts. First, there is a highly significant increase in cardiovascular disease as CKD develops. Indeed, decreasing eGFR or increasing urine albumin level leads to increasing risk for cardiovascular events and cardiovascular mortality.[2] Both declining eGFR and rising urine albumin level are directly associated with increasing cardiovascular events and cardiovascular death. And a combination of decreased GFR and increased urine albumin level has a synergistic effect on the development of cardiovascular events and cardiovascular death. Indeed there is a better chance that a person with diabetes mellitus and CKD will die from a cardiovascular event than progress to end stage renal disease (ESRD). Illustrating this was a very interesting study from 2014 that analyzed deaths in people with type 2 diabetes mellitus using the National Health and Nutrition Examination Survey (NHANES) database.[3] These researchers found that the presence of albuminuria (>30 mg/g) without an associated decrease in eGFR led to increased death rates as compared to people with type 2 diabetes mellitus and no evidence of CKD. In addition, those with a decreased eGFR (<60 mL/min) without an increase in urine albumin level led to even greater increase in death rates as compared to increased albuminuria alone. The combination of decreased eGFR and increased urine albumin level led to the highest death rates. But of greatest interest was that those people with type 2 diabetes mellitus and no signs of CKD, had death rates similar to the age-matched population who did not have type 2 diabetes mellitus. This finding suggested that all excess deaths in type 2 diabetes mellitus patients was associated with the presence of CKD. Second, death rates for people on dialysis range from 10% to 20% per year depending on the center and modality of dialysis. When considering that most people with CKD will die from a cardiovascular death before reaching ESKD and that the death rates for people on dialysis (who comprise most of the ESKD population—in 2013 about 468,000 were on dialysis and 193,000 had a transplant) are so high, the CKD number must in the millions for the population to keep increasing.

This dramatic increase in CKD and ESRD is occurring worldwide. Indeed China and India have the greatest number of cases and the rise in both countries is continuing. It is also important to note that different populations have different relative risks. For example, there is a significantly higher rate of CKD and ESRD amongst African-Americans, Hispanics, American-Indians, Middle Eastern areas, and Asians (especially Asians from Southern areas) as compared to the Caucasian population in the United States.[1] There are likely different rates of kidney disease amongst many other ethnic and racial groups around the world that have yet to be determined. Hence, all physicians need to have a higher suspicion for DKD in groups at increased risk so that appropriate screening and interventions are done.

It is very important for all physicians to diagnose DKD as early as possible and to start treatment as early as possible. Early treatment will not only help to prevent progression to ESRD but also slow the development of cardiovascular disease. Indeed it is important for all physicians to view CKD patients at being high risk for cardiovascular disease so that appropriate monitoring is done and appropriate interventions are initiated in order to prevent the development of cardiovascular disease. A surprising statistic illustrates the need for early diagnosis and treatment. In the United States, as many as 40% of people starting dialysis met a nephrologist for the first time when they start dialysis.[1] Of course some of these are acute kidney injury patients but not all. And another 30% meet the nephrologist only within the last 12 months before starting dialysis. Thus, about 70% of the people with ESKD meet the nephrologist within the last 12 months before starting dialysis. This data suggests either that primary care doctors and endocrinologists are not recognizing the declining eGFR or they do not think that nephrologists can do more than they are already doing. As will be discussed here, there are aggressive interventions and management that may slow progression of DKD. If the primary care doctors and endocrinologists are comfortable treating to goals then a referral may not be needed. But if not, then co-management with a nephrologist or learning what needs to be done is required to best care for the patients with DKD.

HOW TO SCREEN FOR AND DIAGNOSE DIABETIC KIDNEY DISEASE

The screening for DKD has two main components: (1) Evaluation for increased urine albumin levels and routine measurement of serum creatinine, and (2) Calculation of eGFR (Box 8.2). The urine albumin level should be measured at least once per year ideally using the albumin/creatinine ratio. A 24-hour urine is acceptable if there is no machine available for the albumin/creatinine ratio test but the albumin/creatinine is preferable. The advantage of the albumin/creatinine ratio is that it is very accurate and easy to obtain. Ideally the first morning specimen is most accurate (and that is what is used in clinical studies) but in routine clinical practice that is not needed. Just obtain the sample at the time of the visit. Normal is less than 30 mg/g. If the level is elevated it should be repeated as there are reasons for transient elevations as shown in Box 8.3. If the level is persistently elevated then the person has kidney disease. It is likely DKD but other causes of kidney disease may also increase urine albumin level and/or lead to a decrease in eGFR as discussed here. Of note, the typical urine dipstick is not a good screening tool as it is a qualitative (not quantitative test) and it is not sensitive enough to determine low

Box 8.2: Screening for diabetic kidney disease.

- Yearly evaluation of urine albumin level ideally with spot urine albumin/creatinine ratio (normal <30 mg/g). Repeat 1 month later if abnormal to verify it is elevated
- The routine urine dipstick is not an adequate screening tool as it is not sensitive enough to measure low level but significant increase in the urine albumin level
- Yearly measurement of serum creatinine and calculation of eGFR using one of the formulae (e.g. CKD-EPI equation).

(CKD-EPI: Chronic Kidney Disease-Epidemiology Collaboration; eGFR: Estimated glomerular filtration rate)

Box 8.3: Reasons for transient elevations of urine albumin level.

- Urinary tract infection
- Recent strenuous exercise
- Pregnancy
- Congestive heart failure
- Recent increase in blood pressure
- Significant hyperglycemia.

level increase in the urine albumin level. The other test that must be done to screen for DKD is the measurement of the serum creatinine level and calculation of eGFR. It is essential to calculate eGFR as factors such as age and gender that greatly affect eGFR. There are a number of formulae that have been developed to calculate eGFR. The three most common are: (1) The Cockcroft–Gault equation, (2) The Modification of Diet in Renal Disease (MDRD) formula, and (3) The Chronic Kidney Disease-Epidemiology Collaboration (CKD-EPI) formula. All of these are routinely available online. At this time, the CKD-EPI is considered to be the most accurate for predicting outcomes. But all of them provide useful information as to the true GFR. And in studies comparing these formulae to true GFR, the accuracy is within 10–20%. Even with this disparity with true GFR, within each person, these formulae do provide accurate information on the rate of change. The eGFR should be calculated at least yearly and more often in a person with established kidney disease.

In general, the diagnosis of DKD may be made in a patient with diabetes mellitus and the onset of increased urine albumin level and/or a decline in eGFR associated with a relatively bland urinalysis (Box 8.4). But it is important to remember that just because a person has diabetes mellitus and has kidney disease does not mean that they have DKD. Hence, one needs to know what signs point to causes of kidney diseases other than diabetes mellitus. Box 8.5 shows reasons to consider other causes. These include the development of kidney disease in a person with type 1 diabetes mellitus who was diagnosed less than 5 years ago. It is unusual for DKD to develop in a person with type 1 diabetes mellitus of less than 5 years duration. On the other hand, people with type 2 diabetes mellitus may have DKD at the time of diagnosis as these people, on average, have diabetes mellitus for 10 years or so before the diagnosis is made. Another reason to consider a kidney disease other than diabetes mellitus is the lack of diabetic retinopathy especially in a person with type 1 diabetes mellitus. It used to be said that the absence of diabetic retinopathy in a patient with kidney disease was a clear indication that the person did not have DKD. This is definitely not true, but the complete absence of eye disease should

Box 8.4: Diagnosis of diabetic kidney disease.

- Either increased urine albumin/creatinine ratio (>30 mg/g) and/or decreased eGFR (<60 mL/min) in a person with diabetes
- Relatively unremarkable urine sediment analysis.

(eGFR: Estimated glomerular filtration rate)

Box 8.5: Reasons to consider a kidney disease other than diabetes.

- Development of kidney disease in a person with type 1 diabetes of less than 5 years duration
- Active urinary sediment (e.g. many red blood cells, many white blood cells, or casts)
- Lack of diabetic retinopathy especially in a person with type 1 diabetes
- Rapidly declining estimated glomerular filtration rate (eGFR) or a change in pattern from a slow rate of decline to a rapid rate of decline in eGFR
- Normal urine albumin level.

at least raise the possibility of a nondiabetic cause for kidney disease. Thirdly, the presence of an active urinary sediment should also be of concern. An active sediment may include many red blood cells (RBCs) (as much as 5–10 RBCs per high-power field though are seen in people with DKD but not more usually), white blood cells, and casts. Thus, a urinalysis with sediment analysis should be part of the initial evaluation (and any time there is a significant change in kidney parameters—eGFR or urine albumin level). Fourth, DKD patients may have a decline in eGFR as much as 10–20 mL/min per year but a more common rate of decline is 2–5 mL/min/year. Thus, if a person is losing eGFR at a rate faster than 2–5 mL/min/year then another kidney disease should be considered. Of significant concern is an unexpected acceleration in the rate of eGFR decline. Another reason to consider a disease other than DKD is a normal urine albumin level as most people with DKD have an increased urine albumin/protein level. This is not a hard and fast rule as many studies have shown that some people have even very advanced DKD (as determined by kidney biopsy) and normal urine albumin levels.[4] So, the absence of increased urine albumin level should certainly alert the physician to another cause for kidney disease but often the person is found to have DKD. Lastly, rapidly rising urine albumin/protein levels should stimulate a search for other causes. Rapidly rising urine albumin levels do occur in people with diabetes mellitus even after many years of stable albumin levels. So, alone this may be simply a sign of worsening diabetic kidney damage, but this should stimulate a search for possible other kidney diseases.

Logical next questions are, should a patient see a nephrologist for diagnosis and should a kidney biopsy be done? For most people, there is no need to see a nephrologist at the time of diagnosis unless there is a possibility of another kidney disease and/or the physician wants assistance in achieving optimal care. If the primary care physician or endocrinologist feels confident there is no reason to consider another kidney disease and is confident about the goals and how to attain them then a referral is not indicated. But if there is any concern about diagnosis or treatment then a referral for at least a one-time evaluation is indicated. Also in a patient with established DKD and the patient is not being followed by a nephrologist, then if one of the issues in Box 8.5 appear, a referral to a nephrologist is indicated. A nephrologist evaluation will likely include a detailed history, an examination of the urine, possibly a kidney ultrasound, and possibly a number of serologic and other laboratory tests. The nephrologist will also consider whether a kidney biopsy should be done. There are two reasons to perform a biopsy, diagnosis, and prognosis. In general, biopsies are not done solely for prognostic purposes due to the invasiveness of the test. Diagnostic biopsies should be done if there is a possibility of finding a nondiabetic treatable cause of kidney disease. The two most common causes of kidney disease in diabetic people other than diabetes mellitus are: (1) Hypertension, and (2) Immunoglobulin A (IgA) nephropathy. Hypertension should be being treated anyway so there is no need to biopsy to diagnose hypertension. IgA nephropathy is often not treated (as treatment options are limited) although there are specific clinical scenarios where treatment might be indicated. Hence, kidney biopsy should be performed in patients with DKD if issues shown in Box 8.5 arise and there is a likelihood of a treatment other than treatments for diabetes mellitus and hypertension being started.

PRIMARY PREVENTION OF DIABETIC KIDNEY DISEASE

Ideally it is best to prevent the development of DKD. About 10–30% of people with diabetes mellitus will develop DKD as defined as decreased eGFR (<60 mL/min) and/or increased urine albumin/creatinine ratio (>30 mg/g). People with type 1 diabetes mellitus develop DKD at higher incidence than people with type 2 diabetes mellitus. But considering there are many more people with type 2 diabetes mellitus than type 1 diabetes mellitus, the rapid rise in DKD worldwide is primarily due to type 2 diabetes mellitus. At this time, there is no way to distinguish those at risk for developing DKD. It is an area of great research interest though as if a particular test could identify who is likely to develop DKD, then those people could be targeted with especially aggressive management of diabetes mellitus and blood pressure for example. Many possible candidate markers have been identified in the last 10 years including such markers as tumor necrosis factor-alpha receptor and kidney injury molecule-1 (KIM-1).[5] At this time though, the clinical utility of these markers have not been verified, so it is best to treat all diabetic patients as if they are at risk for the development of DKD and other diabetic complications.

There is a great deal of evidence supporting a role for glucose control for primary prevention of DKD. The importance of tight control was definitively shown for patients with type 1 diabetes mellitus in the Diabetes Control and Complications Trial (DCCT) study.[6] In this study, 1,441 patients with type 1 diabetes mellitus were evaluated for a mean of 6.5 years and treated either conventionally or intensively. Conventionally treated people had an average hemoglobin A1c of 9.1 and intensively treated people had a median hemoglobin A1c of 7.2. Intensive treatment led to a decrease in the development of microalbuminuria by 39%. Since the conclusion of the original DCCT study, there has been a follow-up study called Epidemiology of Diabetes Interventions and Complications (EDIC) and the 25-year follow-up was recently reported.[6] During the EDIC study, all patients were treated to an A1c of about 8.0%. So, for the past 25 years, the main difference between the two groups occurred only during the first 6.5 years. Very importantly, the originally intensively treated group had 50% less development of microalbuminuria and 50% less development of an eGFR of less than 60 mL/min as compared to the original conventionally treated group. This difference has been seen throughout the follow-up period. These findings stress the great importance of glucose control (generally aiming for a hemoglobin A1c of 7%) for the primary prevention of DKD. Similar findings have been found for people with type 2 diabetes mellitus in studies such as the United Kingdom Prospective Diabetes Study (UKPDS).[7] Thus, we are not doing our patients any favors by waiting to get their glucose levels under control.

Blood pressure control has also been shown to be of major importance in the primary prevention of DKD. As much as 60% of people with type 2 diabetes mellitus and hypertension will develop DKD. Although there is universal agreement that blood pressure control is needed to prevent the development of DKD, there is much controversy over the blood pressure goal.

At this time, it is quite challenging to determine the appropriate goal as already noted, only 10–30% of people with diabetes mellitus will develop DKD. Hence, all of these studies require very large cohorts. In the UKPDS study, a reduction of systolic blood pressure from 154 mm Hg to 144 mm Hg led to a 29% reduction in the development of increased albumin levels. But current guidelines suggest lowering blood pressure more than 144 mm Hg. Over the past 10 years, there have been many hypertension trials directed mainly toward individuals with type 2 diabetes mellitus and high-risk cardiovascular disease [e.g. The Action to Control Cardiovascular Risk in Diabetes (ACCORD)].[8] With respect to cardiovascular disease in people with diabetes mellitus, it appeared that a systolic blood pressure of 120 mm Hg was not better than 135 mm Hg. This led many guidelines committees to change their recommendations for optimal blood pressure control from less than 130/80 to less than 140/80 or less than 140/90. But more recent studies have not been as clear. So at this time, the optimal prevention target is unclear. Almost every expert would agree that the goal should be at least less than 140/80. Aiming for 130/80 seems to be indicated in my opinion for prevention of DKD as this will prevent the clinician from being satisfied with levels close to but higher than 140/80.

Another issue for prevention is whether there are specific drugs that are uniquely valuable for primary prevention. In most of the primary prevention studies, there were no major differences between antihypertensive classes. So at this time, there are no specific recommendations as to which antihypertensive medications to use. Choose based on cost, potency, convenience, comorbidities, and side effects as one would do with any medication. Of course there is a unique class of medications, renin-angiotensin-aldosterone system (RAAS) inhibitors such as angiotensin converting enzyme inhibitors (ACEIs) and angiotensin receptor blockers (ARBs) that are recommended to be first-line agents for blood pressure control in people with diabetes mellitus (Box 8.6). There is strong evidence for activation of the RAAS in people with diabetes mellitus and RAAS inhibitors have been shown to have benefits not only for blood pressure lowering but also for protection against the development of cardiovascular disease and retinopathy. Thus, in people with hypertension perhaps using RAAS inhibitor as the initial drug is a logical choice. But should everybody with diabetes mellitus receive an RAAS inhibitor (regardless of blood pressure) to prevent the development of DKD. A meta-analysis from 2012 suggested that ACEIs but not ARBs did reduce the development of increased urine albumin levels.[9] But an important study from 2009 in the New England Journal of Medicine showed no

Box 8.6: Prevention of diabetic kidney disease.

- *Blood glucose control*—Aim for a hemoglobin A1c of less than 7%
- *Blood pressure control*—Aim for less than 140/80 but ideally closer to 130/80 is likely best
- No clear unique role for renin-angiotensin-aldosterone system (RAAS) inhibitors.

benefit for ACEIs or ARBs for the prevention of pathological changes in the kidney.[10] In this study, the authors gave each participant (type 1 diabetic patients without kidney disease) enalapril, losartan, or placebo. All participants were biopsied before the study started and after 5 years. There was no difference amongst the treatment groups as to the development of pathological changes in the kidney. These findings do not support using ACEIs or ARBs for primary prevention in people with type 1 diabetes mellitus. In large studies in people with type 2 diabetes mellitus, some studies showed a benefit but others did not.[11] An important difference, though, were the baseline blood pressures in all studies. The studies that showed a benefit had higher baseline blood pressures as compared to the other studies. Hence, the beneficial effect may have been due to lowering blood pressure rather than to a unique effect of the RAAS inhibitors. At this time, there is no unique role for RAAS inhibitors for the primary prevention of DKD. On the other hand, there are very strong indications to use these drugs in the treatment of established DKD as discussed in the next section.

TREATMENT OF DIABETIC KIDNEY DISEASE (BOX 8.7)

There are three major goals in treating DKD: (1) Blood sugar control, (2) Blood pressure control, and (3) Lowering urine albumin level. Many studies have validated the importance of blood sugar control for people with DKD. In general, the hemoglobin A1c goal is 7% but any improvement in blood sugar control has beneficial outcomes. There are no clear studies at this time that suggest that the any particular drug used to achieve blood sugar is of unique benefit for treating DKD. There are ongoing studies using dipeptidyl peptidase-4 (DPP-4) inhibitors and sodium-glucose co-transporter-2 (SGLT-2) inhibitors to determine if these classes of medications slow progression of DKD. These studies are likely to be reported in the years 2018–2020.

Blood pressure control is of great importance in slowing progression of kidney disease. But as with primary prevention, the specific goal is controversial. As mentioned previously the studies showing no benefit of lower than 140/80 in the high-risk cardiovascular disease patients have dominated the blood pressure goal-setting conversation for both prevention and treatment of DKD. But a recent analysis of the Veterans Affairs Nephropathy in Diabetes (VA NEPHRON-D) study suggest that less than 130/80 does lead to better outcomes for DKD patients.[12] The VA NEPHRON-D study was intended to study whether a combination of ACEI and ARB are beneficial in slowing progression of DKD. The study was stopped early (as discussed here). But further analysis of the slope of decline in eGFR was slower in patients who had blood

Box 8.7: Treatment of diabetic kidney disease.

- *Blood glucose control*—Aim for hemoglobin A1c of 7%
- *Blood pressure control*—Aim for 130/80
- Use RAAS inhibitors if urine albumin level is elevated
- Consider using combination of ACEI or ARB with aldosterone antagonist
- Little to no role for low protein diet (<0.8 g/kg/day)
- Avoid high protein diets (>1.5–2.0 g/kg/day)
- Screen patients for anemia and measure iron stores
- Screen patients for hyperparathyroidism.

(ACEI: Angiotensin converting enzyme inhibitor; ARB: Angiotensin receptor blocker; RAAS: Renin-angiotensin-aldosterone system) pressures of a systolic blood pressure of at least less than 140 mm Hg. And there was a clear trend to slower rates of decline in eGFR with lower systolic blood pressures. Current recommendations are to aim for less than 140/80 if there are low levels of urine albumin/creatinine ratio (<300 mg/g) and less than 130/80 if there are higher levels of the urine albumin/creatinine ratio. It is quite possible that 130/80 or better will be the target for DKD for all patients as more studies are done.

For controlling blood pressure, any antihypertensive may be used. But of course there is a unique role for ACEIs and ARBs in lowering the urine albumin level. Many studies have shown a benefit for slowing progression if the urine albumin level is reduced at least if the patient has high levels of urine albumin/creatinine ratio (>300 mg/g). Lowering urine albumin likely not only helps to slow progression of DKD but likely also lowers the risk of cardiovascular events. Blood sugar control and/or blood pressure control will lower the urine albumin level. But there is a unique role for RAAS inhibitors in treating DKD patients as these drugs have been clearly proven to be effective in lowering urine albumin levels and for slowing decline in eGFR in people with increased urine albumin levels. It is recommended that all patients with an elevated urine albumin level should be on an RAAS inhibitor even if the blood pressure is well controlled. The dose should be increased as needed to try to lower the urine albumin level. And a serum potassium level should be checked about 1 week after starting an RAAS inhibitor and any time the dose is increased as elevated potassium is the main reason for decreasing or stopping these medications. In addition to ACEIs and ARBs, one may use the renin inhibitor, aliskiren or an aldosterone antagonist such as spironolactone or eplerenone. All of these have been shown to be effective in lowering urine albumin levels.

Considering the utility of RAAS inhibitors in slowing progression of DKD, there has been much interest in combining these agents for even greater effect. Some major studies have questioned the usefulness and safety of combining ACEIs and ARBs.[13,14] In these studies, the combination was not more effective than either agent alone and there were more adverse events in the combination group (e.g. increased acute kidney injury and high potassium levels). This led many medical guideline groups to not recommend using the combination. But there are questions about the inclusion criteria in these studies that may have led to higher adverse events. For example, in VA NEPHRON-D, patients with a serum potassium level as high as 5.5 mM were included. It is quite likely that putting a participant with this level on both ACEI and ARB might lead to a very high level of potassium. Despite these important trials, there may well be circumstances where the combination is beneficial. A recent meta-analysis determined that with respect to progression to ESKD, the combination of ACEI and ARB was more protective than either agent alone.[15] Also, there is an ongoing study called VALID, which is evaluating benazepril and valsartan in combination that is to be reported on by 2017. Thus, when to use the combination of ACEI and ARB is evolving. At this time, it is not clear what recommendation to make as regards combination of ACEIs and ARBs.

A combination of growing interest is using an aldosterone antagonist with an ACEI or ARB. The combination appears to be beneficial but there are no long-term studies. A new nonsteroidal aldosterone antagonist, finerenone, is currently under investigation and should provide some answers as to the efficacy and safety of this combination as there is an ongoing trial with this drug in combination with either an ACEI or ARB. Of note, the renin inhibitor, aliskiren, should not be used in combination as combination studies showed increased adverse events as compared to the single agents.[16]

In addition, there are some other medications to consider for lowering urine albumin level. Some studies have shown that the nondihydropyridine medications diltiazem and verapamil have a modest urine albumin lowering effect. If a patient cannot take an RAAS inhibitor for some reason (e.g. high potassium, allergy, etc.) then one of these agents may be considered. A new medication that was recently approved in the USA is the drug patiromer that may change how the RAAS are prescribed.[17,18] Patiromer is an oral potassium binder that may be taken chronically. Hence, if high potassium is limiting use of an RAAS inhibitor, possibly taking patiromer will allow continued use of the RAAS inhibitor. But it is not clear how safe it is to use this drug for a prolonged period. More long-term studies need to be done to determine if this medication can be taken safely.

Lastly, it has been suggested that low protein diets are of use in slowing progression of DKD. A low protein diet is defined as less than 0.8 g/kg/day. Although there is excellent evidence in animal models of DKD that low protein diets do slow progression, the evidence in humans is much less compelling. At this time, routine use of a low protein diet cannot be recommended. But if other treatment options have been maximized then the implementation of a low protein diet may be indicated. On the other hand, it is best to avoid a high protein diet in people with DKD as many studies (mostly in animals though) suggest high protein intake may accelerate decline in eGFR. It is not clear how high is too high but perhaps higher than 1.5–2.0 g/kg/day should be avoided.

COMPLICATIONS OF CHRONIC KIDNEY DISEASE

Two complications of CKD need to be screened for in people with DKD: (1) Anemia, and (2) Hyperparathyroidism. Anemia occurs for two main reasons: (1) Decreased production of the growth hormone erythropoietin, and (2) Decreased absorption of iron. Hyperparathyroidism in early stage CKD occurs due to loss of proximal tubular cells that have the enzyme (1 alpha-hydroxylase) that produce the activated form of vitamin D. Activated vitamin D works in concert with parathyroid hormone (PTH) to maintain bone health. Each affects the other's production. Low levels of activated vitamin D lead to increased levels of PTH and possible bone disease and vascular calcification. Both anemia and hyperparathyroidism might occur at higher eGFRs in people with DKD as compared to people with non-DKD. A possible reason for this is that the main reason for developing these complications is loss of kidney tissue. But people with DKD have both a loss of kidney tissue and they have the negative effect of elevated glucose on the metabolic processes that produce erythropoietin and that activate 1 alpha-hydroxylase. Indeed studies in cell culture where proximal tubular cells were exposed to high glucose, 1 alpha-hydroxylase activity was significantly reduced. So, all patients with DKD should be routinely screened for anemia and hyperparathyroidism.

When to refer to nephrology?

Referral to a nephrologist is most dependent on the knowledge and expertise of the primary care physician. Possible reasons for referral to a nephrologist include: (1) Initial evaluation to determine if there is a kidney disease other than diabetes mellitus, (2) A change in kidney

Box 8.8: Reasons to refer to a nephrologist.

- Initial evaluation to determine if there is a kidney disease other than diabetes. And if the estimated glomerular filtration rate (eGFR) is less than 45 mL/min (<60 mL/min if the patient is <50 years old)
- A significant change in the rate of decline in eGFR
- Assistance in optimizing management
- Continuously rising urine albumin level
- Difficult to control hypertension
- Evaluation and management of anemia and/or hyperparathyroidism
- Electrolyte abnormalities, particularly management of high potassium.

function as noted in Box 8.5 that might indicate a kidney disease other than diabetes mellitus, (3) If the eGFR is less than 45 mL/min (and <60 mL/min if the patient is <50 years old) should at least prompt a screening visit to a nephrologist to see if any treatments should be optimized or new ones started, (4) If urine albumin levels are rising, (5) Difficult to control hypertension, (6) Evaluation and management of anemia and/or hyperparathyroidism, and (7) Electrolyte abnormalities, particularly high potassium (Box 8.8).

CONCLUSION

There is an ongoing epidemic rise of the number of people with DKD. Currently, there are multiple treatments for both the prevention and treatment of DKD. It is essential for all physicians caring for diabetic patients to optimal implement treatments to prevent the development of DKD. It is also critical to screen for signs of DKD on a routine basis and to aggressively implement treatments to slow progression. Current treatments do not cure DKD but current treatments if implemented early and aggressively used to treat to goals can significantly prevent DKD and slow worsening of DKD.

REFERENCES

1. United States Renal Data System (USRDS). (2016). Survey USRDS. [online] Available from www.usrds.org. [Accessed February, 2018].
2. Ninomiya T, Perkovic V, de Galan BE, et al. Albuminuria and kidney function independently predict cardiovascular and renal outcomes in diabetes. J Am Soc Nephrol. 2009;20(8):1813-21.
3. Afkarian M, Sachs MC, Kestenbaum B, et al. Kidney disease and increased mortality risk in type 2 diabetes. J Am Soc Nephrol. 2013;24(2):302-8.
4. Dwyer JP, Parving HH, Hunsicker LG, et al. Renal dysfunction in the presence of normoalbuminuria in type 2 diabetes: results from the DEMAND Study. Cardiorenal Med. 2012;2(1):1-10.
5. Macisaac RJ, Ekinci EI, Jerums G. Markers of and risk factors for the development and progression of diabetic kidney disease. Am J Kidney Dis. 2014;63(2 Suppl 2):S39-62.
6. Group DE, de Boer IH, Sun W, et al. Intensive diabetes therapy and glomerular filtration rate in type 1 diabetes. N Engl J Med. 2011;365(25):2366-76.
7. Intensive blood-glucose control with sulphonylureas or insulin compared with conventional treatment and risk of complications in patients with type 2 diabetes (UKPDS 33). UK Prospective Diabetes Study (UKPDS) Group. Lancet. 1998;352(9131):837-53.
8. Group AS, Cushman WC, Evans GW, et al. Effects of intensive blood-pressure control in type 2 diabetes mellitus. N Engl J Med. 2010;362(17):1575-85.

9. Lv J, Perkovic V, Foote CV, et al. Antihypertensive agents for preventing diabetic kidney disease. Cochrane Database Syst Rev. 2012;12:CD004136.
10. Mauer M, Zinman B, Gardiner R, et al. Renal and retinal effects of enalapril and losartan in type 1 diabetes. N Engl J Med. 2009;361(1):40-51.
11. Bilous R, Chaturvedi N, Sjølie AK, et al. Effect of candesartan on microalbuminuria and albumin excretion rate in diabetes: three randomized trials. Ann Intern Med. 2009;151(1):11-20.
12. Leehey DJ, Zhang JH, Emanuele NV, et al. BP and renal outcomes in diabetic kidney disease: the veterans affairs nephropathy in diabetes trial. Clin J Am Soc Nephrol. 2015;10(12):2159-69.
13. ONTARGET Investigators, Yusuf S, Teo KK, et al. Telmisartan, ramipril, or both in patients at high risk for vascular events. N Engl J Med. 2008;358(15):1547-59.
14. Pham JT, Schmitt BP, Leehey DJ. Effects of dual blockade of the renin-angiotensin system in diabetic kidney disease: a systematic review and meta-analysis. J Nephrol Therapeutic. 2012;2(1-8):003.
15. Palmer SC, Mavridis D, Navarese E, et al. Comparative efficacy and safety of blood pressure-lowering agents in adults with diabetes and kidney disease: a network meta-analysis. Lancet. 2015;385(9982):2047-56.
16. Parving HH, Brenner BM, McMurray JJ, et al. Cardiorenal end points in a trial of aliskiren for type 2 diabetes. N Engl J Med. 2012;367(23):2204-13.
17. Bakris GL, Pitt B, Weir MR, et al. Effect of patiromer on serum potassium level in patients with hyperkalemia and diabetic kidney disease: the AMETHYST-DN randomized clinical trial. JAMA. 2015;314(2):151-61.
18. Weir MR, Bakris GL, Bushinsky DA, et al. Patiromer in patients with kidney disease and hyperkalemia receiving RAAS inhibitors. N Engl J Med. 2015;372(3):211-21.

CHAPTER 9

The Diabetic Foot

David R Campbell, Arturo R Rolla

INTRODUCTION

The feet accomplish a great deal of mechanical and dynamic functions in our daily ambulation sustaining very high vertical and torque pressures, and they are at a long distance from the heart and central nervous system. To do this mechanical work they precise good innervation (pain, position and temperature sensations, motor strength, and coordination), vascular supply, and a dynamic osteoarticular architecture that helps to distribute evenly the pressures. Unfortunately, these requirements are frequently compromised by long-term diabetes.

Diabetic foot problems are very common and expensive, ending in amputations, and have a high mortality rate, comparable or worse than many cancers. The sine-qua-non pathogenic factors are neuropathy, ischemia, and abnormal architecture. It is very rare to have a serious foot problem in a person with diabetes who does not have these three factors. There are other secondary or triggering factors that appear frequently (trauma, friction, infection, unrelated deformities, etc.). Prevention with education and frequent feet examinations by experienced physicians are extremely important to avoid prolonged, expensive treatments, and amputations (Boxes 9.1 and 9.2).

Neuropathy is an important pathogenic factor acting by many different mechanisms. Some of them are due to peripheral sensory neuropathy: (a) Decreased pain sensation that does not allow the patient to perceive lesions in the foot, (b) Decreased position sensation causing incoordination, falls, or abnormal walking, and, (c) Decreased coordination in the foot muscles that can lead to unusual articular movements. Autonomic neuropathy may cause increased blood flow but with arteriovenous shunts that steal effective circulation, and dryness of the

Box 9.1: Prevention.

There are very few better examples in medicine of how prevention can help the feet of persons with diabetes

- Ongoing education about foot care
- The moment the diagnosis of peripheral neuropathy is made in a patient, a plan of prevention of foot problems should be initiated
- Every clinic visit the patients should remove shoes and socks to permit a thorough examination of the feet

Box 9.2: Bacteriology of diabetic foot infections.

- They usually start with the normal skin flora (*Staphylococcus* and *Streptococcus*)
- As it gets more chronic, resistant organisms (MRSA), then gram negative, and later anaerobic germs appear
- Most of them are polymicrobial
- Superficial cultures are of no value to select antibiotics
- There is no particular antibiotic alone or in combination that has been proven more effective than others

skin that facilitates its disruption. There is also research data indicating that the neuropathy also interferes with the normal local inflammatory response to trauma and infection.

Peripheral vascular disease is another important pathogenic factor because it decreases the offer of oxygen, white cells, and nutrients to fight against infections, and also impairs the healing process once the infection has been controlled. Some patients may have a history of intermittent claudication, although the majority do not have it (see Chapter on Peripheral Vascular Disease).

FOOT DEFORMITIES

Chronic glycation of the collagen leads to shortening and stiffness of tendons, ligaments, and connective tissue that alters the normal architecture and biodynamic forces, increasing pressures over certain areas of the foot, instead of allowing for a more even distribution. Glycation of proteins is a slow, nonenzymatic process that depends on the increased glucose concentration and time. Collagen has a very long half-life (6–8 years) that increases its chances of glycation, so that it may appear over long periods of time even in normoglycemic individuals. The glycation of the collagen fibrils cause 'cross-linking' with thickening and shortening of the fibers, and make them more difficult to digest with an increase in the volume of the older collagen. The effects of collagen glycation are better known in the hands (Dupuytren's contractures, stenosing tenosynovitis, cheiroarthropathy, etc.) where it tends to affect more the flexor tendons decreasing the dorsal extension of the fingers. In the feet, it affects more the extensor tendons that first start to protrude on the dorsum of the feet, and later cause the elevation of the first interphalangeal joints of the toes (hammer toes) and plantar protrusion of the metatarsal-phalangeal joint (Fig. 9.1). There is also glycation of the Achilles tendon with shortening and decreased elongation that impairs the normal dorsiflexion of the feet which is very important for normal walking. The foot muscles may also be affected by the neuropathy increasing the imbalance of the tendon forces and the osteoarticular protrusions (Figs. 9.2 and 9.3).

There may also be changes in the foot architecture, intrinsic to the person's feet and unrelated to diabetes (flat feet, bunions, etc.) that could lead to protrusion of areas of the foot that get irritated by the extra pressure or friction. The most common one is under the head of the metatarsal bones frequently associated with pronation of the foot (Fig. 9.4). Charcot's neuroarthropathy is also a cause of severe deformities that frequently leads to ulcerations and infections.

Other factors are frequently present:

- *Diabetic factor* consists of the duration of diabetes and degree of poor glycemic control. Many years with diabetes and poor control increase the severity of the main pathogenic factors, and tend to worsen the presentation and the prognosis. Part of the overall management of

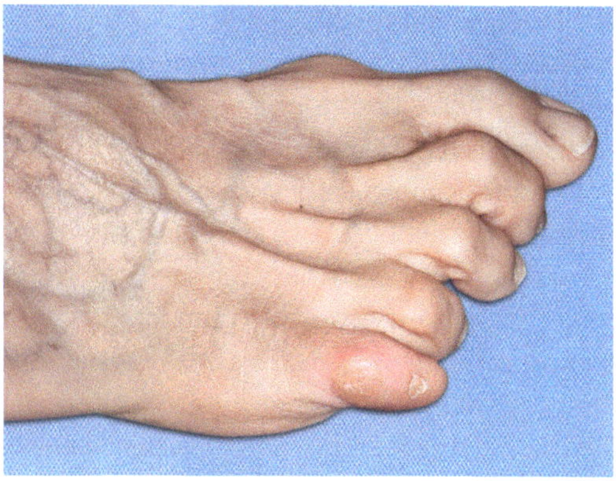

Fig. 9.1: Shortening and protrusion of the extensor tendons in the dorsum of the feet causing the upward deviation of the proximal phalanxes and the first interphalangeal joint of the toes (hammer toes).

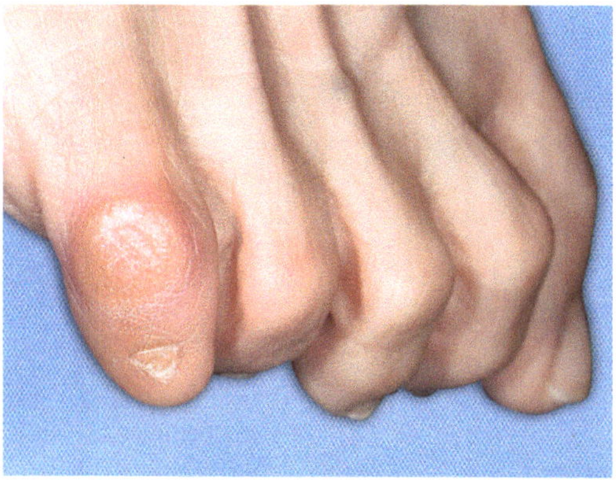

Fig. 9.2: Hammer toes with protrusion of the first interphalangeal joint leading to increased pressure against the shoes and callus formation, like seen in the fifth toe.

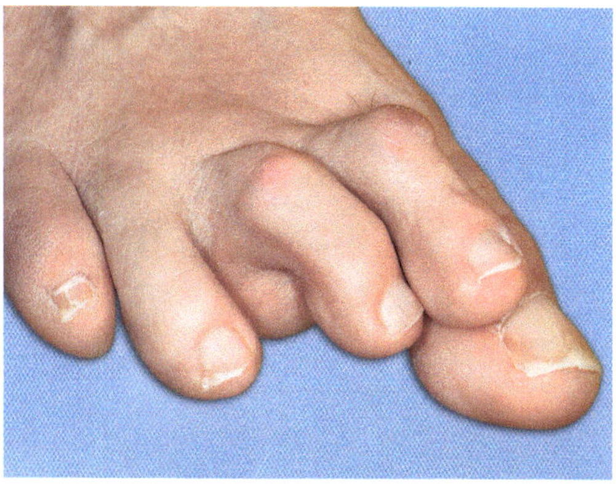

Fig. 9.3: Hammer toes with medial deviation of the second and third toes showing calluses over the raised first interphalangeal joints.

a patient with a diabetic foot is to obtain the best possible glycemic control to help with the infection and healing process—before, during, and after the foot problem. Persons with diabetes are more frequently carriers of *Staphylococcus* in the skin, and hyperglycemia interferes with the bactericidal effect of the leukocytes.

- *Skin irritation* is due to abnormal pressures on areas of altered foot architecture and mechanical forces or friction against the shoes when the toes or other areas are protruding. It usually starts as an area of skin erythema that progresses to a callus of variable dimensions (Fig. 9.5). The continuous ambulation starts causing lineal fissures on the callus that continue to deepen until they reach beyond the skin. By then, a blister may appear in the area of greater pressures, and if the outer cover breaks it becomes an ulcer (Fig. 9.6). The ulcer becomes easily infected, first with the usual skin germs, and then the ulcer slowly gets deeper breaking through the skin into the subcutaneous tissue where it may cause a cellulitis (Fig. 9.7).
- *Trauma* from daily walking, ill-fitted shoes, thickened and ingrown nails, punctures, foreign bodies inside of the shoes that go unnoticed, socks with folds, etc. They are easily found

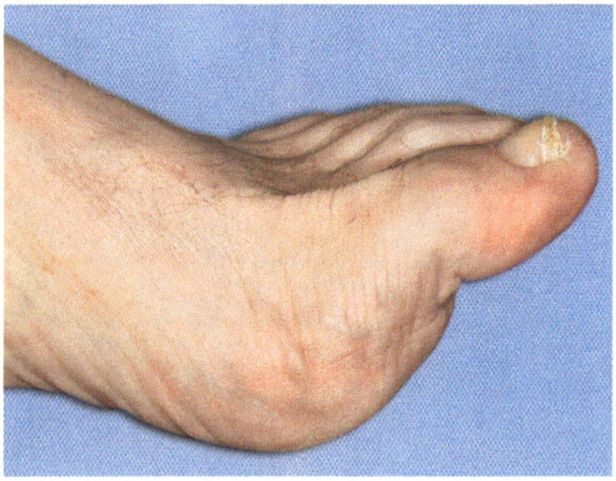

Fig. 9.4: The upward deviation of the toes because of the extensor tendon retraction tends to increase the pressure over the metatarsal-phalangeal joint and the heads of the metatarsal bones. In pronated feet there is a marked increase in the pressures over the head of the first metatarsal bone.

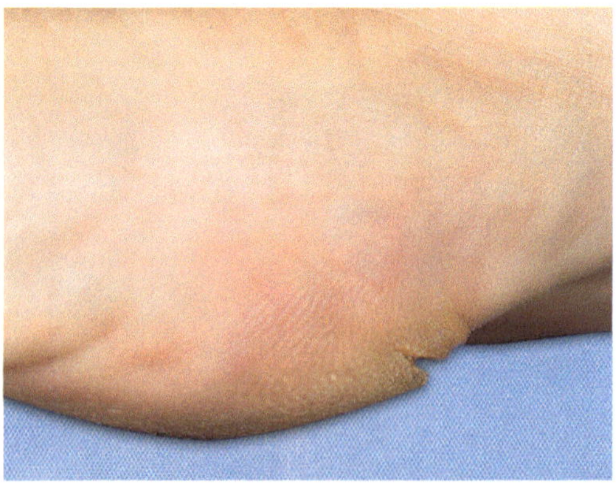

Fig. 9.5: Callus formation under the head of the first metatarsal and first metatarsophalangeal joint.

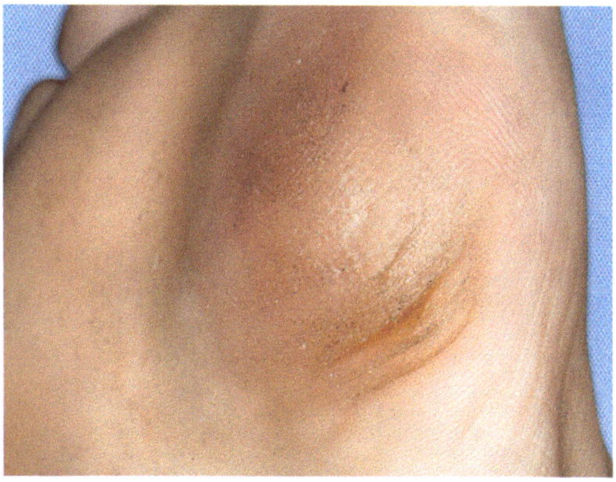

Fig. 9.6: Fissure formation in the callus that will lead to infections.

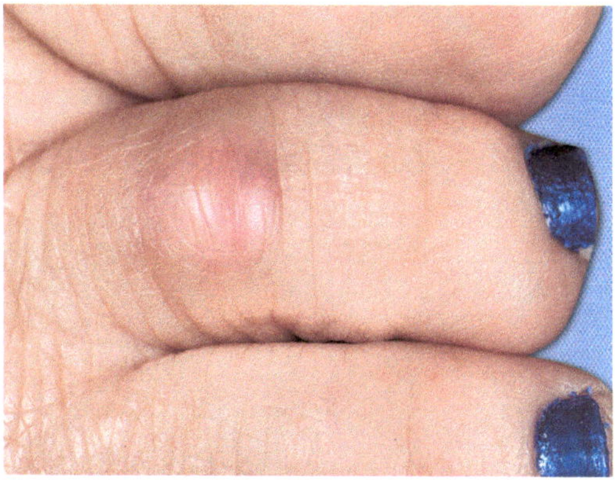

Fig. 9.7: Early thickening of the skin and redness over a protruding interphalangeal joint.

because of the initial erythema they cause, and they should be corrected and/or protected at all cost to avoid progression of the lesions.

- *Infection* is the beginning of more serious problems. Initially it is confined to the thickened epidermis and the superficial ulcer. Once the infection reaches into the subcutaneous tissue the situation is more serious as it progresses to cellulitis, abscess, sinus tracts, and osteomyelitis (Fig. 9.8). To make things worse, the infection increases the ischemia and may lead to gangrene of the area (Fig. 9.9). An old diagnostic difference may still be used today: dry and wet gangrene. Dry gangrene is called when there is only ischemia and necrotic tissue without infection. Wet gangrene appears when there is an infection in and around the gangrenous tissues (Warning 1) (Box 9.3).

WARNING 1

"3 I's

- Infection
- Increases
- Ischemia

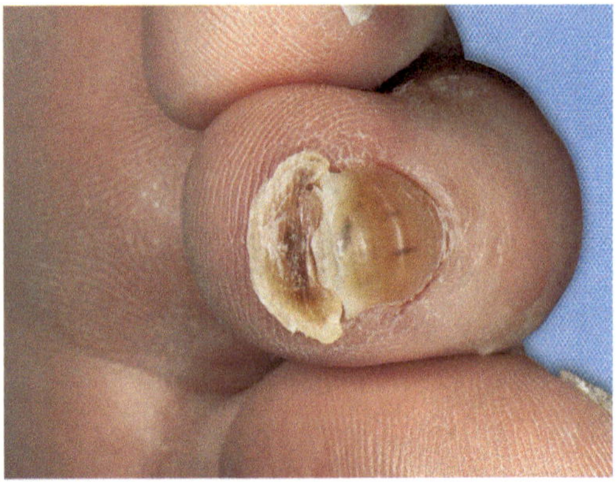

Fig. 9.8: At times the dorsal retraction of the hammer toes causes pressure on the tip of the toes with callus formation and possibility of infections.

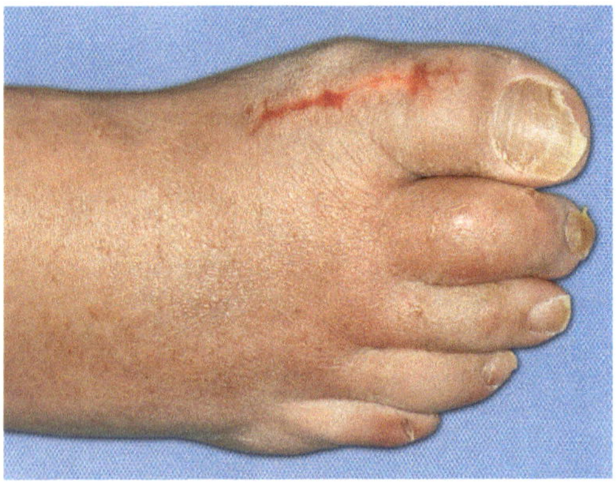

Fig. 9.9: The toe with a callus and fissure at the tip caused this infection of the second toe that was starting to expand into a cellulitis of the entire foot.

Box 9.3: Sites of increased pressure or friction more frequent in the feet.

- Head of the metatarsals—over the first in pronated feet, or more lateral in supinated feet
- Top of the interphalangeal joints or at the tip in hammer toes
- Heels
- Areas of foot deformity or bone protrusions
- Any other areas that may have continuous friction or pressures

- *Psychosocial factors* are frequently present initially and during the follow-up, starting with the lack of appropriate education about foot care, poor hygiene, and inability to follow instructions. The cure of these lesions is usually slow, and the patients tend to get frustrated, abandoning treatments, or looking for other alternatives. The best way to deal with these types of problems is patience, closer follow-up, and repeated education.
- *Older age and male sex* are also known factors for diabetic foot problems.

- *Cardiovascular risk factors* like hypertension, dyslipidemia, and smoking increase the prevalence and severity of both peripheral vascular disease and neuropathy.
- *Visual impairment* interferes with the daily foot inspection, increases the chances of foot trauma, and is frequently associated with other systemic complications.
- *Chronic renal failure* especially if the patient is on the chronic dialysis.
- *History of previous foot problems and amputations:* All types of amputations change the areas of increased pressure in the same or the other foot.
- *Previous skin infections,* often interdigital mycoses (tinea pedis) that break the skin and facilitate the entrance of the bacteria.
- *Decreased plantar subcutaneous tissue,* most likely due to arterial insufficiency, decreases the cushion protection on the protruding surfaces, and increases the effect of direct pressures on these areas (Warnings 2 and 3).

WARNING 2

"In diabetes, the complications complicate the complications"

WARNING 3

"Diabetic patients should remove shoes and socks at every visit"

FOOT INSPECTION

It should be done frequently at the time of every visit by somebody with experience and removing shoes and socks. Start by observing carefully both feet looking for areas of erythema, calluses, ulcers, bone deformities and protrusions, changes in the arch, and comparing with the other foot, etc. The toenails and interdigital spaces should be inspected as well. Lateral deviation of toes like with valgus deformities, may cause calluses and ulceration in between the toes. The range of motion of the metatarsal-phalangeal joint of the first toe may become limited (hallux limitus or rigidus) so that it cannot bend up with normal walking leading to increased plantar pressures. Occasionally it may be important to watch the patient walk, and observe the shoes to see how they are being worn particularly at the heels. The presence of cellulitis, abscesses, and gangrene, is usually quite apparent, and at times it may present with systemic symptoms (Fever, chills, etc.) and increased glucose levels. Always look in the inflamed areas for ulcerations or, at times, puncture lesions that may not have been noticed by the patient. The differential diagnosis of a swollen and painful foot—without ulcerations—is with an acute attack of gout or pseudogout, simple trauma, or a stress fracture. Plantar warts may be confused with calluses but they are not usually in the areas of increased pressure and tend to be more painful (Fig. 9.10).

NEUROLOGICAL EXAMINATION

- *Vibratory sensation* using a tuning fork of 128 Hz applied to the tip of the first toe and others, over the first metatarsal head, and at the heel. If these areas do not show good vibratory sensation the examination should continue up in the leg at the malleoli, shin, and even knee cap. The tuning fork should be stroked lightly, and if the patient perceives vibrations he should be asked when he stops feeling them. At that point the examining professional checks on his knuckles to see if he is still able to perceive the vibrations. The results should

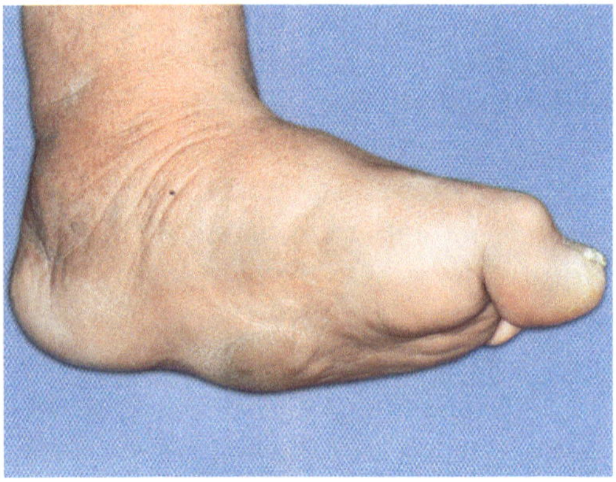

Fig. 9.10: Outside of the usual areas of pressure, other areas may appear from previous deformities or like in this case from Charcot's neuroarthropathy.

be posted as normal, decreased, or absent followed by the areas in question. Vibratory sensation is thought to be the first modality to disappear in diabetic neuropathy but it is not necessarily the case in some patients.

- *Touch sensation with a monofilament* of 10 g is the next clinical test to do. The filament is pressed against similar areas in the foot until it bends. The patient should not be looking and respond if he feels the touch sensation or not. Most of the times this test is reported present or absent. If necessary it can be repeated with a pin (*pinprick* sensation) but usually the monofilament test is sufficient.
- *Deep tendon reflexes* starting with the Achilles tendons and then at the knees. Both reflexes may be absent in elderly individuals without diabetes or with other forms of neuropathies, so their absence only helps to corroborate the diagnosis, and their presence makes the possibility of peripheral diabetic neuropathy unlikely.
- *Temperature discrimination* could be done with the test tubes with warm or cold water but they are usually not a part of simple examinations.

There are several electrodiagnostic tests, like nerve conduction velocity and electromyogram, that may be used but their need, reliability, and advantages have not been clearly demonstrated. They should be reserved for special cases in which the differential diagnosis is not clear (see Chapter on Neuropathy). The neurological deficits of diabetic peripheral neuropathy are bilateral and symmetrical. If one side appears to be more involved another diagnosis needs to be found (previous surgeries in that lower extremity or the spine, disk problems, etc.). On the other hand, the foot lesions initially are usually unilateral because of the associated local factors. Remember that very often there is a discrepancy between the severity of the lesions and the pain symptomatology in these patients.

In very advanced cases the intrinsic muscles of the foot may appear atrophic and may even have spontaneous fasciculations mostly in the legs. This is because of diabetic peripheral neuropathy is more of a sensory than a motor neuropathy. Long tract signs should be absent (flexor Babinski's response).

VASCULAR EXAMINATION

Initially look for skin color changes, hair growth in toes and dorsum of the feet. Then the two foot pulses to palpate are the dorsalis pedis and the posterior tibialis. In the majority of patients with a diabetic foot they will be absent but in some forms of advanced neuropathies, particularly in Charcot's neuroarthropathy, the pulses may be increased because of decreased sympathetic innervation that increases the blood flow with the formation of arteriovenous shunts. Next comes the palpation of the popliteal and femoral arteries, trying to ascertain the levels of arterial blockages. Both at the femoral and popliteal levels bruits may be heard with the stethoscope (more specific tests can be found in the Peripheral Vascular Disease Chapter) (Warning 4).

WARNING 4

"Patients with Charcot's neuroarthropathy may have increased pedal pulses"

MANAGEMENT OF ACUTE DIABETIC FOOT PROBLEMS

Once a cutaneous foot inflammation is found it becomes important to find the degree and depth of the infection (superficial, cellulitis, abscess, or osteomyelitis) because the treatment will be different. Always bear in mind that the inflammatory process in these patients is frequently diminished because of the peripheral vascular disease and the neuropathy. So, many times it is better to overreact than ignore the problem. Some patients have fever and are toxic but it is not uncommon to find patients with the serious foot infections completely asymptomatic or only with unexplained hyperglycemia. If there is a large area of inflammation, the patient should be immediately hospitalized, the infected foot should be debrided by an experienced podiatrist or surgeon and deep tissue cultures should be taken, followed by a deep probe with a sterile instrument to see if it reaches the bone, trying to find if there is or not osteomyelitis or not.

Laboratory Tests

Severe deep infections will show an increased white blood cell count with a shift to the left, and increased serum C-reactive protein and sedimentation rate. Remember that in some persons with diabetes the sedimentation rate may be chronically elevated because of nephropathy and/or age.

Bacteriology Cultures

Even though the majority of severe diabetic foot problems have an infectious component, their exact diagnosis and treatment are usually broad based. Most foot infections are multibacterial, and the superficial cultures are often misleading because they do not represent the germs growing inside especially in the cases of deep abscesses and osteomyelitis. Ideally then cultures should be obtained from deep tissues at the time of debridement and drainage.

Initially the germs involved are the usually skin contaminants, *Staphylococcus* and *Streptococcus* which respond very well to the usual antibiotics. Later on, resistant species and enteric pathogens appear. The more chronic the foot infection, the more mixed and the more resistant pathogens appear. It is not clear the pathogenicity of each one of the germs in the mixed cultures obtained, and they should be only a rough indication for the administration of antibiotics. The presence of resistance, on the other hand, should be taken into consideration especially if the patients have been admitted to hospital or chronic care facilities. On the other hand, if the secretions are fetid or there is a gas present on X-rays the presence of anaerobes should be suspected.

The risk of osteomyelitis increases with ulcers larger than 2 cm, an increased sedimentation rate, positive probe to the bone with a sterile instrument, and abnormal plain X-rays. The best imaging modality to confirm the diagnosis of osteomyelitis by now is a magnetic resonance imaging (MRI). If the MRI results are negative the chances are that there is no osteomyelitis. The gold standard for the diagnosis of osteomyelitis is a bone biopsy with cultures, although it is done infrequently.

Radiological Studies

Any severe ulceration with signs of infections requires plain X-rays films of both feet. It gives an overall idea of the bone and joint structures. Unfortunately plain X-rays may be normal in the early stages of osteomyelitis. Occasionally, they may show gas in the area of inflammation, or the presence of a foreign object. On the other hand, it they may show changes of neuroarthropathy of Charcot's, a more severe form of diabetic neuropathy (see Chapter on Diabetic Neuropathies). In general, neuroarthropathy of Charcot is more frequent in the tarso-metatarsal and the metatarsal-phalangeal joint, while osteomyelitis tends to be more common in the fore foot, and it is almost always associated with a deep skin ulcer in the area.

If osteomyelitis or a deep infection is suspected an MRI of the foot is the best imaging technique with very good sensitivity and specificity. Nuclear studies like the technetium-99m bone scan and an indium-111 labeled WBC scan may be indicated as well, although they have many false-positive findings. An MRI is also helpful in the difficult differential diagnosis between osteomyelitis and Charcot's osteoarthropathy, although to make things complicated, a Charcot's foot may be complicated with osteomyelitis if the bone deformities lead to ulceration and sinus tract formation.

The MRI in cases of osteomyelitis show basically low signal intensity in the marrow on T1-weighed images, high signal intensity on T2-weighed images, and marrow enhancement after the administration of contrast. Two caveats should be remembered with these studies. The first is that the administration of gadolinium to patients with a glomerular filtration rate (GFR) of less than 30 cc/min may cause gadolinium-induced nephrogenic systemic fibrosis. The other one is that because of the poor perfusion of the diabetic foot, the marrow enhancement after the administration of contrast may take a longer time than usual, and for that reason delayed images may be indicated.

Osteomyelitis usually appears in a single bone with diffuse bone marrow involvement, in weight-bearing regions. Other MRI changes of osteomyelitis are periosteal reaction, location

Table 9.1: Advantages.

Plain X-rays	*MRI*
▪ Very accessible ▪ Low cost ▪ Show bony abnormalities well ▪ May show foreign objects and gas	▪ May show preoperative mapping of ischemic and infected areas allowing a better delineation of the area of amputation ▪ Earlier and better detection of osteomyelitis ▪ May follow sinus tracts from the skin ulcer to the bones ▪ May show foreign objects and gas

Table 9.2: Disadvantages.

Plain X-rays	*MRI*
Takes longer to show changes of osteomyelitis	▪ Not always accessible ▪ Much higher cost

close to a deep ulcer, a sinus tract leading to the bone, and cellulitis or an abscess in the area. If the ulcer is rather superficial it may not appear clearly in the MRI, and for that reason it may be necessary to put skin markers close to the ulcer (Tables 9.1 and 9.2).

TREATMENT

The most effective treatment is prevention. Careful examination at every clinic visit after removing shoes and socks is essential. As soon as the diagnosis of diabetic neuropathy is ascertained, immediately a program of foot protection should be organized, starting with education. Daily examination of the feet and application of lubricant lotions or creams are very important. The dry skin tends to break more easily and the skin gets to be more resilient when lubricated properly. New shoes should be broken-in over several days. Podiatric care, protective shoes, reduction of pressure, nail, and calluses care, and, at times, prophylactic surgery to reduce areas of increased pressure are indicated. Temporary offloading of the area may also be indicated. Bathroom surgery of calluses and nails should be clearly discouraged. The patients should be taught not to soak the feet, not to 'pop' blisters, and to call immediately if there is any new foot lesion. The earlier a lesion is treated appropriately the better results obtained, and the shorter the treatment (Fig. 9.11).

The initial therapeutic decisions depend on the severity of the lesions that will determine how aggressive the treatment should be, the need for consultations and hospital admission. Again, this decision should be made by a professional with experience keeping always in mind that severe diabetic foot problems require more than one doctor, they require an entire experienced team!.

General and Local Treatment

The first measure is to unload the pressure on the foot, even if that requires complete bed rest. Local dry, sterile dressing, changed daily is usually all that is needed. Expensive 'biological' dressings have not been critically proven better so far, and should be reserved for chronic,

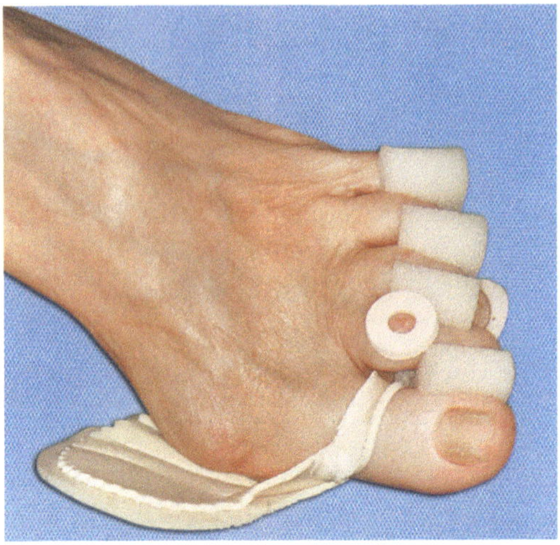

Fig. 9.11: Protection of the areas with increased pressure and calluses is very important.

recalcitrant lesions. Diabetic control is very important, and, at times, temporary insulin administration may be required until the stress hyperglycemia normalizes.

The key to local wound care is adequate surgical debridement. If the wound remains mucky a wet to dry dressing will continue the process of debridement. Once granulation tissue appears inside of the wound a nonadherent dressing is helpful. Negative pressure dressings are useful in large wounds, before and after skin grafting. Many other types of more expensive dressings and treatments have been advocated (hyperbaric oxygen, honey, maggots, silver ointments, etc.) but the benefits are not clear.

Minor infections can be managed as outpatients if the patient is able to stay off his foot and take an oral antibiotic. Local debridement with sterile technique may be useful to assess the full extent of the lesion. The majority of minor infections are due to *Staphylococcus aureus*, with increasing prevalence in the community of methicillin-resistant *Staphylococcus aureus* (MRSA) that may be sensitive to minocycline, clindamycin, or Bactrim (SMX/TMP).

Moderate and severe infections need to be evaluated and debrided by a surgeon or podiatrist, to ascertain the depth of the wound and the possible involvement of the underlying bone. If a sterile probe touches the bone inside of the wound then the diagnosis of osteomyelitis is established, and the patient needs to be hospitalized for bed rest and intravenous broad-spectrum antibiotics. Deep cultures of the wound should be taken at the time of debridement.

Antibiotic Treatment

It continues to be rather empiric, and should be as broad spectrum as the situation requires, keeping in mind the rate of *Staphylococcus* methicillin resistant in the area. The first decision is to determine if the antibiotics may be given by mouth or intravenously. In early cases of 'community-acquired' lesions that are not very severe oral cephalexin, dicloxacillin, clindamycin, amoxicillin/clavulanic acid (if *Staphylococcus*-resistant suspected or found), SMX/TMP (Bactrim), or quinolones may be recommended. If anaerobes need to be treated metronidazole may be added. Many antibiotics can be successful with early foot infections, and the selection should be guided by the local germs, previous experience, antibiotic cost, and early results.

Intravenous antibiotics are used for more severe infections usually requiring initial hospitalization, and again the initial selection is empirical but broad spectrum, in general covering Gram-positive and negative plus anaerobic bacilli. Later on the deep cultures results may indicate some changes. The usual intravenous antibiotics are ticarcillin/clavulanic acid, piperacillin/tazobactam, or vancomycin again depending on previous local experience, availability, and cost. The next question is the duration of the antibiotic treatment, and that should always depend on the degree of improvement of the foot problem. In the cases of osteomyelitis, antibiotic treatment may be required for months. In general, the patients and family should be warned about the prolonged duration of these treatments. Most of the patients with diabetic foot problems have already serious compromises with their health and prolonged bed rest and infections usually take a serious toll on them with poor quality of life and a high mortality. For that reason, at times, surgical treatments like revascularization or amputations may be indicated, even though the patients are always very reluctant to have them.

OSTEOMYELITIS

If an ulcer develops over a prominent bone in the forefoot such as a metatarsal head or toe with evidences of osteomyelitis the simplest and most effective treatment is to remove the infected bone. If this simple surgery is not done the chances are that the bone infection will recur as soon as the patient starts to ambulate. Ulcers with osteomyelitis of the calcaneus are a more difficult because the required extensive debridement may result in an ulcer that cannot heal well and soon enough to give a functional foot. A very long trial of rest and antibiotics may be indicated, although this may be debilitating for the patient and at times a below-the-knee amputation is the best answer.

Amputations

If the patient presents with a life-threatening infection and extensive tissue loss, then an open amputation may be required as the initial treatment. This could be an open toe amputation, a transmetatarsal amputation, or a guillotine amputation of the ankle. Once the infection is controlled and the circulation optimized, then still an amputation may be required to close the foot. The toe amputation is the simplest one of these, and it can be done under local anesthesia. The transmetatarsal amputation is a frequent choice because it leaves the patient with a walking foot that does not require a prosthesis, and prevents possible future problems in the resected forefoot. This surgery is particularly useful when there is an extensive infection of metatarsal heads. Many patients live long for a long time after these Transmetatarsal amputations ambulating, with the usual foot care, and free of problems. The Symes amputation at the ankle has never been found very effective as it requires two operations, has a high failure rate, and requires a prosthesis.

The below-the-knee amputation is performed usually in patients who cannot be revascularized. With the new, lighter prosthesis walking requires only an extra 10% of energy. Most patients learn to walk with the prosthesis after a short period of physical therapy and

Flowchart 9.1: Pathogenic factors of a diabetic foot

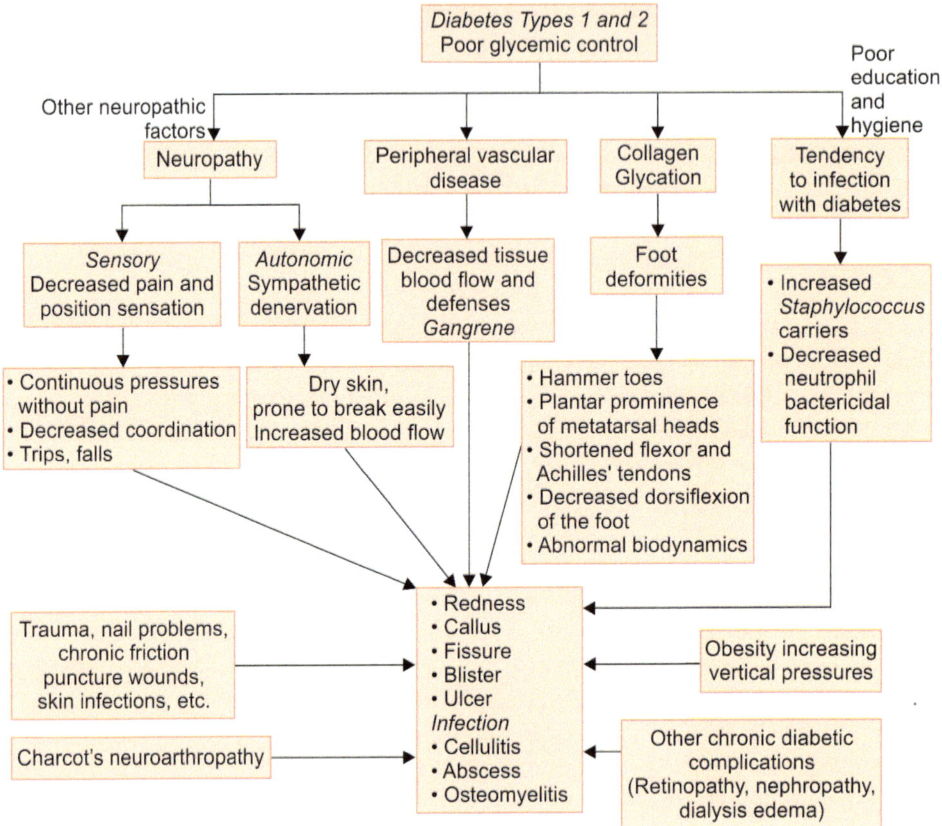

education, even after bilateral below-the-knee amputations. Above-the knee amputation may be required in some patients but they lose the knee function which requires 65% extra energy to ambulate. The above-the-knee amputation should mostly be considered in patients deemed to be poor candidates to walk anymore. Failure of closure of a below-the-knee amputation is associated with very high mortality.

Charcot's disease of the ankle and extensive osteomyelitis of the calcaneus may best be treated early with a below-the-knee amputation as the success of any other approach is so poor, the amputation is well tolerated, and allows the patient to start ambulating much sooner. It has been said that it is more important to save the foot than to save the knee. This should be remembered when considering major revascularizations that are unlikely to succeed and may result in an above-the-knee amputation rather than a below-the-knee amputation.

The order of treatment in severe cases is first to treat the infection with incision and drainage plus antibiotics and offloading. If a wound fails to heel promptly then a consultation with a vascular surgeon is needed. Digital subtraction arteriography and angioplasty or stenting can be done at this time if appropriate. If the endovascular procedures are not feasible, a vascular bypass should be considered (see the Chapter on Peripheral Vascular Disease).

Once the foot starts improving the patient may start getting out of the bed but always with 'offloading,' non-weight bearing of the affected area. Different types of casts, orthotic devices, and custom-made shoes may be used along with crutches and walkers. The aim is to prevent any pressure over the ulcer or incision site, trying to distribute the pressure over a wider area of the soles. Total contact casts with ankle support may be used, but in all of these situations the affected and nonaffected foot should be examined regularly.

BIBLIOGRAPHY

1. Donovan A, Schweitzer ME. Use of MR imaging in diagnosing diabetes-related pedal osteomyelitis. Radiographics. 2010;30:723-36.
2. Game FL. Osteomyelitis in the diabetic foot: diagnosis and management. Med Clin North Am. 2013;97(5):947-56.
3. Lipsky BA. Treating diabetic foot osteomyelitis primarily with surgery or antibiotics: have we answered the question? Diabetes Care. 2014;37(3):593-5.
4. Low KTA, Peh WCG. Magnetic resonance imaging of diabetic foot complications. Singapore Med J. 2015;56(1):23-34.
5. Peters EJ, Lipsky BA. Diagnosis and management of infection in the diabetic foot. Med Clin North Am. 2013;97(5):911-46.
6. Sumpio BE. Foot ulcers. N Eng J Med. 2000;343(11):787-93.

CHAPTER 10

Peripheral Vascular and Cerebrovascular Diseases

David R Campbell, Arturo R Rolla

INTRODUCTION

Atherosclerosis is a chronic inflammatory process of medium and large arteries caused by an accumulation of lipids that leads to the progressive narrowing of their lumen. Peripheral vascular disease (PVD) or peripheral arterial disease (PAD) is the clinical name of the atherosclerosis of the extracardiac vessels. Diabetes is an important independent risk factor in most arteries but the sites that cause the most frequent clinical problems are the heart, lower extremities and cerebral circulation. Aortic, renal, and upper extremity circulation may occasionally be impaired. The arteriosclerotic process is more frequent and severe in diabetic patients because hyperglycemia is frequently associated with other cardiovascular risk factors, and because diabetes mellitus type 2 (DM-2) aggravates them. An arterial thrombosis in the heart or the brain is the most frequent cause of death in patients with diabetes. In a way, diabetes is 'a cardiovascular disease initially characterized by the increased blood sugar levels'. Before the onset of DM-2 there are many years of 'metabolic syndrome' with increased activity of the other cardiovascular risk factors so some patients may already have vascular abnormalities at the time of diagnosis as it was shown in the United Kingdom Prospective Diabetes Study (UKPDS).

- Patients with diabetes live with high blood sugar but die of a clot in the heart or the brain
- Diabetes type 2 attracts and potentiates all the cardiovascular risk factors

PERIPHERAL VASCULAR DISEASE

Of all the patients with PVD about one-third have diabetes, and of all the patients with diabetes also a third have PVD. The prevalence increases with age, duration, and lack of control of diabetes plus the presence and severity of other risk factors (smoking, hypertension, and hyperlipidemia). Patients with DM-2 have a two to four fourfold increase in the incidence of PVD compared to nondiabetic individuals depending on the way that PVD is diagnosed. PVD is asymptomatic in many patients until it presents usually as intermittent claudication, although this manifestation may be decreased or absent in persons with diabetes because of the frequent presence of concomitant neuropathy and decreased walking due to obesity and associated complications (arthrosis). Patients with DM tend to have more PVD obstructions below than above the knees. Another characteristic of the diabetic PVD is the presence of arterial media calcifications, more frequent in the femoral and tibial arteries although they may also be seen in the pedal arteries. Arterial calcifications may not interfere with the blood flow but create problems in the determination of distal blood pressures, Duplex scanning, and during vascular surgery (Box 10.1).

The clinical diagnosis is usually made by diminished or absent pulses in the lower extremities, or by the use of the ankle-brachial index (ABI) that requires the use of a Doppler probe. There are stages in the clinical appearance of PVD:

- Asymptomatic with diminished or absent pedal pulses. This stage may be prolonged by decreased physical activity or neuropathy.
- Intermittent claudication that slowly progress to shorter walking distances.
- Disabling intermittent claudication that interferes severely with daily life.
- Resting ischemic pain.
- Gangrene, usually of the toes.

Intermittent claudication is an important manifestation of PVD, and is the result of an imbalance between the decreased blood flow and the increased oxygen muscular demands of exercise. The discomfort or pain is confined to a particular muscular group, is induced by exercise, and is relieved by rest. It may be uni or bilateral. The severity of the symptoms of claudication depends on the degree of ischemia, the presence of collateral circulation, and the intensity of the exercise. The patient may describe the claudication from a simple discomfort to a severe pain frequently associated with weakness of the affected muscles, and it should disappear in minutes after resting. Location of the pain helps to find the sites of obstruction. In diabetes, it is usually in the calves, but claudication pain in the thighs or buttocks may also happen indicating a higher level of obstruction. Buttock or hip pain is indicative of aortoiliac disease, and is frequently associated with erectile dysfunction (Leriche's syndrome). Thigh claudication is usually due to common femoral artery obstructions, while the most frequent, calf claudication may be due to lesions of the superficial femoral, popliteal, and/or tibialis arteries.

The walking distance that causes the claudication should be documented and followed because it tends to decrease with time, and it is an indication of progression of the obstruction. The patients should also be asked about the time to recover and the presence of a 'second wind' that allows them

Box 10.1: Differences in the PVD among persons with diabetes

- Arteries below the knee are affected more than the arteries above the knee
- Calcification of the arterial media
- Thickening of the capillary basement membranes and some other poorly known mechanisms that tend to worsen the manifestations of PVD
- No evidence of "small artery disease" in DM
- Concomitant diabetic neuropathy that decreases the pain sensation and increases the chances of ulcerations and infections
- Increased thrombogenicity and infection tendency
- Concomitant cardiovascular disease and nephropathy

to continue walking usually for the same distance that caused the claudication initially. Sudden aggravation of these symptoms may be an indication of a thrombotic or embolic complication.

The ischemic manifestations of PVD in individuals with DM are complicated by the presence of neuropathy, the increased tendency to infections plus decreased collateral circulation, and probably decreased oxygen diffusion due to thickening of basement membranes that is worse in the lower extremities. Infections further interfere with the blood supply, and are frequently the cause of gangrenous complications. For all these reasons diabetes is a major risk for amputations around the world. Atherosclerosis is a generalized disease worsened by diabetes, so every diabetic patient with PVD should be suspected of also having cardiac or cerebral vascular disease particularly if they are going to be subjected to major surgical procedures.

Peripheral vascular disease and severe limb ischemia are more prevalent among women than men, and tend to affect them at a younger age. Hormone replacement therapy in postmenopausal women does not protect them, and may even increase the prevalence of symptomatic PVD. African ancestry also tends to increase this prevalence, while it tends to be lower among Hispanic and Asian individuals. The progression of PVD tends to be accelerated in patients with concomitant chronic renal failure.

A careful history of the intermittent claudication and all the cardiovascular risk factors and complications should be obtained. Duration, control, treatments, and complications of the diabetes are also important details. After a complete physical examination a careful examination of the lower extremities circulation should be done. Skin lesions and pigmentations, hair growth, changes in the toenails, dependent rubor, and pallor after elevation of the extremity should be examined. If the patient has resting ischemic pain the elevation of the extremity may aggravate the pain. Detailed neurological examination of the lower extremities is also important because of the frequent association with diabetic neuropathy that tends to complicate the prognosis. Finally, careful examination of the dorsalis pedis, posterior tibialis, popliteal, and femoral pulses should be done. In patients with severe edema of the feet from congestive heart failure and/or nephropathy palpation of pedal pulses may be difficult, and should be repeated after bed rest and diuresis or with a Doppler instrument. Auscultation over the femoral and popliteal arteries and over the upper portion of the anterior tibialis muscle (tibialis artery underneath) may disclose bruits.

Doppler

Ankle-brachial index is the ratio of the ankle systolic blood pressure divided by the brachial systolic pressure detected with a continuous wave Doppler probe that unfortunately is not widely available. The patient should be resting for at least 10 minutes, then the cuff is inflated just above the ankle level to obtain the ABI. Both dorsalis pedis and posterior tibialis systolic pressures should be measured along with the brachial artery in both arms. The higher values of the systolic pressures in the ankle and arm are then taken for the calculations. Under normal circumstances both systolic pressures should be at the same level with an index close to 1. If the index is less than 0.90 it is an indication that there may be PVD. The problems obtaining the ABI may be increasing pain with the inflation of the cuff, pedal pulses too weak to be detected, and calcified arteries that cannot be compressed by the cuff causing systolic pressure levels that are very high and ABIs of more than 1.40.

The differential diagnosis of intermittent claudication especially among the elderly is with lumbar spinal stenosis caused by degenerative changes (neurogenic claudication). The claudication of spinal stenosis is aggravated by lumbar extension, improved by stooping, is not relieved by resting in the standing position, and it requires sitting. Lumbar pain and more marked leg weakness are indicative of spinal stenosis. Some patients with spinal stenosis may have absent pedal pulses and concomitant PVD. Changes in deep tendon reflexes may also be due to diabetic neuropathy. At times, a magnetic resonance imaging (MRI) of the lumbar spine and/or vascular images may be necessary to ascertain the nature of the claudication. Diabetic neuropathic pain is quite different. It does not appear, or even gets better with ambulation, and tends to worsen at night while the patient is sleeping.

Routine laboratory tests should include fasting and/or random blood glucose level, lipid profile, blood urea nitrogen (BUN) and creatinine, sedimentation rate, C-reactive protein (CRP), and a complete blood count. Fever, leukocytosis and elevations of the sedimentation rate, CRP, and glycemic levels are the indications of the possibility of an infection. Plain X-ray films may show arterial calcifications.

Transcutaneous oxygen measurements may be used occasionally usually in the conjunction with hyperbaric oxygen treatments. There are other similar techniques and their importance is not clear at the present time.

'Stress peripheral vascular studies' are becoming more common in laboratories with experience. Similar to the cardiac stress tests, the patient is put to walk or run on a treadmill and the ankle pressures are measured. If exercise causes a decrease in the ankle pressures it is an indication of PVD. This test is particularly useful for the differential diagnosis between PVD and spinal stenosis.

TREATMENT OF ASYMPTOMATIC PATIENTS WITH PERIPHERAL VASCULAR DISEASE OR WITH MODERATE INTERMITTENT CLAUDICATION (STAGES 1 AND 2)

It aims to improve symptoms, and try to slow down the progression. The rate of progression from asymptomatic PVD or with intermittent claudication to critical limb ischemia is very low even after many years, so there is no need to obtain vascular images initially unless there are questions about the diagnosis or a sudden aggravation of the symptoms. On the other hand, because of the increased rate of coronary and cerebrovascular problems a program of exercise and aggressive risk factors treatments are mandatory. Of all the known medical treatments for the prevention of cardiovascular problems, the 4S trial (Scandinavian Simvastatin Survival Study) showed a significant drop in the new cases of PVD among the patients treated with that statin medication but they did not report data specific for patients with DM. There are no clear data on the benefit of the different treatments of hyperlipidemia, hypertension, or hyperglycemia on the prevention or treatment of PVD in diabetic individuals.

Since PVD is frequently associated with a marked increased of cardiovascular morbidity and mortality it paradoxically requires at this stage more diagnostic and therapeutic attention to the heart and cerebral circulation than the feet. All the cardiovascular risk factors should be treated aggressively, while the glycemic control does not seem to be that effective halting the progression of the PVD. A stress EKG and carotid ultrasound should be considered in these patients particularly before starting an exercise program.

The best long-term results for the patients with mild to moderate intermittent claudication are obtained with a supervised program of increasing ambulation, frequently starting on a treadmill. The ambulation distances progressively increase, and the quality of life improves over a period of several months. The mechanisms of this improvement are not very clear since there is no improvement in the ABI but may be due to increased collateral circulation, improvement in capillary distribution, and/or better mitochondrial oxidative capacity in the muscles.

Several medical treatments have been proposed for the improvement of intermittent claudication, but all of them with minimal and questionable results. Pentoxifylline, a xanthine derivative, thought to improve the blood rheology was the first one, but well-controlled studies showed over the years not to be more effective than placebo, and its use has been almost abandoned by now.

Cilostazol, a vasodilator and antagonist of the 5-HT2 receptor, has shown antiplatelet and type III phosphodiesterase inhibitor has shown some benefits in improving walking distances mostly accompanied by an exercise program. The dose is 100 mg twice a day, and should be taken 30 minutes before or 2 hours after a meal. It may cause headache, diarrhea, dizziness, palpitations because of reflex tachycardia, and it may worsen congestive heart failure. As a matter of fact, cilostazol has a black box warning regarding its use in patients with congestive heart failure of any severity.

Naftidrofuryl, a vasodilator and antagonist of the 5-HT2 receptor also has an indication for the treatment of intermittent claudication, and has been approved in Europe but not in USA. As with other vasodilator agents its benefits are controversial at this point. The usual dose is 100 mg three times a day. Side effects consist of nausea, abdominal pain, rash, and hepatic dysfunction.

TREATMENT OF PATIENTS WITH SEVERE, DISABLING PERIPHERAL VASCULAR DISEASE (STAGE 3)

Once intermittent claudication starts being disabling and interfering with daily life the need for more invasive studies appear, starting with vascular imaging (see below). In the last decades the imaging and vascular procedures have improved rapidly. Endovascular interventions especially are being used now more frequently than the classical open surgical bypass operations. The critical questions are at what stage a more invasive approach to the patient with intermittent claudication should start, patient selection considering age, lifestyle and overall health, and what type of procedure is indicated? The answer to the last question depends on the experience and possibilities of the different medical centers and vascular surgeons or interventionists.

The initial goals are to decrease the claudication symptomatology and improve the overall mobility and quality of life. A secondary goal is the prevention of amputations that has significantly decreased over the years. It is very difficult to compare the benefits of supervised exercises and surgical procedures in the literature because of the patients' selection with more severe cases receiving more aggressive treatments. Endovascular and surgical procedures have the advantage of more prompt and slightly better results but are significantly more costly, have associated morbidity and mortality plus the risk of restenosis, and also requires a prolonged plan of physical therapy. Open surgery compared with endovascular procedures is associated with longer hospital stay and recovery time, higher complications rates but more durable patency. If a revascularization procedure fails the subsequent procedures have a lower rate of improvement and increased overall morbidity.

Without any doubts, in the selected patients that require interventions the combination of endovascular or surgical treatments combined with a structured exercise program gives the best results. Some studies have also indicated that adding antiplatelet medications there is an improvement in at least short-term results, although with the risk of increasing bleeding especially when they are combined with aspirin. There is a great need for data at longer-term not only in relief of claudication symptoms but also on amputations and cardiovascular morbidity and mortality with these combined treatments.

TREATMENT OF RESTING PAIN, ACUTE LIMB ISCHEMIA, AND GANGRENE (STAGES 4 AND 5)

Sudden aggravations or acute presentations with an ischemic, threatened limb may be due to thromboembolism (especially in patients with atrial fibrillation), sudden thrombotic occlusion of a previously narrowed artery, atheroembolic (*cholesterol*) embolization usually from an ulcerated plaque, and less commonly from an arterial dissection. In patients who had previous vascular surgery the acute closing of the venous or prosthetic bypass graft is a more likely possibility. Ischemic pain at rest is usually in the toes and anterior foot very severe and poorly responsive to even opiates analgesics. It tends to get aggravated by the elevation of the extremity, and gets better by hanging the feet at the side of the bed. Focal areas of discoloration usually around the toes are indicative of impending gangrene. This is usually an emergency that requires urgent admission and consultation with vascular surgery. The concomitant presence of infection (*wet gangrene*) calls for initial intravenous antibiotics and drainage of the abscessed areas.

Vascular imaging is clearly indicated in anticipation of surgery to ascertain the levels of obstruction, feasibility of improvement, and after vascular interventions to ascertain the patency of grafts. Ultrasound vascular studies (B-mode and Duplex) are the least invasive and less expensive modalities since they do not require injection of contrast. Ultrasonography may show the location and extent of the lesions plus some morphologic and hemodynamic details. Contrast arteriography remains the gold standard although at times computed tomography (CT) angiograms may be indicated. CT angiograms with digital subtraction give very detailed arterial images but it also involves radiation exposure, arterial punctures, catheter damage, and the need for contrast injections that may compromise the renal function. MR angiograms are being used less frequently specially in patients with renal failure. The results of these vascular studies will indicate the location, severity collateral circulation, and best possible treatment for the lesion and the individual patient taking into account age and general health status.

The recent decades brought the possibility of intervening on smaller arteries and the utilization of endovascular procedures (angioplasty plus stents). At the present time in many centers these endovascular procedures are three times more common that the classical bypass surgeries. The procedure selection depends on the experience of the team, the type of lesion, and overall health of the patient. The use of synthetic versus venous materials is also an important technical consideration. Also in all of these patients we have to consider the frequent concomitant complications of neuropathy and infections, the need for prolonged follow-up and physical therapy, and that the long-term results of these procedures tend to be worse in individuals with DM.

Frequently, at the time of these interventions the patients are frequently placed on antiplatelet therapies and supervised physical therapy. The advantages and disadvantages of each antiplatelet therapy after vascular procedures are quite controversial. In a large Cochrane meta-analysis of almost 6,000 randomized patients after bypass surgery, aspirin alone, or with dipyridamole, was shown to be more effective in graft patency and limb salvage at 1 and 2 years compared to other medical adjuvant treatments, and equally as effective as clopidogrel plus aspirin although with more bleeding complications in the last type of treatment. Hyperbaric oxygen therapy (*chambers*) is an expensive and controversial way to improve healing specially in wounds. Unfortunately, the trials so far have not been well designed and the improvements shown have been mostly for short, not long terms.

Cholesterol embolization or Blue toes syndrome causes painful gangrene and cyanosis of the toes from embolic material of ulcerated plaques usually in the lower aorta or large arteries going to the lower extremities. It may start spontaneously, or after anticoagulation, trauma, or arterial catheterizations. If the ulcerated plaque is in the aorta the manifestations are usually bilateral. Unilateral manifestations suggest the ulcerated plaques are in the iliac artery or below. If they are above the kidney they may cause hypertension or an acute decrease in renal function. Some cholesterol embolization may go to the muscles causing myalgias as well. The toes may have a clear demarcation between the ischemic and normally perfused areas, or areas of livedo reticularis. A paradoxical and confusing finding is the frequent presence of pedal pulses indicating that the ischemia is at the level of smaller arterioles. The differential diagnosis is with some unusual forms of vasculitis (palpable petechiae) and with calciphylaxis (may affect other parts of the body and upper extremities). The diagnosis and localization of the arterial ulcerations is made with vascular imaging. The treatment is the removal of the ulcerated plaques to prevent further embolization followed by localized amputations if necessary (prolonged ischemia). The overall mortality during and after episodes of cholesterol embolization is quite high indicating severe, generalized arteriosclerosis.

AMPUTATIONS

In the last decades the number of lower limb amputations in patients with DM has decreased significantly but they are still necessary. Emergency initial amputations are rarely done nowadays, and mostly they are necessary when the vascular procedures have failed. The most common amputations are of one or several toes, transmetatarsal, and below or above the knee. The decision to amputate has to consider the natural patient's resistance and the fact is that very prolonged bed rest or minimal ambulation with chronic infections can be very deleterious to the overall health of the patient. At times, an amputation followed by one of the new prosthesis and physical therapy gets the patient on his feet with rapid improvement in quality of life in a faster and safer way.

CEREBROVASCULAR DISEASE

It is a major cause of morbidity, disability, and mortality among patient with DM that may cause transient ischemic attacks (TIAs), cerebrovascular accidents (strokes), and multi-infarct dementia. Carotid atherosclerosis is the cause of about 20% of these problems, and has the same pathogenic factors of the atherosclerosis in other parts of the body. The carotid bifurcation is the most frequent site, but intracerebral arteries are also frequently involved. The diagnosis is made by finding a bruit over a carotid artery or after obtaining a routine ultrasound showing an obstruction of over 75% of the lumen, although more frequently they present as a symptomatic complication.

Ulcerated plaques in the carotid arteries may cause embolizations to the retinal or cerebral arteries. 'Amaurosis fugax' or transient unilateral blindness may be a manifestation of retinal embolization, although at times they may be an asymptomatic finding during an ophthalmologic examination. The strokes may occur in any part of the brain but are more common in the territory of the middle cerebral artery. About half of the patients having a stroke had a previous TIA with motor or sensory symptoms. The strokes may be due to embolizations, luminal stenosis of the carotid arteries affecting areas of the brain with borderline (*watershed*) perfusion, local thrombosis of cerebral arteries, or hypertensive hemorrhages. Patients with diabetes have increased frequency, mortality, and recurrence of strokes plus an increase in the associated dementia. Atheromas of small vessels may cause 'lacunar strokes' that at times are subclinical but may lead to multi-infarct dementia and/or a pseudo-bulbar state.

- Patients with diabetic retinopathy more marked in one eye compared with the other should be suspected of having a carotid lesion on the side with less retinopathy
- This clinical finding emphasizes the pathogenic importance of hypertension in diabetic retinopathy

The most common screening test is carotid ultrasonography which is very accurate in identifying stenosis and severity, calcifications, and plaque ulcerations. CT and MR angiograms are frequently obtained to help in the management of these lesions, and to study the collateral circulation. Cerebral angiography may be indicated although rarely nowadays. Medical management of patients with a significant carotid stenosis (>60–75%) consists of smoking cessation, blood pressure control avoiding hypotensive episodes, and the use of statins to control the hypercholesterolemia. The therapeutic effect of glycemic control has not been clearly established. Aspirin, alone, with dipyridamole or clopidogrel, are antiplatelet agents commonly used in primary and secondary prevention. The decision when to use and which one of the more invasive treatments (carotid endarterectomy or stenting) is still controversial considering their periprocedural morbidity in relation to the possibility of having a stroke in the future, especially in asymptomatic patients. Patients with a TIA or a stroke plus a significant carotid stenosis on the same side seem to have a more clear indication for invasive procedures in centers with experience. There is an ongoing controversy at the present time about endarterectomy versus angioplasty with stenting awaiting for more definitive trials. While we wait for results of these investigations, the most important factor in the decision is the expertise of the team doing these particular procedures. In general angioplasty tends to have a higher rate of periprocedural strokes, and endarterectomy have a higher rate of myocardial infarctions.

The treatment of an acute stroke requires control of the blood pressure trying not to lower it too much to avoid increasing the area of ischemia. Thrombolysis may be used within the first 3 hours from the onset of symptoms. Strokes in diabetic and nondiabetic individuals frequently increase the blood sugar levels because of stress hyperglycemia, and it is an indication of increased severity, morbidity, and poor outcomes. The benefits of intensive glycemic control during acute strokes are presently a matter of controversy. Common sense indicates the prevention of extremes of high and low blood glucose levels during acute strokes, while we await for the results of future trials.

- Hypoglycemias may mimic transient ischemic attacks and vice versa
- And patients with hyperosmolar comas are frequently diagnosed initially as having an stroke

Venous insufficiency of the lower extremities is not necessarily a 'diabetic' complication but being associated with obesity, it is relatively common in patients with DM-2, and it may cause or aggravate problems in the lower extremities. There are two systems of veins in the extremities: (1) Superficial and (2) Deep. Superficial veins are located between the skin and the deep muscular fascia. The deep veins tend to follow the trajectory of the arteries, and are communicated with the superficial system by 'perforating or communicating veins.' In the standing position the column of blood from the heart to the lower legs has a high hydrostatic pressure that is compensated by the contraction of the muscles pushing the blood upward. The superficial system does not have the muscle protection and requires to be isolated from the deep pressures by a system of valves that are present mostly in the perforating veins. When these valves or the veins themselves are incompetent the high pressure applied to the superficial veins causes extravasation of blood and hypoxia in the area. Chronic venous hypertension then decreases the subcutaneous tissue in the lower parts of the legs (*lipodermatosclerosis*), and thinning of the skin that facilitates the formation of 'venous ulcers' and cellulitis. Different from neuropathy and ischemia, the venous ulcers tend to appear around the malleolus, they are more superficial, surrounded by thin, pigmented skin, are very slow to heal, and frequently leave a scar. It also causes hemosiderin pigmentation below the area of thinning of the subcutaneous tissue. Frequently, the patients complain of dull aches and heaviness sensation, and they may or may not present dilated varicose veins.

The venous insufficiency may be 'primary' and related to family history, aging, pregnancies, prolonged standing, or obesity. It may also be secondary to trauma or previous phlebitis that interferes with the function of the perforating veins and valves. Accordingly, the problem it may be uni or bilateral. Some patients not all develop chronic edema that does not respond very well to diuretics, but improves with leg elevation and compressing stockings. Daily lubrication and mechanical protection prevents ulcerations. Infected ulcers and cellulitis may require topical and systemic antibiotics plus bed rest.

BIBLIOGRAPHY

1. Antoniou GA, Fisher RK, Georgiadis GS, et al. Statin therapy in lower limb peripheral arterial disease: Systematic review and meta-analysis. Vascul Pharmacol. 2014;63(2): 79-87.
2. Bedenis R, Lethaby A, Maxwell H, et al. Antiplatelet agents for preventing thrombosis after peripheral arterial bypass surgery. Cochrane Database Syst Rev. 2015;192:CD000535.

3. Bedenis R, Stewart M, Cleanthis M, et al. Cilostazol for intermittent claudication. Cochrane Database Syst Rev. 2014;10:CD003748.
4. Criqui MH, Aboyans V. Epidemiology of peripheral artery disease. Circ Res. 2015;116(19):1509-26.
5. de Backer TL, Vander Stichele R, Lehert P, et al. Naftidrofuryl for intermittent claudication. Cochrane Database Syst Rev. 2012;12:CD001368.
6. Diehm C, Allenberg JR, Pittrow D, et al. Mortality and vascular morbidity in older adults with asymptomatic versus symptomatic peripheral artery disease. Circulation. 2009;120(21):2053-61.
7. Fakhry F, Spronk S, van der Laan L, et al. Endovascular revascularization and supervised exercise for peripheral artery disease and intermittent claudication: a randomized clinical trial. JAMA. 2015;314(18):1936-44.
8. Gardener AW, Poehlman ET. Exercise rehabilitation programs for the treatment of claudication pain. A meta-analysis. JAMA. 1995;274(12):975-80.
9. Garimella PS, Hirsch AT. Peripheral artery disease and chronic kidney disease: clinical synergy to improve outcomes. Adv Chronic Kidney Dis. 2014;21(6):460-71.
10. Grotta JC. Clinical practice. Carotid stenosis. N Engl J Med. 2013;369(12):1143-50.
11. Hiramoto JS, Katz R, Weisman S, et al. Gender-specific risk factors for peripheral artery disease in a voluntary screening population. J Am Heart Assoc. 2014;3(2):e000651.
12. Jauch-Chara K, Oltmanns KM. Glycemic control after brain injury: boon and bane for the brain. Neuroscience. 2014;283:202-9.
13. Koga M, Yamagami H, Okuda S, et al. Blood glucose levels during the initial 72 h and 3-month functional outcomes in acute intracerebral hemorrhage: the SAMURAI-ICH study. J Neurol Sci. 2015;350(1-2):75-8.
14. Kranke P, Bennett MH, Martyn-St James M, et al. Hyperbaric oxygen therapy for chronic wounds. Cochrane Database Syst Rev. 2015;6(4):CD0004123.
15. Lane R, Ellis B, Watson L, et al. Exercise for intermittent claudication. Cochrane Database Syst Rev. 2014;7:CD000990.
16. Luchsinger JA, Tang MX, Stern Y, et al. Diabetes mellitus and risk of Alzheimer's disease and dementia with stroke in a multiethnic cohort. Am J Epidemiol. 2001;154(7):635-41.
17. Malgor RD, Alahdab F, Elraiyah TA, et al. A systematic review of treatment of intermittent claudication in the lower extremities. J Vasc Surg. 2015;61(3 Suppl):54S-73.
18. McDermott MM. Erasing disability in peripheral artery disease: The role of endovascular procedures and supervised exercise. JAMA. 2015;314(18):1921-3.
19. Neel JD, Kruse RL, Dombrovskiy VY, et al. Cilostazol and freedom from amputation after lower extremity revascularization. J Vasc Surg. 2015;61(4):960-4.
20. Stevens JW, Simpson E, Harnan S, et al. Systematic review of the efficacy of cilostazol, naftidrofuryl oxalate and pentoxifylline for the treatment of intermittent claudication. Br J Surg. 2012;99(12):1630-8.
21. Timaran CH, Mantese VA, Malas M, et al. Differential outcomes of carotid stenting and endarterectomy performed exclusively by vascular surgeons in the Carotid Revascularization Endarterectomy versus Stenting Trial (CREST). J Vasc Surg. 2013;57(2):303-8.
22. Tight blood pressure control and risk of macrovascular and microvascular complications in type 2 diabetes: UKPDS 38. UK Prospective Diabetes Study Group. BMJ. 1998;317:703-13.
23. Vazquez-Benitez G, Desai JR, Xu S, et al. Preventable major cardiovascular events associated with uncontrolled glucose, blood pressure, and lipids and active smoking in adults with diabetes with and without cardiovascular disease: a contemporary analysis. Diabetes Care. 2015;38(5):905-12.

CHAPTER 11

Diabetes Mellitus and Infection

Sanjay Agarwal, Ashwin Pillai

INTRODUCTION

Diabetes mellitus (DM) comprises a gamut of metabolic disorders, characterized by an absolute or relative insulin deficiency, with consequent hyperglycemia.

Diabetes is considered one of the largest emerging threats to health in the 21st century. As a measure of the magnitude of the problem, India currently ranks 2nd in the world with an estimated diabetic population of 72.9 million, nearly half that of China at 114.4 million. However, it is estimated that by the year 2045, this number would rise to a staggering 134.3 million, overtaking China at its projection of 119.8 million.[1]

Besides the complications induced by glycemic variability itself, diabetic patients are especially vulnerable to infections. The two factors perpetuate one other, culminating in a vicious cycle. It is commonly known that diabetes adversely influences the outcome of various infections. For instance, diabetes triples the risk of hospitalization in cases of H1N1 and increases the risk of intensive care unit (ICU) admission nearly fourfold amongst the hospitalized cases.[2]

Diabetes is also associated with higher mortality, both due to infections, and all-cause mortality. Females appear to be at a greater risk, with an age-adjusted relative risk (RR) of deaths due to infections of 2.4 [95% confidence interval (CI), 1.2–4.7] versus an age-adjusted RR of 1.7 (95% CI, 0.8–4.7) for males.

Diabetes inherently increases the risk of contracting infections, and their subsequent severity, by two broad mechanisms (Flowchart 11.1):

1. *Immune perturbation:* This includes inflammation perpetuating DM, and DM impairing an appropriate immune response.
2. Hyperglycemia creating a favorable milieu for pathogen growth.

IMMUNE PERTURBATION[3]

Immune perturbation refers to disruption of host defenses at virtually every level, from the cellular and humoral level, to the microcellular level, in the form of organ dysfunction.

- *Effects on various metabolic and signaling pathways* (Table 11.1):[4] Hyperglycemia affects various metabolic pathways. Chief mechanisms include: shunting through the polyol

Flowchart 11.1: An overview of causes predisposing to infection.

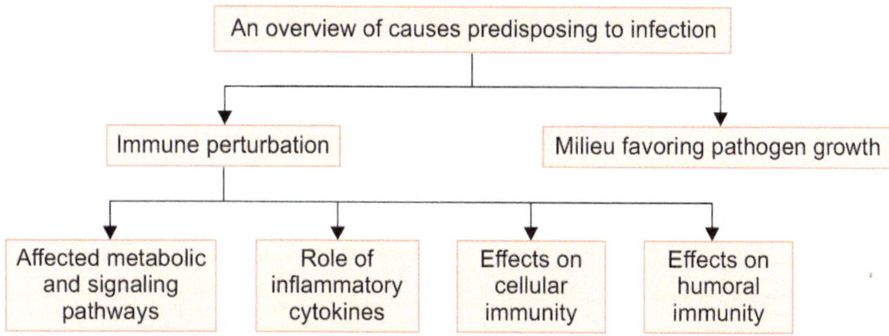

Table 11.1: Affected parameters along with functional pathology in immune perturbation.

Affected parameters	*Functional pathology*
Polyol pathway shunting	Increases formation of reactive oxygen species and advanced glycation end products
Oxidative stress	Direct membrane damage Increased cytokine production.
Elevated protein kinase C	Stimulates release of reactive oxygen species from neutrophils
Advanced glycation end products	Alters signaling properties and activates proapoptotic and inflammatory activity
Inflammatory cytokines	Reduced IL-1,6 from monocytes Reduced IFN-γ and TNF-α by T cells.
Cell-mediated immunity	Impaired membrane transmigration, chemotaxis, and phagocytosis by neutrophils
Humoral immunity	Complement C4 deficiency

(INF-γ: Interferon-γ; IL-1: Interleukin-1; TNF-α: Tumor necrosis factor-α).

pathway, enhanced oxidative stress, increased activation of protein kinase C (PKC), and increased formation of advanced glycation end products (AGEs).

- *Shunting through the polyol pathway:* Excess glucose is converted to sorbitol and fructose via sorbitol dehydrogenase and aldose reductase. This polyol pathway shunting leads to increased formation of AGEs, as well as reactive oxygen species. Innate immunity is further affected, as this shunting leads to hampered opsonophagocytosis by neutrophils.[5]
- *Oxidative stress:* In a hyperglycemic state, there is excessive production of superoxides, with a concomitant decrease in antioxidant capacity.[6,7] One of the ways this occurs, is by an overload of the mitochondrial electron transport chain. There is a release of electrons which, in turn, interact with oxygen, producing superoxides. Reactive oxygen species can cause direct damage to the cell and organelle membranes, as well as nucleic acids. They can additionally stimulate the production of cytokines via mitogen-activated protein (MAP) kinase signaling.[8,9]
- *Elevated protein kinase C:* Hyperglycemic states are associated with increased levels of glycolysis, and subsequent metabolic products. Significant in this respect, is the increased

production of dihydroxyacetone phosphate (DHAP). In some tissues, this is reduced to glycerol phosphate and converted into diacylglycerol (DAG). DAG is a second messenger in the inositol 1,4,5-triphosphate (IP3)-DAG pathway and activates PKC. Increased PKC activation in neutrophils stimulates the release of reactive oxygen species.[10]

- *Advanced glycation end products:* Hyperglycemia, and the subsequent increase in the formation of AGEs, can alter tissue functions by binding to proteins at the subcellular level, for instance, causing cross-linking of the basement membrane.[11-13] Other examples of altered functional properties include those of albumin and collagen. These tissues acquire signaling properties, such that they possess proinflammatory and proapoptotic activity.[14-18]

- *Effects on inflammatory cytokines:* In response to lipopolysaccharide stimulation, monocytes and mononuclear cells in diabetic patients secrete less interleukin-1 (IL-1) and IL-6.[19,20] This is apparently due to an intrinsic cellular defect.[21] Increased glycation inhibits the production of IL-10 by myeloid cells, and reduces the expression of class I MHC on their surface,[22] thereby impairing cellular immunity. Interferon-gamma (IFN-gamma) and tumor necrosis factor-alpha (TNF-alpha) production by T cells are also impaired.
- *Effects on neutrophils and lymphocytes:* Polymorphs are affected on various fronts. There is impaired mobilization, membrane transmigration, chemotaxis, and phagocytic activity.[21,23,24] The hyperglycemic environment also impairs glucose-6-phosphate dehydrogenase (G6PD), and increases apoptosis of polymorphs. Additionally, in cells with insulin-independent glucose transport mechanisms, the hyperglycemic environment leads to increased influx of glucose. This leads to increased consumption of nicotinamide adenine dinucleotide phosphate (NADPH) as a part of glucose metabolism. The resultant decrease in the levels of NADPH results in a decrease in the regeneration of the molecules that play a vital role in protection against oxidative damage.
  Notably, studies have shown that even in diabetic patients, the proliferative function and antigenic response activity of CD4 T-lymphocytes is not impaired at hemoglobin A1c (HbA1c) levels less than 8%.[4]
- *Effects on humoral immunity:* The complement system and immunoglobulins are both affected by hyperglycemia. The main role of the complement system is to opsonize and promote phagocytosis of antigens, and their subsequent lysis by neutrophils and macrophages. Additionally, they provide the second signal for B-cell activation and antibody production. Studies have found a deficiency of the C4 complement in diabetic patients, probably secondary to polymorph dysfunction and reduced cytokine response.[25,26]
  Immunoglobulins are also subject to increased glycation in a hyperglycemic environment. However, antibody responses after vaccinations and common infections have been found to be adequate in patients with diabetes mellitus.[4]

CREATION OF A MILIEU FAVORING PATHOGEN GROWTH

Some organisms are known to be more virulent in a hyperglycemic environment. One of the potential reasons for this is increased adherence of microorganisms to diabetic cells as opposed to nondiabetic ones. The carbohydrate composition of receptors is believed to play a significant role in this. This has been particularly described in the case of *Candida albicans*.

Macro- and microvascular pathologies leading to impaired local circulation result not only in delayed wound healing, but also to a delayed and suboptimal response to infection.[27]

Sensory neuropathy may contribute to increased risk of infection due to unawareness of trivial trauma and subsequent inadequate attention to the wound.

Autonomic neuropathy is also contributory to infection. For instance, a bladder that is not completely emptied due to autonomic dysfunction predisposes to urinary colonization by microorganisms.[28]

DIABETES AND SPECIFIC INFECTIONS

Numerous studies have detailed varying degrees of association between the presence of diabetes and certain infections.

The graph here provides a useful frame of reference with respect to the strength of association between diabetes and specific infections found by various studies (Fig. 11.1).

- *Head and neck infections:* A modest increased association between DM and head and neck infections has been observed. Pooled data from cohort studies have shown a crude odds ratio (OR) of 1.33 (95% CI 1.08–1.65) and an adjusted OR of 1.17 (95% CI 1.13–1.22).[29]

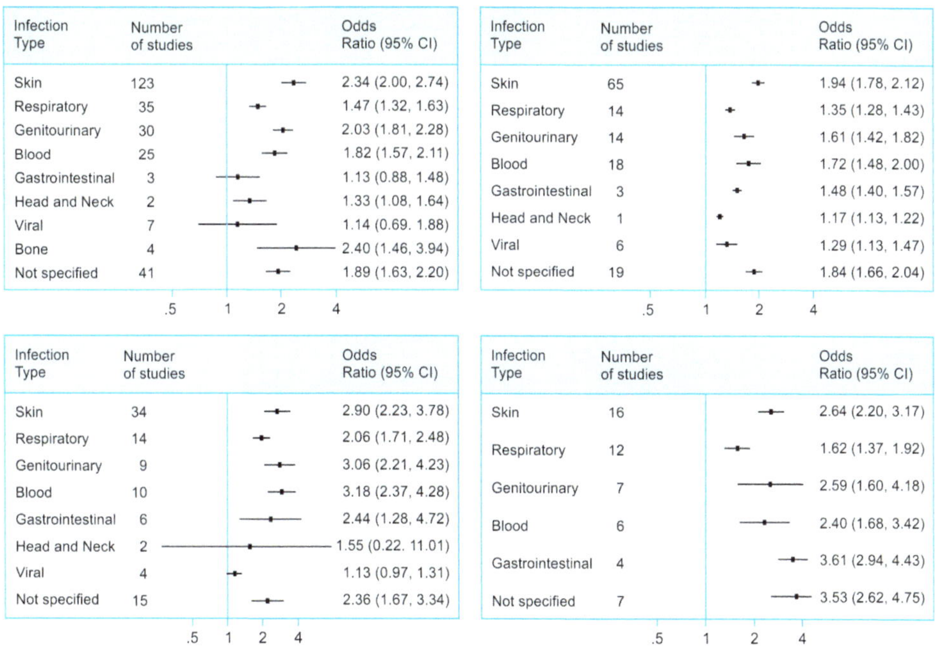

Fig. 11.1: Strength of association between diabetes and specific infections found by various studies. (CI: Confidence interval).

Source: Abu-Ashour W, Twells L, Valcour J, et al. The association between diabetes mellitus and incident infections: a systematic review and meta-analysis of observational studies. BMJ Open Diabetes Res Care. 2017;5:e000336.

- *Malignant otitis externa:* Otitis externa is called malignant when it spreads rapidly from the external ear to the adjacent soft tissue, mastoid and the skull base, and potentially to the central nervous system (CNS) (Figs. 11.2A to C).

  Skull base osteomyelitis is a key feature.

  Etiologic agents include *Pseudomonas aeruginosa*, or less commonly, aspergillus.

  The exact incidence is not known. However, diabetes is a known risk factor for its development.

  - *Key investigations*:

    Radionuclide scanning: Technetium 99m and gallium scans show increased uptake and are useful in differentiating regular otitis externa from the malignant, necrotizing variant.

  - *Management*: Primarily medical, with anti-pseudomonal antibiotics. Oral ciprofloxacin has been found to be effective. It may require to be continued for months until a gallium scan shows a significant reduction in inflammatory activity.

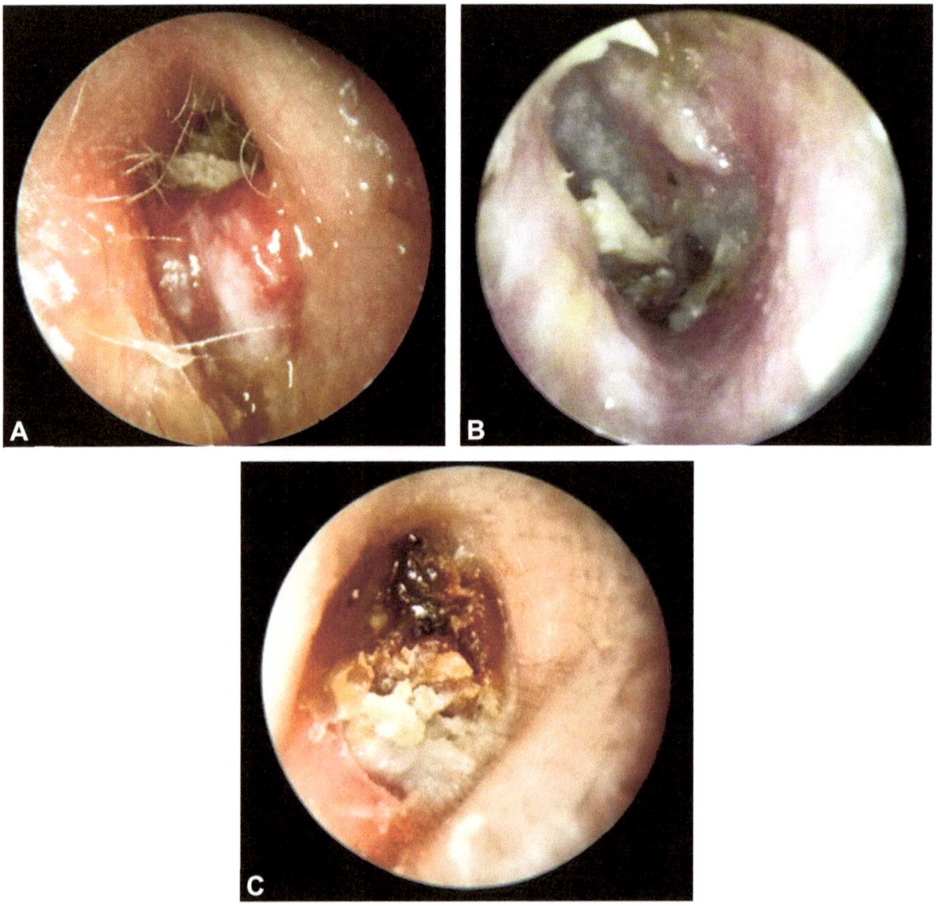

Figs. 11.2A to C: Intraoperative images of malignant otitis externa.
Source: Dr Murarji Ghadge, Consultant ear-nose-throat (ENT) surgeon, Ruby Hall Clinic, Pune.

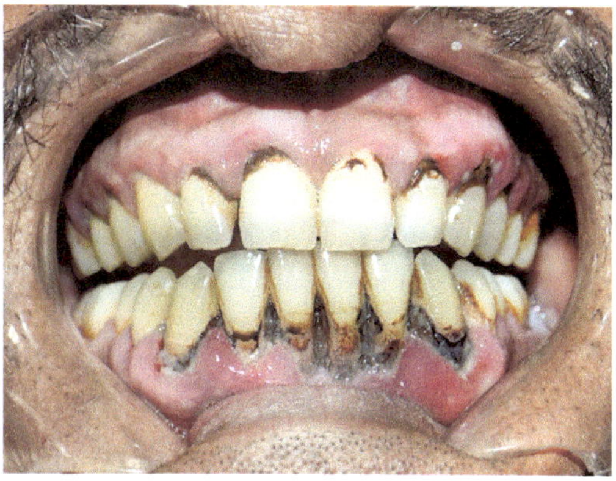

Fig. 11.3: Periodontitis.
Source: Dr Nihar Pillai, BDS, Mumbai.

Surgical debridement is reserved for patients with infected bone who deteriorate despite medical therapy.

- *Periodontitis:* Periodontitis refers to a state of chronic inflammation of the periodontal tissue, associated with loss of connective tissue, alveolar bone resorption, and may result in tooth loss (Fig. 11.3).

  It has been found to be four times more common in patients with DM and has been reported as the sixth most common complication.[4]

  The inflammatory state may start, perpetuate, and/or exacerbate insulin resistance. The subsequent poor glycemic control may further worsen the periodontitis, resulting in a vicious cycle.

  Apart from immune perturbation, other risk factors propounded include: altered collagen metabolism, altered oral vascularization, hereditary factors, and subgingival microbiota aspects.

  Management consists primarily of supra and subgingival scaling. Curettage and flap surgeries may be indicated in some cases. Antibiotic coverage for both Gram-positive organisms and anaerobes, such as amoxicillin-clavulanic acid and metronidazole are frequently employed.

  Maintenance of oral hygiene is of paramount importance.

- *Respiratory tract infections:* Meta-analyses have shown a positive association between diabetes and respiratory tract infections. Cohort studies have shown a crude OR of 1.47 (95% CI 1.32–1.63) and an adjusted OR of 1.35 (95% CI 1.28–1.43). Pooled results from CCS suggest a stronger association with a crude OR of 2.06 (95% CI 1.71–2.48) and an adjusted OR of 1.62 (95% CI 1.37–1.92).[28]

  The increased risk may be due to diabetic autonomic neuropathy-associated gastroparesis, impaired cough reflex, and a disrupted sleep pattern.[29]

  - *Tuberculosis:* Since as early as the early 1,000s CE, the relationship between tuberculosis (TB) and DM has been known. DM has been recognized as a significant risk factor for TB. Although human immunodeficiency virus (HIV) is a more potent risk factor, due to a far greater prevalence of DM, its effect on the burden of TB is less than that due to DM.

Approximately 70% of the world population of diabetics lives in TB endemic countries. In the 22 countries with the highest burden of TB, the prevalence of DM in the general population ranged from 2% to 9%.[30] Out of the ten countries with the highest incidence of DM, eight were listed as having a high TB burden by the World Health Organization (WHO).[31] For instance, Indonesia, listed at number 3 among countries with a high TB burden, was listed as 4th amongst the countries with a high prevalence of DM.[32] The scenario in India is quite similar.

The exact pathophysiology is unknown. However, proposed mechanisms include: impaired cellular immunity, depressed function of alveolar macrophages, reduced levels of IFN-gamma, pulmonary microangiopathy, and micronutrient deficiency. It has been found that, in diabetics, monocyte chemotaxis is significantly impaired.[33] This was not found to improve with administration of insulin.

- *Diabetes mellitus as a risk factor for tuberculosis*:
  - *Latent infection*:[34] Reports have mentioned a higher prevalence of latent TB infection among diabetics. However, these have been confounded by the absence of control groups. Results of one study showed the reaction to purified protein derivate (PPD) is significantly correlated to the degree of hyperglycemia. However, this was not confirmed by other studies after adjusting for other variables. Therefore, it appears that diabetic patients are not at greater risk for latent infection with *Mycobacterium tuberculosis*.
  - *Active disease*: A definite correlation between diabetes and active TB has been reported by studies.[35] In a review of four cohort studies, the pooled OR was found to be 2.52 (95% CI 1.53–4.03) and in ten case-control studies, the pooled OR was found to be 2.2 (range 1.16–7.81).[35]

    This relationship between DM and TB was found to be more prominent in patients with type 1 DM, who usually fall into the young age demographic.[36] This higher susceptibility may be because achieving good glycemic control is more difficult in patients with type 1 DM. Poor glycemic control has been positively correlated with the occurrence of TB.[37]
- *Effects of diabetes mellitus on the clinical features of tuberculosis*:
  - *Age*: Diabetic patients with TB tend to be older than those without. This is likely a reflection of the fact that type 2 DM becomes more common with age.
  - *Sex*: Men may be at greater risk, but conclusive evidence is lacking.
  - *Sites*: Extrapulmonary TB has been reported as being less common in diabetics.[38]
  - *Sputum positivity:* Contrasting reports appear in literature. Currently, there is no concrete evidence for or against higher rates of sputum positivity.
- *Effects on the radiological manifestations*: The effects of DM on the radiological presentation of TB have been a matter of controversy with numerous studies providing conflicting findings. A review by Parvaneh Baghaei, Majid Marjani et al. have suggested that these differences are likely to be due to differences in patient selection and the definition used for diabetes.

  No difference in the incidence of isolated pleural TB and pleural effusions have been reported between patients with and without diabetes mellitus.

Some studies have reported a higher incidence of involvement of the lower lobe in diabetics.

Cavitatory lesions, in particular cavitatory nodular lesions have been reported more commonly in diabetics.

A study of the computed tomography (CT) findings of TB has shown a high prevalence of nonsegmental distribution (30%) and multiple small cavities among diabetic patients. However, unusual locations of lesions such as lower lobes, anterior segment of upper lobes, or the right middle lobe were equally infrequent in diabetics and nondiabetics (Fig. 11.4).

- *Effects of diabetes on the treatment response in tuberculosis*: There have been conflicting reports with respect to the treatment outcome in diabetes. At present, although there is no irrefutable evidence in favor of either better or worse prognosis, some studies show a tendency toward a worse prognosis.[35] Studies have shown a higher mortality (up to six times greater)[39] and a higher risk of treatment failure (OR of 7.65)[40] after accounting for confounding factors such as noncompliance and drug resistance.

  Drug resistance has been proposed as a possible reason for this. Reviews regarding the subject[41] have reported that despite no conclusive evidence, some studies have reported a higher incidence of multidrug-resistant tuberculosis (MDR-TB) in diabetic patients, and have suggested that diabetic patients are at an increased risk of relapsing with MDR strains. A proposed mechanism for this revolves around the *katG* gene. The *katG* gene is ordinarily involved in protecting mycobacteria against oxidative stress.

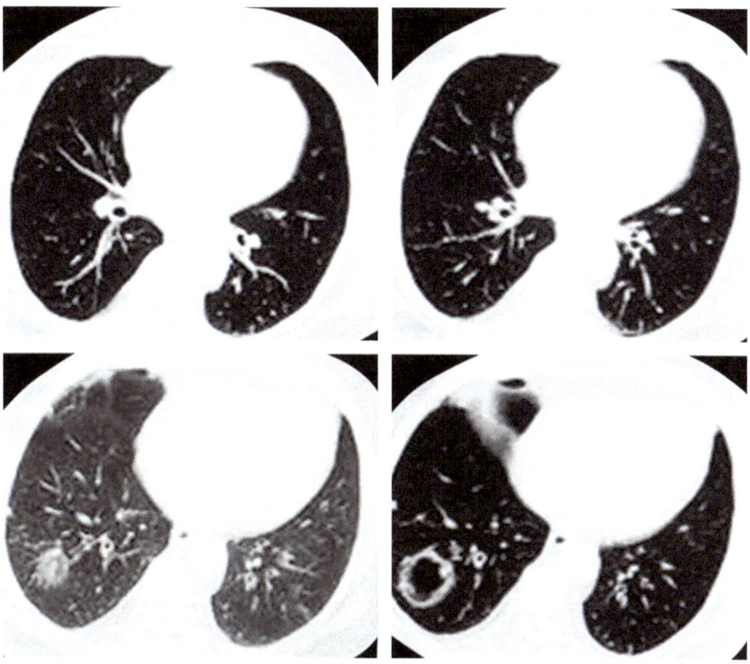

Fig. 11.4: Right lower lobe apical segment cavitation.
Source: Dr Vaishal Sheth, Fellow, Dept. of Chest Medicine, Ruby Hall Clinic.

It also codes for an enzyme that converts INH into its active form. In type 2 DM, the production of reactive oxygen species is impaired, so strains with *katG* mutation may be able to survive better.

Another reason proposed is lower area-under-the curve (AUC) of plasma concentrations of antitubercular drugs. This was particularly noted with rifampicin. A study in Indonesia found the AUC to be almost 53% of that seen in nondiabetics.[42] However, the exact mechanism of this reduction in plasma concentration was not defined. Interestingly, no differences in the pharmacokinetics of rifampicin, pyrazinamide, and ethambutol were noticed during the intensive phase. One of the reasons proposed for the earlier, is that drug doses during the maintenance phase do not account for the increased weight of the patient as treatment progresses.

- *Effects of tuberculosis on diabetes mellitus and glycemic control*: Glucose intolerance has been reported in between 16.5% and 49% of patients with active TB.[35] Patients have been shown to have glucose intolerance at the time of diagnosis that was seen to resolve after completion of treatment. This has been termed "transient hyperglycemia". It has been noted that the control of glucose levels is most difficult in the intensive phase, with many patients requiring insulin.

  Multiple factors have been proposed to be responsible for this.

  An excess of inflammatory cytokines such as IL-6 and TNF-alpha may play a role in increasing insulin resistance.

  INH and rifampicin have been found to have direct hyperglycemic effects.

  Rifampicin is an inducer for cytochrome P450 enzymes. Thus, it further aggravates matters by inducing the metabolism of sulphonylureas and subsequently, lowering their serum levels.[43] Thiazolidinediones are also metabolized to a greater extent. Pioglitazone levels have been found to be lower by up to 54%.[41] Interestingly, although the levels of meglitinides were reduced due to increased metabolism, their glucose lowering capacity was not significantly altered.[41]

  However, rifampicin does not affect the metabolism of metformin or insulin.

- *Pneumonia and influenza:* The respiratory infections most frequently associated with diabetic patients were influenza, and those caused by *Streptococcus pneumoniae.*[4]

  Pneumonia was the most frequent manifestation of pneumococcal infection. Diabetic subjects were 15.8–25.6 times more likely to be hospitalized for pneumonia during the influenza season.[28] However, this may, in part, be due to a lower threshold for hospitalization of diabetic patients.

  Rates of admission for influenza during the epidemic season, were found to be 5.7–6.2 times higher in diabetics than nondiabetics.[28]

  The mortality due to both influenza and pneumonia was found to be 1.7 times greater in diabetics in patients above the age of 30 years, and 7.6 times greater in patients below.[28]

- *Genitourinary infections:* A positive association has been found between DM and genitourinary (GU) tract infections. For cohort studies, the crude OR has been shown to 2.03 (95% CI 1.81–2.28) and adjusted OR of 1.61 (95% CI 1.42–1.82). For case-control studies, the crude OR has been shown to be 3.06 (95% CI 2.21–4.23) and adjusted OR of 2.59 (95% CI 1.60–4.17).[29]

- *Asymptomatic bacteriuria:* Bacteriuria is defined by the presence of an uropathogen in urine, with colony counts exceeding 10^5 colony forming units (CFUs) per mL.

  Commonly implicated organisms include Gram-negative organisms such as Escherichia coli.

  Asymptomatic bacteriuria has been found to occur more frequently in females than males. Reviews suggest that it is the duration of diabetes, and not the degree of glycemic control that correlate with an increased incidence of bacteriuria.[28] The prevalence of bacteriuria was found to increase 1.9-fold for every 10-year increase in the duration of diabetes.[41] Macroalbuminuria and noncircumcised partners were also considered contributory. However, no conclusive evidence of a correlation of risk with HbA1c was found.

  Studies have shown that asymptomatic bacteriuria, whether in type 1 or type 2 DM, is not a risk factor for a faster decline in renal function or the development of hypertension, at least over a 6-year period.[44]

  Clinically, although there is a possibility of progression to upper urinary tract infection (UTI), data for antibiotic prophylaxis in all cases of asymptomatic bacteriuria is controversial.

  Studies have shown no benefit in treating with antibiotics with respect to the development of symptomatic UTI, complications, or mortality.[45]

  This, put together with the numerous antibiotic-associated side effects, cost to the patient, and the risk of subsequent development of resistance altogether do not support the use of antibiotics routinely.

  Notable exceptions to this, however, include:
  - Pregnant women
  - Prior to urological intervention
  - Renal transplant patients.
- *Cystitis:* Emphysematous cystitis has been found to occur more often in diabetics than nondiabetics with women affected more frequently than men.[46] It is characterized by the presence of gas in the urinary bladder due to infection by carbon dioxide (CO_2) producing bacteria. Pathogens frequently isolated include *Escherichia coli,* Enterobacteria, *Proteus, Klebsiella,* and *Candida.*

  In women with good glycemic control who have been diabetic for a short period, the treatment is the same as that of an uncomplicated UTI.

  Current recommendations include the use of nitrofurantoin in the dose of 100 mg thrice a day for 5 days, sulfamethoxazole-trimethoprim in the dose of 960 mg twice a day for 3 days, or a single dose of 3 g of fosfomycin. Second-line medications include fluoroquinolones and beta lactams.
- *Pyelonephritis:* Acute pyelonephritis has been found to occur 4–5 times as often in diabetics.[47] Frequently isolated pathogens include *Escherichia coli* and *Proteus* species. The clinical features are similar to those in nondiabetics. A notable difference, however, is an increased propensity for bilateral renal involvement (Figs. 11.5A and B).[47]

  Emphysematous pyelonephritis is characterized by renal parenchymal necrosis, with collection of gas in the collecting ductules, or in the perinephric tissues. It has

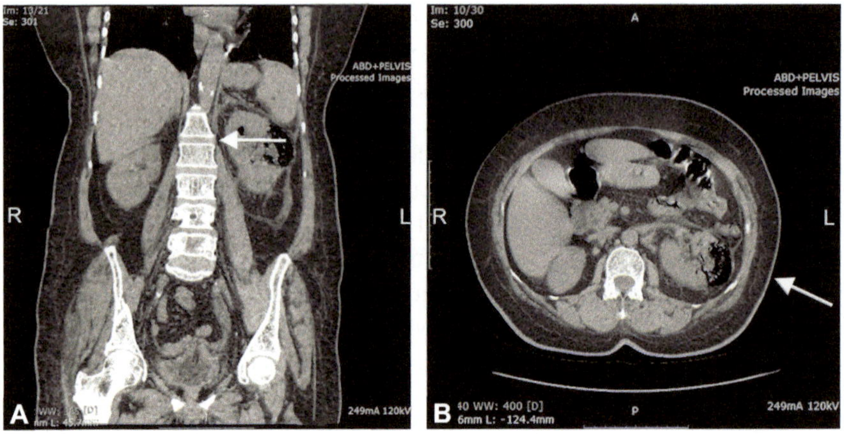

Figs. 11.5A and B: Computed tomography scan of emphysematous pyelonephritis.
Source: Dr Sanjay Agarwal, MD, FACE, Head of Department, Ruby Hall Clinic, Pune.

been observed more commonly in diabetic women.[4] *Escherichia coli* and *Enterobacter aerogenes* are the most frequently isolated pathogens.

Common symptoms include fever, flank pain, nausea, vomiting, and perhaps a mass in the flanks. Crackles in the flanks or thighs are less common.

A CT scan is diagnostic.

Uncomplicated pyelonephritis is managed using antibiotics such as a broad-spectrum cephalosporin, piperacillin-tazobactam or carbapenems, or fluoroquinolones empirically, and subsequent modification as per culture reports.

Emphysematous pyelonephritis additionally requires surgical intervention. Historically, open drainage was preferred. Recently, reports of successful treatment with percutaneous drainage have been published in literature. Certain cases may require a nephrectomy.

- *Perinephric abscesses:* Up to a third of patients of perinephric abscesses are found to be diabetic.[4] The clinical symptoms often overlap with those of acute pyelonephritis. In view of the absence of specific clinical features, the diagnosis is often made late. Therefore, this diagnosis should be borne in mind for all cases of pyelonephritis not improving with antibiotics.

- *Gastrointestinal and hepatobiliary infections:* An increased association between DM and gastrointestinal (GI) tract infections has been noted. A review of cohort studies has shown a crude OR of 1.13 (95% CI 0.86–1.47) with an adjusted OR of 1.48 (95% CI 1.40–1.57). Case-control studies have shown a stronger association with a crude OR of 2.44 (95% CI 1.26–4.71) and an adjusted OR of 3.61 (95% CI 2.94–4.43).[29]
    - *Helicobacter pylori gastritis: Helicobacter pylori* gastritis has been associated with increased insulin requirements in children with type 1 DM.[48] Additionally, reduced efficacy of *Helicobacter pylori* eradication regimens, as well as higher rates of reinfection have been reported in patients with diabetes.[4] Currently, there is no conclusive data proving a causal relationship between *Helicobacter pylori* infection diabetes, as well as its macrovascular complications, neuropathy, and microalbuminuria.

- *Cholecystitis:* Emphysematous cholecystitis has shown an association with diabetes. Emphysematous cholecystitis has been reported more frequently in males with DM.[48]

  Ischemic necrosis of the gallbladder wall, with subsequent infiltration by gas producing organisms culminates in this otherwise infrequent disease. Thus, the primary insult is that of ischemia. The list of implicated organisms includes: *Clostridium welchii, Clostridium perfringens, Escherichia coli, Klebsiella,* Streptococci, *Salmonella enteritidis,* and *Campylobacter*. Clinical signs are consistent with regular cholecystitis, making diagnosis difficult without a high index of suspicion. The presence of crackles on abdominal palpation is a poor prognostic indicator.[49]

  Various imaging modalities assist in the diagnosis. An ultrasound may characteristically show an "effervescent bladder", whereas a conventional X-ray or a CT will reveal gas under the liver, and delineate the gas in the gallbladder wall, respectively.

  The definitive treatment is a cholecystectomy, with an open approach preferred over a laparoscopic. Antibiotics and hyperbaric oxygen therapy have been used as well as adjuncts.
- *Hepatitis C:* Hepatitis C reportedly affects 170 million people worldwide.[50] Various studies have reported a prevalence of DM ranging from 13% to 33% in hepatitis C infected patients,[51] almost three times that of the general population (4–10%).

  Thus, DM is often considered an extrahepatic manifestation of hepatitis C.

Proposed mechanisms for this association include:

- The role of hepatic fibrosis and cirrhosis in impaired glucose tolerance.
- An intense inflammatory response to hepatitis C, and the consequent high levels of circulating inflammatory cytokines including TNF-alpha.
- *Direct effects of hepatitis C virus on insulin signaling*: A disturbed equilibrium with respect to different phosphorylated moieties of the molecule insulin receptor substrate-1 (IRS-1), i.e. stimulatory tyrosine moiety and inhibitory serine moiety is believed to play a central role.
- *Beta cell dysfunction*: Hepatitis C virus (HCV)-infected beta cells show both structural and functional impairment. Studies have demonstrated a blunted infected beta-cell response to glucose.[52]

- *Hepatitis B:* According to data from the US Centers for Disease Control and Prevention (CDC), diabetics in the age group of 23–59 years had 2.1 (95% CI = 1.6–2.8) times the odds of developing acute hepatitis B. For diabetics above the age of 60 years, the odds were 1.5 times (95% CI = 0.9–2.5) greater than nondiabetics.

  With specific reference to immunization, the Advisory Committee on Immunization Practices (ACIP) recommends the administration of the vaccine to all diabetics between the ages of 19–59 years (recommendation category A).

  However, for unvaccinated diabetics above the age of 60 years, the administration of vaccine is to be at the discretion of the treating physician (recommendation category B).
- *Enteroviruses:* Enteroviruses, particularly coxsackie B3 and B4, are purported to play a role in the pathogenesis of type 1 DM in genetically predisposed individuals.[26] While the definitive mechanism is yet to be established, proposed mechanisms include:[4]
  - Persistent viral infection leading to T-cell damage, release of intracellular sequestered antigens, and a subsequent autoimmune response.

    - Molecular mimicry (partial sequence homology) between the 2C viral protease and the GAD65 as well as between the VP1 viral capsid protein and the IA2 protein.
    - Bystander activation of autoreactive T cells.
    - Thymus infection, and
    - Loss of regulatory T cells.

- *Skin and soft tissue infections:* The incidence of skin and soft tissue infections has been found to be greater in diabetics. Cohort studies have shown a crude OR of 2.23 (95% CI 1.67–2.96) and an adjusted OR of 2.03 (95% CI 1.84-2-25). Case-control studies have shown a crude OR of 1.69 (95% CI 1.05-2-72).[29]
  - *Lower extremity infections and ulcers:* This includes diabetic foot infections, which refer to infections of the soft tissue or bone below the malleoli.[53] The estimated lifetime risk of a person with diabetes developing a foot ulcer is 15–25% with an annual incidence of 3–10%.[54] The most commonly implicated organisms are Gram-positive aerobic cocci, mainly staphylococci. Methicillin-resistant *Staphylococcus aureus* (MRSA) is present in 10–32% of diabetic infections[55] and is associated with a higher rate of treatment failure. Anaerobic organisms are more frequently present in necrotic wounds and infections of the ischemic foot (Fig. 11.6).[53]
  - *Tropical hand syndrome:* For any diabetic adult from a tropical country with hand cellulitis, infection, and gangrene, the diagnosis of tropical hand syndrome may be considered (Figs. 11.7A and B).

    The syndrome comprises:[56]
    - Localized cellulitis with swelling and hand ulcers
    - Fulminant hand sepsis
    - Gangrene affecting the whole limb.

    It may rapidly progress to Meleney's (synergistic) gangrene involving the superficial fascia of the entire limb, and can result in death within days of onset of symptoms.

    Unlike diabetic foot, the tropical hand syndrome is a less recognized and less defined complication that may be seen in diabetics. In fact, it is generally not classified as an expected diabetic complication.

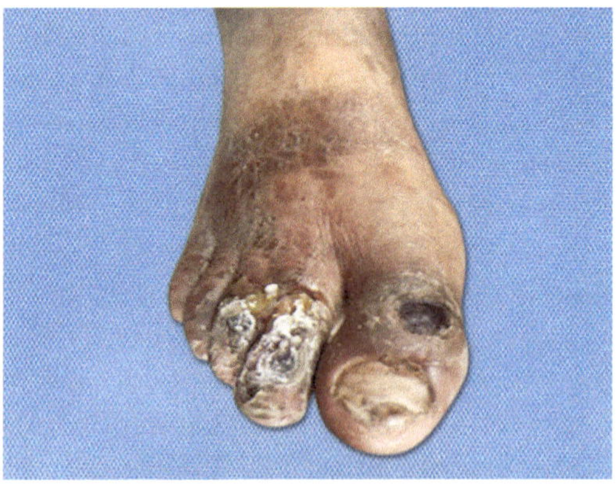

Fig. 11.6: Diabetic foot infections.

Source: Dr Sanjay Agarwal, MD, FACE, Head of Department, Ruby Hall Clinic, Pune.

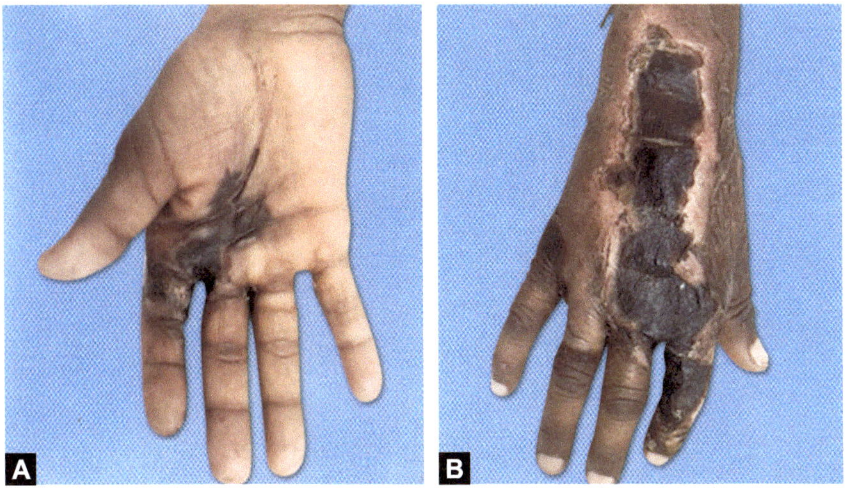

Figs. 11.7A and B: Tropical hand syndrome.
Source: Dr Sanjay Agarwal, MD, FACE, Head of Department, Ruby Hall Clinic, Pune.

Humidity is considered a risk factor for its development, as is supported by its occurrence in coastal and tropical areas. A male preponderance has been noted.[57]

A history of antecedent minor trauma may be elicited.

Peripheral arterial disease and neuropathy do not appear to play a contributory role.[58]

Early institution of culture and sensitivity-guided antibiotics is a must. Tissue biopsy is preferred as the source for culture because the biopsy specimen tends to yield a single organism in more than 75% of cases whereas swabs tended to yield polymicrobial growths.[59]

Wound incision and drainage, debridement, or if required, amputation constitute the surgical aspects of management.

- *Necrotizing fasciitis:*[60] This is a deep-seated infection of subcutaneous tissue resulting in progressive destruction of fascia, muscle, and fat with two broad clinical subtypes:
  1. *Type 1*: Mixed infection with aerobes and anaerobes. Most common in patients with DM and peripheral vascular disease (PVD), postsurgery.
  2. *Type 2*: Spontaneous gangrenous myositis. Associated with Group A Streptococci.

     75% of the cases are found to be diabetic. Mortality is high and has been estimated to be up to 40%. Commonly affected sites include the abdominal wall, perineum, and limbs (Figs. 11.8A and B).

     Management involves simultaneous measures involving good glycemic control, the use of antibiotics like penicillin, cephalosporins, aminoglycosides, clindamycin, and metronidazole, surgical debridement, and the use of hyperbaric oxygen therapy as an adjunct.
- *Fournier's gangrene:* Fournier's gangrene is an uncommon polymicrobial necrotizing infection affecting, most frequently, the male genitalia (86% of cases) (Fig. 11.9).[54]

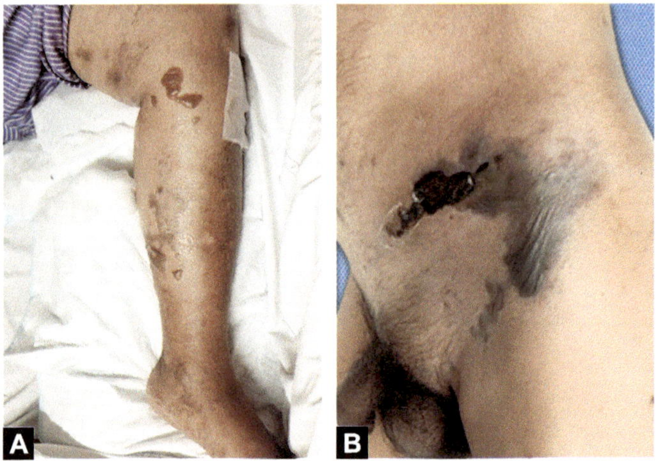

Figs. 11.8A and B: Necrotizing fasciitis.
Source: Dr Sanjay Agarwal, MD, FACE, Head of Department, Ruby Hall Clinic, Pune.

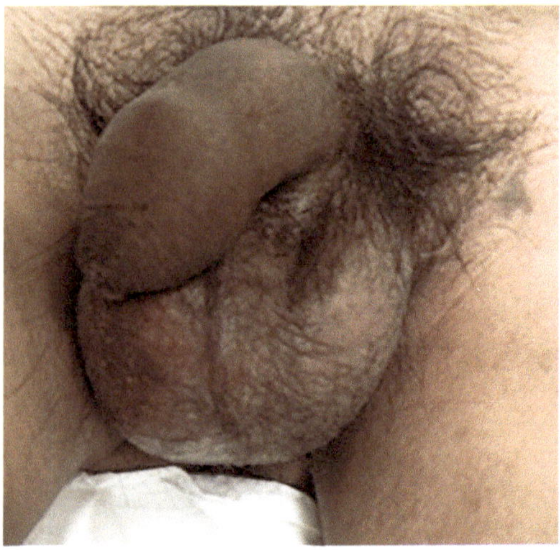

Fig. 11.9: Fournier's gangrene.
Source: Dr Sanjay Agarwal, MD, FACE, Head of Department, Ruby Hall Clinic, Pune

It usually involves the scrotum, but can extend to the penis, perineum, and abdominal wall. The testes are usually spared (Fig. 11.10).

Studies have shown that up to 70% of the people with this condition are found to be diabetic.[4] Diabetic patients are thought to have a higher mortality in this condition, however, convincing data is lacking.[54]

Treatment involves a multifaceted approach[61] including:

- *Use of broad-spectrum antibiotics*: Classically, triple therapy with cephalosporins/aminoglycosides, metronidazole, and penicillin is recommended.
- *Hyperbaric oxygen therapy*: The rationale behind the use of hyperbaric oxygen therapy (HBOT) includes optimization of neutrophil function, inhibition of anaerobes,

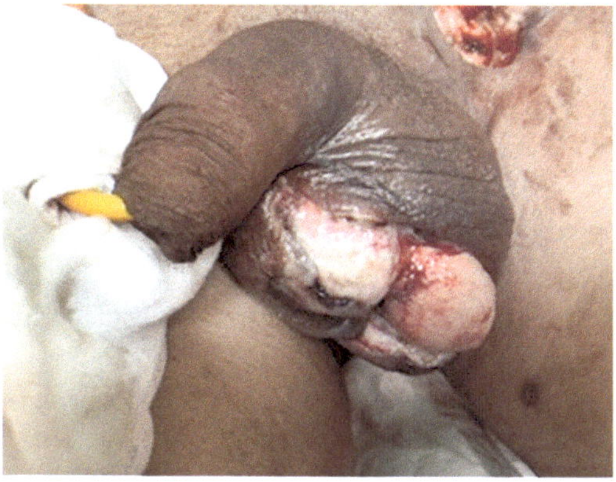

Fig. 11.10: Fournier's gangrene post deroofing. The testicular sparing is noted.
Source: Dr Sanjay Agarwal, MD, FACE, Head of Department, Ruby Hall Clinic, Pune.

increased fibroblast proliferation and angiogenesis, reduction of edema by hyperoxia-induced vasoconstriction, and increased intracellular transport of antibiotics.

- *Radical surgical debridement and subsequent vacuum-assisted closure or plastic reconstruction as appropriate*: Usually, debridement of deep fascia and muscle is not required.

- *Carbuncle:* A carbuncle is essentially an inflammatory mass that results from the coalescence of multiple furuncles. The most common sites are the back, and the nape of the neck. Carbuncles have been historically associated with DM and other immunocompromised states.

  Commonly implicated are bacteria *Staphylococcus aureus* and *Streptococcus pyogenes*.

  Presenting features include local erythema, itching, and tenderness. Systemic symptoms like fever, chills, and prostration may also be seen.

  Soma patients may present in frank sepsis and require urgent institution of antibiotics. Surgical treatment is an essential component of management. Two methods are adopted, based on the preference of the surgeon:
  - Incision and drainage
  - Saucerization.

- *Surgical site and postoperative infections:* Surgical site infections are found more commonly in diabetics. A review of cohort studies has shown a crude OR of 2.35 (95% CI 1.97–2.80) and an adjusted OR of 2.03 (95% CI 1.84–2.25). Data from case-control studies have shown a crude OR of 3.13 (95% CI 2.37–4.15) and an adjusted OR of 2.66 (95% CI 2.18–3.23).[29]
  - A landmark study revealing the relationship between perioperative glycemic status and mortality outcomes came from the Portland Diabetes Project.
  - Mortality was found to be greater in those with both, poor and overly aggressive glycemic.
  - Maintaining blood glucose in the range of 130–180 mg/dL by means of 2 hourly glucose monitoring and insulin was associated with better outcomes.
- *Fungal infections:*
  - *Oral and esophageal candidiasis:*[4] Commonly due to *Candida albicans*. Clinically, it can present in a variety of ways, ranging from median rhomboid glossitis, central papillary

atrophy, atrophic glossitis, denture stomatitis, pseudomembranous candidiasis, and angular cheilitis. Diagnosis is usually clinical, however, esophageal candidiasis requires an endoscopy for diagnosis.

- *Fungal cystitis:* Fungal cystitis caused by *Candida* has been described. Distinguishing colonization and infection is essential. Candida is a dimorphic fungus with both hyphal and yeast forms. Invasive candidiasis is characterized by the presence of hyphal forms of the organism whereas superficial infections characteristically have yeast forms. Further, fungal cystitis may also result in the formation of "fungal balls" which may result in obstruction of the urinary tract.
- *Mucormycosis:* Mucormycosis is a relatively rare, highly angioinvasive fungal infection. Also called zygomycosis or phycomycosis, it is most often caused by the fungal species of *Rhizopus and Mucor,* although it may occasionally occur due to *Absidia* and *Cunninghamella* species. The disease is known to be more common in diabetic patients. A study has found that it occurs in approximately 50% of diabetics.[4] Another study, in their review has reported the prevalence of diabetes in mucormycosis was as high as 70.4% (Figs. 11.11A to C).[62]

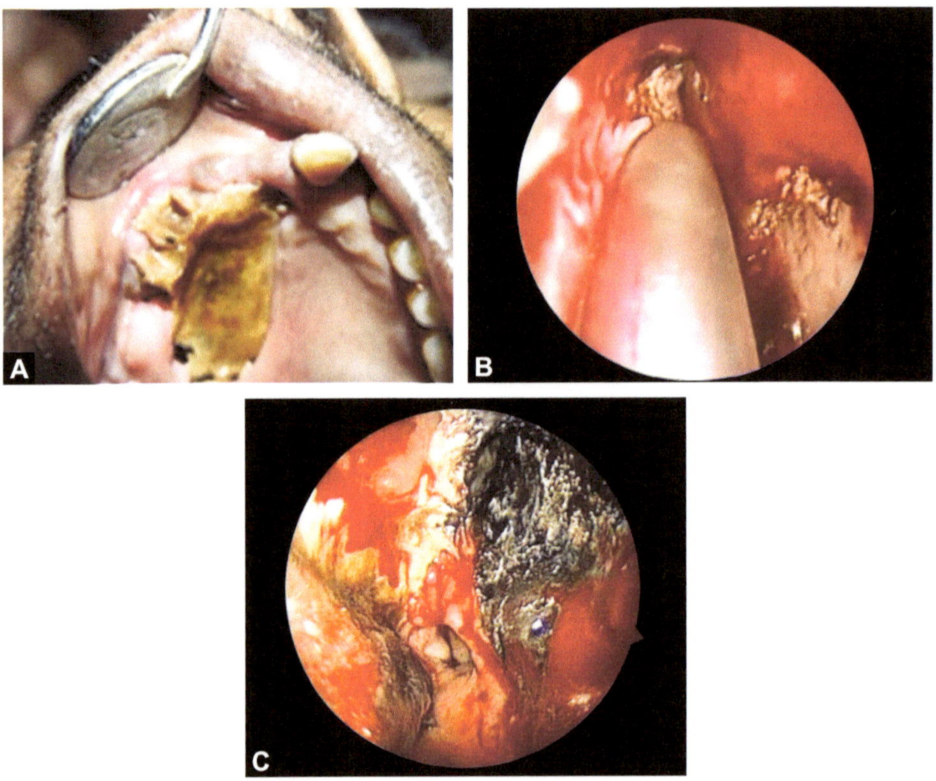

Figs. 11.11A to C: Intraoperative photos of mucormycosis.
Source: Dr Murarji Ghadge, Consultant ear-nose-throat (ENT) surgeon, Ruby Hall Clinic, Pune.

This may be due to the impaired ability of the alveolar macrophages of diabetic patients to attach to the hyphae of the fungi, as demonstrated by immunologic studies with *Rhizopus oryzae*.[63]

Five clinical forms have been described:

1. Rhinocerebral
2. Pulmonary
3. Gastrointestinal
4. Primary cutaneous
5. Disseminated.

Rhinocerebral mucormycosis may present with unilateral proptosis, diplopia, headache, and may often be the first manifestation of previously undiagnosed diabetes.

There appears to be no evidence of increased mortality in diabetics with mucormycosis.

Effective surgical debridement and treatment with amphotericin-B have shown good efficacy. Tight glycemic control is also vital.

- *Magnetic resonance imaging (Figs. 11.12A to D):*
  - *T1 (noncontrast)*: Isointense lesions relative to brain in most cases (approximately 80%).
  - *T2:* Variable with around 20% of patients showing high T2 signal. Fungal elements themselves tend to have low signal on T2.
  - *T1C + (gadolinium)*: The devitalized mucosa appears on contrast-enhanced magnetic resonance (MR) imaging as contiguous foci of nonenhancing tissue, this gives a black turbinate sign.

- *Miscellaneous infections:*
  - *Bacteremia:* Diabetic patients were found to have an increased risk of bloodstream infections and bacteremia. Cohort studies have shown a crude OR of 1.82 (95% CI 1.57–2.12) and an adjusted OR of 1.72 (95% CI 1.48–2.00). Case-control studies have shown a crude OR of 3.18 (95% CI 2.37–4.26) and an adjusted OR of 2.40 (95% CI 1.68–3.42).[29]
  - Human immunodeficiency virus:[64] The effects of HIV on insulin tolerance and glucose homeostasis may be broadly classified into those due to the disease itself, and those associated with its treatment.
    - *Due to the infection, itself:* Evidence suggests that the virus itself does not play a significant role in increasing insulin resistance. In fact, studies in the pre-highly active antiretroviral therapy (HAART) era suggested that in HIV-treatment naive patients with wasting, insulin sensitivity had increased.

      However, the lipodystrophy known to occur in HIV has been linked with increased insulin resistance. The redistribution of subcutaneous fat to visceral fat depots is primarily responsible for this. It is known that visceral fat is associated with the metabolic syndrome, or syndrome X (Figs. 11.13A and B).

      Further, it is to be noted that there are elevated circulatory levels of inflammatory cytokines, particularly TNF-alpha and IL-6. Additional comorbid conditions associated with HIV, such as hepatitis C, contribute to increased cytokine levels.

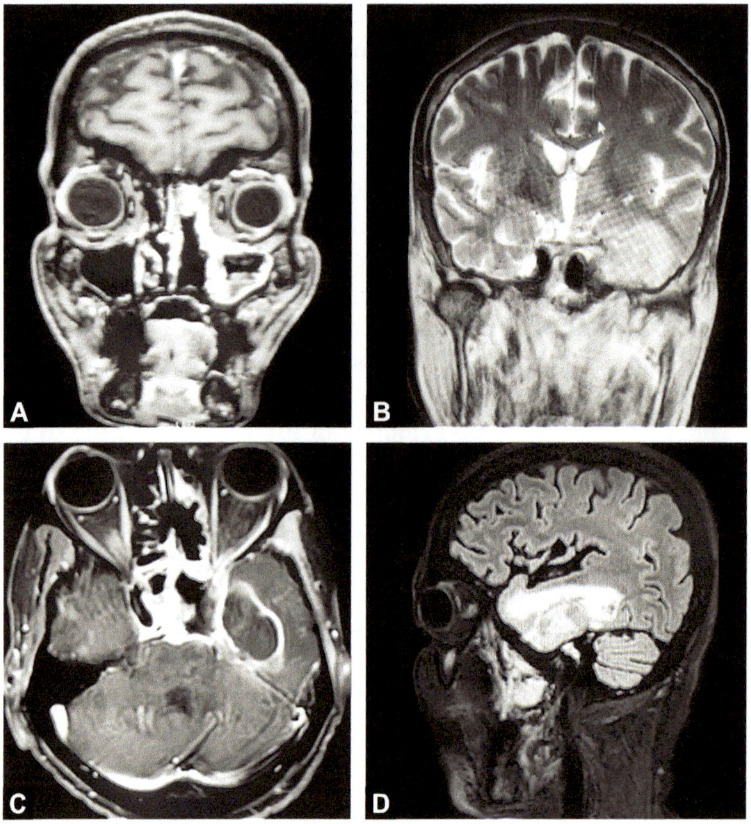

Figs. 11.12A to D: (A and B) show involvement of the paranasal sinuses as well as the left temporal lobe (seen on the coronal T2W image); (C and D) reveal the extent of temporal lobe involvement (seen on the axial view and FLAIR sagittal view) Mucormycosis was subsequently confirmed by FESS and microbiologic examination.
Source: Dr Ashwin Pillai, Fellow, Dept. of Medicine, Ruby Hall Clinic.

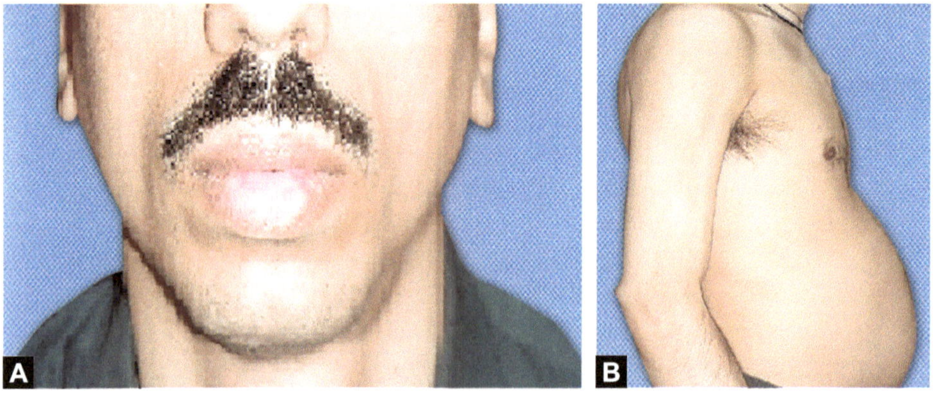

Figs. 11.13A and B: Lipoatrophy and lipohypertrophy with lipodystrophy secondary to stavudine-based ART therapy.
Source: Dr Sanjay Pujari, Director and Chief Consultant, Institute of Infectious Diseases, Pune.

Tumor necrosis factor-alpha can indirectly influence peripheral insulin resistance by stimulating free fatty acid and triglyceride production in the liver.

- *The role of highly active antiretroviral therapy:* Studies have found that the incidence of diabetes in patients on HAART is higher than that of the general population. A study has reported the incidence being four times greater than that of seronegative men.

  Protease inhibitors (PIs) have been particularly implicated in this. The insulin-dependent glucose transporter-4 (GLUT-4) is the first molecule to have been identified as a target for these PIs. Further evidence in this regard is that, after withdrawing PIs, glucose values were found to return to normal.
- *The role of other drugs:* Pentamidine, used in the treatment of Pneumocystis carinii pneumonia, was found to cause beta-cell toxicity in a subset of patients. This was irrespective of the route of administration (inhaled or intravenous). These patients tended to develop hypoglycemia in the short term, followed by late-onset diabetes.

PRINCIPLES OF MANAGEMENT

The management of infections in diabetes varies with the disease itself. However, it is pertinent to bear in mind that a common feature to most infections is poor glycemic control. As such, the management involves two components:

1. *Tight glycemic control:* Achieving tight glycemic control is of paramount importance. Using insulin whether premixed, short or long acting, basal bolus regimens, or even insulin pumps would be useful in achieving this goal.

   However, this may not always be feasible, particularly in the case of an outpatient setting. Real world hindrances such as patient compliance, risk of hypoglycemia due to glycemic variability in the setting of an illness, all create seemingly insidious but formidable challenges.

   Oral hypoglycemic agents (OHAs) will also likely require optimization during the period of infection.

   Both insulin and OHA doses will require review after the infection has subsided as well, reflecting the changed insulin sensitivity status of the patient.
2. *Source control:*
   - Surgical management is often crucial in diabetics. A significant proportion of infections in diabetics tends to be invasive, and may require aggressive management ranging from local care, to debridement, to amputations.
   - Antibiotics may need to be instituted empirically, based on suspected etiologic agents, and national or institutional guidelines, as well as culture and sensitivity patterns.
     The exact duration of antibiotic treatment may be tailored as per the patient's condition and response to treatment.

CONCLUSION

The occurrence of disease in diabetic patients, and their subsequent treatment, poses a greater challenge to physicians today than ever before. As our understanding of the disease process improves, as our therapeutic capabilities improve, so multiply the challenges that we face.

In response to infections, antibiotics were created. For a while the scales tipped in favor of humanity. But then, the pendulum swung the other way, with the emergence of drug-resistant superbugs. However, just as with Heracles against Hydra, the sword of knowledge, and the fire of altruism shall forever be our allies in our labors against these new challenges. A conscious attempt to periodically review, and subsequently refresh, our understanding of the various associated diseases will ensure that, in a country expected to have nearly 80 million diabetic patients over the next decade, we remain comfortably ahead of the curve when it comes to meeting their healthcare needs.

REFERENCES

1. International Diabetes Federation. IDF Diabetes Atlas, 8th edition; 2017.
2. Allard R, Leclerc P, Tremblay C, et al. Diabetes and the severity of pandemic influenza A (H1N1) infection. Diabetes Care. 2010;33(7):1491-3.
3. Casqueiro J, Casqueiro J, Alves C. Infections in patients with diabetes mellitus: A review of pathogenesis. Indian J Endocrinol Metab. 2012;16(Suppl 1):S27-36.
4. Graves DT, Kayal RA. Diabetic complications and dysregulated innate immunity. Front Biosci. 2008;13:1227-39.
5. Mazade MA, Edwards MS. Impairment of type III group B Streptococcus-stimulated superoxide production and opsonophagocytosis by neutrophils in diabetes. Mol Genet Metab. 2001;73(3):259-67.
6. Thornalley P, Wolff S, Crabbe J, et al. The autoxidation of glyceraldehyde and other simple monosaccharides under physiological conditions catalysed by buffer ions. Biochim Biophys Acta. 1984;797(2):276-87.
7. Giugliano D, Ceriello A, Paolisso G. Oxidative stress and diabetic vascular complications. Diabetes Care. 1996;19(3):257-67.
8. Millar TM, Phan V, Tibbles LA. ROS generation in endothelial hypoxia and reoxygenation stimulates MAP kinase signaling and kinase-dependent neutrophil recruitment. Free Radic Biol Med. 2007;42(8):1165-77.
9. Mitra S, Abraham E. Participation of superoxide in neutrophil activation and cytokine production. Biochim Biophys Acta. 2006;1762(8):732-41.
10. Karima M, Kantarci A, Ohira T, et al. Enhanced superoxide release and elevated protein kinase C activity in neutrophils from diabetic patients: association with periodontitis. J Leukoc Biol. 2005;78(4):862-70.
11. Vlassara H. Recent progress in advanced glycation end products and diabetic complications. Diabetes. 1997;46(Suppl 2):S19-25.
12. King GL, Brownlee M. The cellular and molecular mechanisms of diabetic complications. Endocrinol Metab Clin North Am. 1996;25(2):255-70.
13. Stitt AW, He C, Vlassara H. Characterization of the advanced glycation end product receptor complex in human vascular endothelial cells. Biochem Biophys Res Commun. 1999;256(3):549-56.
14. Hiramatsu Y, Sekiguchi N, Hayashi M, et al. Diacylglycerol production and protein kinase C activity are increased in a mouse model of diabetic embryopathy. Diabetes. 2002;51(9):2804-10.
15. Cohen MP, Shea E, Chen S, et al. Glycated albumin increases oxidative stress, activates NF-kappa B and extracellular signal-regulated kinase (ERK), and stimulates ERK-dependent transforming growth factor-beta 1 production in macrophage RAW cells. J Lab Clin Med. 2003;141(4):242-9.
16. Rashid G, Luzon AA, Korzets Z, et al. The effect of advanced glycation end-products and aminoguanidine on TNF alpha production by rat peritoneal macrophages. Perit Dial Int. 2001;21(2):122-9.

17. Alikhani Z, Alikhani M, Boyd CM, et al. Advanced glycation end products enhance expression of pro-apoptotic genes and stimulate fibroblast apoptosis through cytoplasmic and mitochondrial pathways. J Biol Chem. 2005;280(13):12087-95.
18. Alikhani M, Alikhani Z, Boyd C, et al. Advanced glycation end products stimulate osteoblast apoptosis via the MAP kinase and cytosolic apoptotic pathways. Bone. 2007;40(2):345-53.
19. Geerlings SE, Hoepelman AI. Immune dysfunction in patients with diabetes mellitus (DM). FEMS Immunol Med Microbiol. 1999;26(3-4):259-65.
20. Peleg AY, Weerarathna T, McCarthy JS, et al. Common infections in diabetes: pathogenesis, management and relationship to glycemic control. Diabetes Metab Res Rev. 2007;23(1):3-13.
21. Geerlings SE, Brouwer EC, Van Kessel KC, et al. Cytokine secretion is impaired in women with diabetes mellitus. Eur J Clin Invest. 2000;30(11):995-1001.
22. Price CL, Al Hassi HO, English NR, et al. Methylglyoxal modulates immune responses: relevance to diabetes. J Cell Mol Med. 2010;14(6):1806-15.
23. Nirmal J, Caputo GM, Weitekamp MR, et al. Infections in patients with diabetes mellitus. N Engl J Med. 1999;341(4):1906-12.
24. Vardakas KZ, Siempos II, Falagas ME. Diabetes mellitus as a risk factor for nosocomial pneumonia and associated mortality. Diabet Med. 2007;24(10):1168-71.
25. Stoeckle M, Kaech C, Trampuz A, et al. The role of diabetes mellitus in patients with bloodstream infections. Swiss Med Wkly. 2008;138(35-36):512-9.
26. Flyvbjerg A. Diabetic angiopathy, the complement system and the tumor necrosis factor superfamily. Nat Rev Endocrinol. 2010;6(2):94-101.
27. Boyko EJ, Lipsky BA. Infection and diabetes. In: Aubert R (Ed). Diabetes in America, 2nd edition. United States of America: National Institutes of Health; 1995. p. 485.
28. Abu-Ashour W, Twells L, Valcour J, et al. The association between diabetes mellitus and incident infections: a systematic review and meta-analysis of observational studies. BMJ Open Diabetes Res Care. 2017;5(1):e000336.
29. Anntonelli Incalzi R, Fuso L, Giordano A, et al. Neuroadrenergic denervation of the lung in type I diabetes mellitus complicated by autonomic neuropathy. Chest. 2002;121(2):443-51.
30. Lönnroth K, Castro KG, Chakaya JM, et al. Tuberculosis control and elimination 2010-50: cure, care, and social development. Lancet. 2010;375(9728):1814-29.
31. Restrepo BI. Convergence of the tuberculosis and diabetes epidemics: renewal of old acquaintances. Clin Infect Dis. 2007;45(4):436-8.
32. Roglic G, Green A, Sicree R, et al. Global prevalence of diabetes: estimates for the year 2000 and projections for 2030. Wild Diabetes Care. 2004;27(5):1047-53.
33. Moutschen MP, Scheen AJ, Lefebvre PJ. Impaired immune responses in diabetes mellitus: analysis of the factors and mechanisms involved. Relevance to the increased susceptibility of diabetic patients to specific infections. Diabetes Metab. 1992;18(3):187-201.
34. Baghaei P, Marjani M, Javanmard P, et al. Diabetes mellitus and tuberculosis facts and controversies. J Diabetes Metab Disord. 2013;12(1):58.
35. World Health Organization, International Union Against Tuberculosis and Lung Disease. (2011). Collaborative framework for care and control of tuberculosis and diabetes. [online] Available from www.apps.who.int/iris/bitstream/10665/44698/1/9789241502252_eng.pdf. [Accessed February, 2018].
36. Jeon CY, Murray MB. Diabetes mellitus increases the risk of active tuberculosis: a systematic review of 13 observational studies. PLoS Med. 2008;5(7):e152.
37. Leung CC, Lam TH, Chan WM, et al. Diabetic control and risk of tuberculosis: a cohort study. Am J Epidemiol. 2008;167(12):1486-94.
38. Ruslami R, Aarnoutse RE, Alisjahbana B, et al. Implications of the global increase of diabetes for tuberculosis control and patient care. Trop Med Int Health. 2010;12(11):1289-99.

39. Dooley KE, Tang T, Golub JE, et al. Impact of diabetes mellitus on treatment outcomes of patients with active tuberculosis. Am J Trop Med Hyg. 2009;12(4):634-9.
40. Alisjahbana B, Sahiratmadja E, Nelwan EJ, et al. The effect of type 2 diabetes mellitus on the presentation and treatment response of pulmonary tuberculosis. Clin Infect Dis. 2007;12(4):428-35.
41. Keane EM, Boyko EJ, Reller LB, et al. Prevalence of asymptomatic bacteriuria in subjects with NIDDM in San Luis Valley of Colorado. Diabetes Care. 1988;11(9):708-12.
42. Nijland HM, Ruslami R, Stalenhoef JE, et al. Exposure to rifampicin is strongly reduced in patients with tuberculosis and type 2 diabetes. Clin Infect Dis. 2006;43(7):848-54.
43. Dooley KE, Chaisson RE. Tuberculosis and diabetes mellitus: convergence of two epidemics. Lancet Infect Dis. 2009;9(12):737-46.
44. Meiland R, Geerlings SE, Stolk RP, et al. Asymptomatic bacteriuria in women with diabetes mellitus: effect on renal function after 6 years of follow-up. Arch Intern Med. 2006;166(20):2222-7.
45. Zalmanovici Trestioreanu A, Lador A, Sauerbrun-Cutler MT, et al. Antibiotics for asymptomatic bacteriuria. Cochrane Database of Systematic Reviews 2015, Issue 4. Art. No.: CD009534. DOI: 10.1002/14651858.CD009534.pub2.
46. Ludwig E. Urinary tract infections in diabetes mellitus. Orv Hetil. 2008;149(13):597-600.
47. Calvet HM, Yoshikawa TT. Infections in diabetes. Infect Dis Clin North Am. 2001;15(2):407-21.
48. Papamichael KX, Papaioannou G, Karga H, et al. *Helicobacter pylori* infection and endocrine disorders: is there a link? World J Gastroenterol. 2009;15(22):2701-7.
49. Joshi N, Caputo GM, Weitekamp MR, et al. Infections in patients with diabetes mellitus. N Engl J Med. 1999;341(25):1906-12.
50. Jadoon NA, Shahzad MA, Yaqoob R, et al. Seroprevalence of hepatitis C in type 2 diabetes: evidence for a positive association. Virol J. 2010;7:304.
51. Elhawary EI, Mahmoud GF, El-Daly MA, et al. Association of HCV with diabetes mellitus: an Egyptian case-control study. Virol J. 2011;8:367.
52. Masini M, Campani D, Boggi U, et al. Hepatitis C virus infection and human pancreatic beta-cell dysfunction. Diabetes Care. 2005;28(4):940-1.
53. Gemechu FW, Seemant F, Curley CA. Diabetic foot infections. Am Fam Physician. 2013;88(3):177-84.
54. Reiber GE, Vileikyte L, Boyko EJ, et al. Causal pathways for incident lower-extremity ulcers in patients with diabetes from two settings. Diabetes Care. 1999;22(1):157-62.
55. Vardakas KZ, Horianopoulou M, Falagas ME. Factors associated with treatment failure in patients with diabetic foot infections: an analysis of data from randomised control trials. Diabetes Res Clin Pract. 2008;80(3):344-51.
56. Okpara TC, Ezeala-Adikaibe BA, Omire O, et al. Tropical diabetic hand syndrome. Ann Med Health Sci Res. 2015;5(6):473-5.
57. Centers for Disease Control and Prevention (CDC). Tropical diabetic hand syndrome—Dar es Salaam, Tanzania, 1998-2002. MMWR Morb Mortal Wkly Rep. 2002;51(43):969-70.
58. Tiwari S, Chauhan A, Sethi NT. Tropical diabetic hand syndrome. Int J Diabetes Dev Ctries. 2008;28(4):130-1.
59. Abbas ZG, Lutale J, Gill GV, et al. Tropical diabetic hand syndrome: risk factors in an adult diabetes population. Int J Infect Dis. 2001;5(1):19-23.
60. Stevens DL, Bryant AE. Necrotizing soft-tissue infections. N Engl J Med. 2017;377:2253-65.
61. Mallikarjuna MN, Vijayakumar A, Patil VS, et al. Fournier's gangrene: current practices. ISRN Surg. 2012;2012:942437.
62. Blitzer A, Lawson W, Meyers BR, et al. Patient survival factors in paranasal sinus mucormycosis. Laryngoscope. 1980;90(4):635-48.
63. Waldor AR, Ruderman N, Diamon RD. Specific susceptibility to mucormycosis in murine diabetes and bronchoalveolar macrophage defense against Rhizopus. J Clin Invest. 1984;74(1):150-60.
64. Hruz PW. Molecular mechanisms for altered glucose homeostasis in HIV infection. Am J Infect Dis. 2006;2(3):187-92.

CHAPTER 12

Hypertension and Diabetes

Robert C Stanton

INTRODUCTION

There is no debate as to the importance of hypertension management in people with/without diabetes mellitus. For patients with diabetes mellitus, though, hypertension management is of paramount importance for not only prevention of cardiovascular events but also for the prevention of renal and retinal complications. The mechanistic reason for excellent blood pressure control in people with diabetes is likely due to the fact that diabetes mellitus is primarily manifested as a disease of endothelial cells, i.e. the endothelial cell is a central target for elevated glucose levels. Endothelial dysfunction is caused by elevated glucose and subsequent endothelial damage and death leads to the heart attacks, strokes, kidney failure, and retinopathy (a combination of vascular cell damage/death as well as vascular proliferative changes). Considering that hypertension is primarily affecting these same endothelial cells, it is not surprising that hypertension combined with the deleterious effects of high glucose on endothelial cells leads to worse outcomes in people with diabetes mellitus as compared to people who have hypertension alone.

There have been many studies showing that controlling blood pressure has a critical role both for the primary prevention of diabetic complications as well as for the treatment of established complications. But even with the universal understanding of the importance of blood pressure control, there are a number of unresolved issues. These include: (1) What is the blood pressure goal?, (2) What is the best way to diagnose and monitor hypertension?, (3) Is there an ideal medication to use initially?, (4) Is there a specific medication algorithm or regimen to follow?, and (5) When should an evaluation for secondary causes of hypertension being looked for? In this chapter, these issues will be discussed.

DIAGNOSIS AND MONITORING OF BLOOD PRESSURE (BOX 12.1)

At first thought, the diagnosis of hypertension seems obvious. But there are multiple issues surrounding the diagnosis relating to how and where the blood pressure is taken. As with most physiological measurements, the blood pressure needs to be taken in a standardized manner

Box 12.1: Diagnosis and monitoring.

- *Be sure blood pressures are being taken accurately:*
  - Patient should be resting for atleast 5 minutes
  - Cuff should be right size for the patient's arm
  - Arm should be resting (either being held or resting on an armrest)
  - Arm position should be at about heart level.
- *Ideally use home blood pressure monitoring:*
  - Train patients should know how to use a sphygmomanometer or ask them to purchase a machine
  - Verify accuracy of home blood pressure measurement by checking accuracy of machine with office measurement or accuracy of patient's technique with sphygmomanometer
  - Take blood pressure in morning and evening.

under steady state conditions. To achieve this, the blood pressure should be taken with the person at rest (generally at least 5 minutes of rest) with the arm being supported or resting on an armrest, the arm position being at about heart level, and the right-sized cuff being used. The reasons for these conditions are straightforward. Any activity will temporarily increase the blood pressure (normal physiological response). Hence, taking the blood pressure right after someone walks into the office will often be inaccurately high. Secondly, the arm needs to be in a resting position as contracting the muscles will also potentially produce an inaccurately high result as the contracted muscle will possibly require a higher pressure from the cuff to block flow in the artery. Thirdly, if the arm position is too low (e.g. the arm is hanging down) there may be significantly more blood passing through the arm due to gravitational effects that might lead to a falsely high blood pressure reading, whereas if the arm was held up high the opposite would occur. Lastly, if the blood pressure cuff is too small for a person's arm it might produce a falsely high blood pressure due to the need for more pressure to compress the artery, whereas a large cuff may lead to a falsely low blood pressure reading. These comments may all seem obvious, but the vast majority of the time these simple procedures are not followed. Therefore, most blood pressure readings are not accurate. Clearly this is not critical for a person with excellent blood pressure, but for those needing blood pressure control, accurate readings are essential.

There are three ways/settings to monitor blood pressure: (1) Office blood pressure, (2) Home blood pressure, and (3) 24-hour ambulatory blood pressure. The office blood pressure has the potential advantage of being obtained in a controlled setting with expert personnel doing the procedure. In practice though, many of the aforementioned standardized procedures are not done due to time pressures and lack of training. Home blood pressures have the potential of being very accurate if the standard procedures are properly followed. Indeed home blood pressure measurements offer multiple advantages: (1) Many people have some degree of 'white coat' hypertension (elevations in blood pressure when coming to see the physician). Thus, accurate home blood pressures provide the physician with both accurate readings and avoid potential complications caused by treating someone for high blood pressure measured in the office and later causing dizziness or even syncope because the home blood pressures are actually much lower. On the other hand, a small but significant percentage of patients have masked hypertension (defined as normal blood pressure in the office but high blood pressures at home). Hence, home blood pressure monitoring will reveal if a patient has masked hypertension and lead to better outcomes by instituting proper treatment; (2) Blood pressure follows a normal circadian rhythm where it is higher in the morning and lower in the afternoon. This degree of change can be determined if the patient takes multiple readings (morning and afternoon). The physician can then adjust medication dosing and dosing schedule to optimize blood pressure management to prevent the blood pressure from getting too high or too low; and (3) Home blood pressure readings are certainly more accurate than office blood pressures as there are multiple readings on a daily basis as compared to an occasional reading in the office. This also allows the physician to make appropriate medication changes at shorter time intervals as long as the patient provides the physician with the information and achieve optimal blood pressure control faster. Lastly, at this time, there is only a limited role for 24-hour blood pressure monitoring. In USA, it is approved mainly to diagnose 'white coat' hypertension. A clear use for 24-hour blood pressure monitoring is to determine if a patient is a dipper or a nondipper. Normally in the early morning hours, the blood pressure declines significantly (dipping). People whose blood pressure does not dip in the early mornings have been shown to have higher risk for cardiovascular disease. Amongst diabetic patients, nondipping is relatively common and is associated with autonomic dysfunction. And there have been small studies showing possible ways to restore for dipping. For example, in salt sensitive subjects, salt restriction led to restoration of dipping. In another study, switching the angiotensin converting enzyme inhibitor (ACEI) quinapril from the morning to the evening led to restoration of dipping. But no study has yet shown that restoration of dipping has clinical utility. So at this time, it is not critical to determine if a person is a dipper or nondipper.

There are a number of excellent reviews about the various ways to measure blood pressure.[1-4] As noted in the review by Drawz et al.[3] studies comparing home blood pressure monitoring as compared to office blood pressure monitoring, the home blood pressure had significantly better prognostic accuracy as compared to office blood pressure. Of note though, it needs to be reiterated that the patient needs to be trained properly to obtain the accurate blood pressure. If the patient is willing to use a cuff and stethoscope and proper technique, this is the most accurate and least expensive approach. In practice, though, most patients prefer to use a blood pressure machine. It is very important for the patients to bring the machine into a visit to check the accuracy of the blood pressure machine as they may well be giving inaccurate readings for a variety of reasons.

In conclusion, ideally for both confirming diagnosis and for optimal monitoring and management of blood pressure, home blood pressure readings (ideally twice a day—morning and later afternoon or evening) are ideal. Patients need to be trained in proper technique and they need to maintain records to review with the physician. Lastly if using a blood pressure machine, the accuracy of the machine need to be checked with simultaneous reading at an office visit.

BLOOD PRESSURE GOALS (BOX 12.2)

The question of what is defined as hypertension has been a very volatile subject in the past 10 years. Ideally the definition of hypertension would be based on large randomized controlled epidemiologic studies. Although there have been many excellent blood pressure studies, each of them by necessity are focused on a specific subset that may or may not be generalizable to everyone. Indeed large studies often become influential even though their results are only meaningful for the targeted subset of the population that was studied. On the other hand,

Box 12.2: Blood pressure goals.

- Hypertension is defined as more than 140/90 for the office blood pressure
- Hypertension is defined as more than 135/85 for the home blood pressure
- My blood pressure goal recommendation—aim for 130/80
- Guideline Committees recommend less than 140/80 or less than 140/90
  - Also some guidelines recommend less than 130/80 if there is proteinuria
- Avoid systolic blood pressure of less than 120 mm Hg.

guidelines committees often ignore multiple small studies even if there is a clear trend. This is not a criticism of the studies, but rather a criticism of the way guidelines and common practice ideas develop. Within the diabetes population, there has been a great deal of debate as to optimal blood pressure as it may be different depending on whether a particular patient has cardiovascular disease, kidney disease, or eye disease. Indeed within each of these complications there have been studies suggesting different targets. For example, the target for preventing stroke is not necessarily the same as for preventing myocardial ischemia or infarction. The target for kidney disease may be different depending on the degree of proteinuria. In this section, some of the major trials are examined and a recommendation is provided at the end of the section.

There have been a number of large trials published in the last 10 years that have a major impact on the recommendations for blood pressure goals in people with type 2 diabetes mellitus. For an overview of blood pressure studies, please read the following articles.[5-8] For this chapter, two trials will be discussed that reflect both the design and outcomes of these studies: (1) The Action to Control Cardiovascular Risk in Diabetes (ACCORD),[9] and (2) The International Verapamil SR-Trandolapril Study (INVEST).[10] As noted in the published paper, ACCORD was a study of 4,733 participants with type 2 diabetes who were randomly assigned to intensive therapy, targeting a systolic pressure of less than 120 mm Hg, or standard therapy targeting a systolic pressure of less than 140 mm Hg. The primary composite outcome was nonfatal myocardial infarction, nonfatal stroke, or death from cardiovascular causes. The mean follow-up was 4.7 years. After 1 year, the mean systolic blood pressure in the intensive therapy group was 119, while the standard therapy had a mean systolic blood pressure of 135. By the end of the study it was clear that there were no significant differences between the standard and intensive treated group with the respect to cardiovascular outcomes. This led many guideline agencies to change the blood pressure goals for diabetic patients from less than 130/80 to less than 140/80 or less than 140/90. But it is important to understand the inclusion criteria for the study. As stated in the study, participants were eligible if they had type 2 diabetes mellitus and a glycated hemoglobin level of 7.5% or more and were 40 years of age or older with cardiovascular disease or 55 years of age or older with anatomical evidence of a substantial amount of atherosclerosis, albuminuria, left ventricular hypertrophy, or at least two additional risk factors for cardiovascular disease (dyslipidemia, hypertension, smoking, or obesity). Exclusion criteria included a body mass index of more than 45, a serum creatinine level of more than 1.5 mg per deciliter (132.6 μmol/L), and other serious illness. Thus, the participants were at the high-risk for cardiac outcomes and did not have significant kidney disease. Hence, these results are certainly meaningful for people older than 40 are at high-risk for cardiovascular disease but do not reflect goals for those without cardiovascular disease and those with other complications such as kidney disease or retinopathy.

At about the same time the INVEST study was published.[10] As noted in the article, participants in this study received first-line treatment of either a calcium channel blocker or β-blocker followed by ACEI, a diuretic, or both to achieve systolic blood pressure of less than 130 mm Hg and a diastolic blood pressure of less than 85 mm Hg. Patients were categorized as having tight control if they could maintain their systolic blood pressure at less than 130 mm Hg, usual control if it ranged from 130 mm Hg to less than 140 mm Hg, and uncontrolled if it was 140 mm Hg or higher. All participants had hypertension and coronary artery disease. As in the ACCORD study, there was no cardiovascular benefit from having blood pressure less than 130/85. The clear strengths of these studies are that for those people with diabetes, hypertension, and cardiac disease and there was no benefit of blood pressure control lower than 135 to 140/80–85. These studies do not address what is the best blood pressure to prevent the development of diabetic complications. Nor do they address the best blood pressure control for those with retinopathy and/or kidney disease. Indeed many people with diabetes mellitus may well have a combination of complications and are certainly at risk for all complications. So what do other studies report?

First of all the ACCORD study did report a very significant reduction in all stroke and in nonfatal stroke in participants in the intensively treated group (those with mean systolic blood pressure of about 119 mm Hg). Similar results have been found from other studies with respect to stroke. Hence, it certainly can be argued that lower blood pressures are protective against stroke.

People with diabetic kidney disease also have potentially different blood pressure targets. The Randomized Olmesartan and Diabetes Microalbuminuria Prevention (ROADMAP) was a study intended to show that the angiotensin receptor blocker (ARB) olmesartan was a protective against the development of microalbuminuria.[11] Indeed participants treated with olmesartan did have significantly lower rates of the development of microalbuminuria. But of greater importance was the blood pressure of less than 130/80 that was achieved in the treated group. The more likely explanation is that blood pressure control prevented the development of microalbuminuria rather than a specific effect of the ARB, as other ARB studies where blood pressure was controlled in both groups or the initial blood pressures were already well controlled did not show a unique benefit for the ARB in preventing the development of microalbuminuria. But it does point to the idea that a blood pressure of less than 130/80 helps to protect against the development of microalbuminuria. For those with established diabetic kidney disease (as defined as persistent elevated urine albumin level and bland urinalysis in a person with diabetes), a number of studies suggest that atleast less than 140/80 should be the goal for those with proteinuria (a urine albumin/creatinine ratio > 300 mg/g) likely less than 130/80 is the goal. A recent analysis of the Veterans Affairs Nephropathy in Diabetes (VA NEPHRON-D) study was initially done to determine whether combined ACEI and ARB was better than either alone.[12] Blood pressure levels were analyzed with the respect to decline in glomerular filtration rate (GFR). Less than 140/80 clearly showed a highly significant improvement slowing the rate of decline in the estimated glomerular filtration rate (eGFR). There was a strong trend to even more improvement in eGFR with lower blood pressures. Moreover, another recent meta-analysis[13] has suggested that blood pressure is atleast less than 140/80 and possibly less than 130/80 is indicated for optimal outcomes.

Lastly a recent Cochrane review analyzed multiple studies with respect to retinopathy.[14] Their conclusions were that there is a good evidence for intensive blood pressure control to prevent the development of retinopathy but less good evidence as to what is the goal of blood pressure for those with established retinopathy.

So, what should the ideal blood pressure goal be? Everyone agrees on less than 140/80 or less than 140/90. All of the large studies suggest that this goal is what is needed to reduce cardiac events although not stroke events. So, why not make 130/80 the goal? There are few reasons guidelines committees have not selected this goal: (1) The best and largest studies have focused on cardiac outcomes. There have not been similarly large, randomized controlled studies for the other complications. So, with the lack of large studies, the committees have decided to select less than 140/80 as the goal; (2) It takes multiple medications to achieve 130/80. So convenience, cost, and side effects become an important management issue. So, why add more medications if the benefit is not definite?; and (3) Lower blood pressures have been associated with worse outcomes for those people with diabetes mellitus and cardiac disease. For example, further analysis of the INVEST study showed that cardiac deaths increased when the systolic blood pressure was less than 115 mm Hg.[10] Hence, it seems that a systolic blood pressure of less than 115 mm Hg is a risk factor for those people who are at a high-risk for a cardiovascular event.

Considering everything the following conclusions may be drawn: With respect to stroke, kidney disease, and retinopathy it appears that the blood pressure closer to 130/80 is likely beneficial, and that there appears to be no increased risk for those people who are at high-risk for a cardiovascular event at this level. So, it may be best to aim for a blood pressure of 130/80 rather than a goal of less than 140/80. The reasons behind this recommendation are as follows: (1) All of the cardiovascular studies showed benefits in the 130–140 systolic range. The benefits with lower levels than this were not clearly better; (2) This range of blood pressure appears to be at an ideal level for all possible diabetic complications; (3) The risk for worse cardiovascular outcomes did not occur until the systolic blood pressure was less than 115–120 mm Hg; and (4) For psychological reasons, when physicians use a goal of less than 140/80, many use the 140/80 as the mean not as the upper limit such that a number of patients may well have blood pressures somewhat higher than 140/80. Hence, for purely psychological motivation for physicians and the patient, 130/80 is an ideal level that may provide the appropriate motivation to achieve the best outcomes.

A few other studies deserve comment. The United States Joint National Committee 8 (JNC 8) blood pressure guidelines were released in 2014.[15] The guidelines suggested that less than 140/90 was the goal for all (including those with diabetes mellitus) except in people older than 60 years old and without diabetes mellitus, less than 150/90 was the goal. The entire guideline was greeted with considerable controversy including by a minority of the committee members who wrote a dissenting report. In general the dissenters thought that the committee blood pressure guidelines are too high. The committee defended its report by stating that they included only large, randomized controlled studies. And as there are many blood pressure goals yet to be clearly determined, the committee could not make recommendations to use lower goals. Recently the Systolic Blood Pressure Intervention Trial (SPRINT) study has been published.[16] SPRINT studied 9,361 persons older than 50 years old with a systolic blood pressure of 130 mm Hg or higher and an increased cardiovascular risk to a systolic blood pressure target of less than

120 mm Hg (intensive treatment) or a target of less than 140 mm Hg (standard treatment). The primary composite outcome was myocardial infarction, other acute coronary syndromes, stroke, heart failure, or death from cardiovascular causes. The study clearly showed that a systolic blood pressure of less than 120 mm Hg had significant beneficial effects. This study will clearly affect the next JNC guidelines. Of note though, people with diabetes mellitus were excluded from the study. A recent analysis of this according to study using SPRINT criteria showed beneficial effects of lower blood pressure in people with diabetes. Lastly, does older age affect blood pressure goals? There is no definite answer, but a trial in the very elderly (defined as > 80 years old) where blood pressure was lowered to less than 150/80 from a systolic blood pressure of more than 160 mm Hg showed highly significant improvement in the heart failure and improvement in survival.[17] Whether even lower blood pressure is better remains to be determined.

TREATMENT

There are many studies comparing classes of drugs and specific drugs in people with diabetes mellitus with/without complications. Many of these studies are directed to specific drugs usually with the hope that a particular drug or class of drugs will show a specific benefit in patients with diabetes. Considering the often specific focus of these studies, it is best to use these reports as guideposts but not directives as to what drug to use or not to use. The physician needs to apply clinical judgment and individualized treatment. The choice of blood pressure medications for people with diabetes should follow the basic mechanistic understanding from physiology that the blood pressure level is equal to the heart rate × stroke volume × vascular peripheral resistance (Flowchart 12.1). Antihypertensive medications can be classified into each of these categories. In general, physiology leads to maintaining steady state. Hence, the addition of a medication from a specific class may result in a response from another mechanism to maintain steady state. For example, addition of a medicine that causes vasodilation will lead to a compensatory increase in the heart rate or sodium reabsorption to maintain the blood pressure. So, if a single medication is ineffective in lowering the blood pressure, it is most rational to select a medicine from another mechanistic category (e.g. vasodilator and diuretic or beta blocker). Using this structure, one can rationally choose medicines based on a mechanistic rationale. In addition to

Flowchart 12.1: Mechanistic approach to treatment.

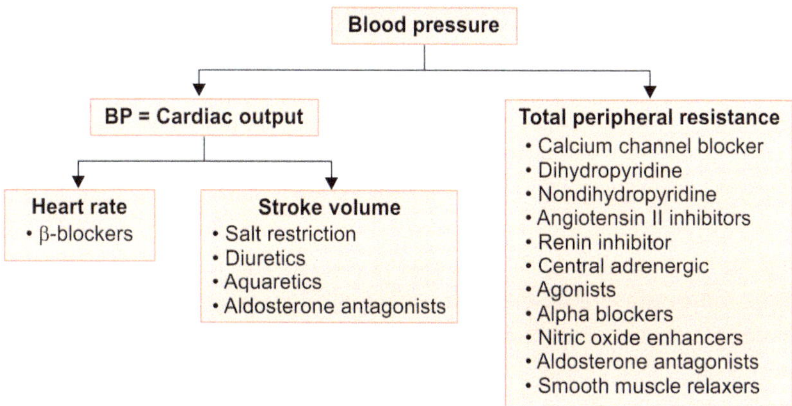

Table 12.1: Possible indications for specific drug classes.

Conditions	***Drug class***
Heart failure	ACEI/ARB, BB, CCB, and spironolactone
Post MI/clinical CAD	ACEI/ARB, BB
CAD	ACEI/ARB, BB, diuretic, and CCB
Diabetes	ACEI/ARB, CCB, and diuretic
CKD	ACEI/ARB
Recurrent stroke prevention	ACEI, diuretic

(ACEI: angiotensin converting enzyme inhibitor; ARB: angiotensin receptor blocker; BB: beta blocker; CAD: coronary artery disease; CCB: calcium channel blocker; CKD: chronic kidney disease; MI: myocardial infarction).
Source: Adapted from James PA, Oparil S, Carter BL, et al. 2014 evidence-based guideline for the management of high blood pressure in adults: report from the panel members appointed to the Eighth Joint National Committee (JNC 8). JAMA. 2014;311(5):507-20.

this basic mechanistic approach, there are other aspects that need to be considered, including cost, convenience, efficacy, side effects, and comorbid conditions (Table 12.1). This rationale is applicable to anyone with hypertension.

Many guidelines suggest that an ACEI or ARB should be the initial drug used to treat hypertension in people with diabetes mellitus. Indeed a large number of studies have determined that people with diabetes have activation of the renin-angiotensin-aldosterone system (RAAS). Activation of the RAAS is associated with worse cardiovascular and kidney outcomes. Hence, the recommendation to use an ACEI or an ARB, in general, is logical. But, in practice, an individualized approach is best. If the patient's starting blood pressure is well above the goal of 130/80, perhaps starting with the medicine most likely to lower the blood pressure most effectively is indicated. For example, dihydropyridine calcium channel blockers are often very effective antihypertensive medications and usually more effective for lowering the blood pressure as compared to RAAS inhibitors. It may be more logical to start with one of these medications first then add an ACEI or ARB as a second or third-line drug. In other words, lowering the blood pressure is the first and most important goal and inhibiting a specific mechanism for increased blood pressure is a secondary goal. In addition to the blood pressure level, comorbidities, past medical and family history, and other medications should all be taken into account when choosing the next medication or to increase a specific medication. Such factors as risk for or history of cardiac disease, stroke, and kidney disease will all inform the decision-making. Current clinical factors such as edema, serum potassium level, serum creatinine level, and drug interactions all need to be taken into account. In total, the blood pressure studies have definitely shown the great importance of controlling blood pressure to maintain and improve health. Of course there are studies showing a unique benefit for particular classes of drugs for particular conditions such as beta blockers for people with myocardial infarction or RAAS inhibitors for people with proteinuria (Table 12.1) but blood pressure control is of paramount importance and the specific indications for a particular comorbidity is a secondary concern.

Other factors in controlling blood pressure are diet, weight loss, and exercise. There is no question that all of these will improve blood pressure and should be the part of any antihypertensive regimen. Diet is not only important for weight loss but also for salt intake.

In general, about 50% of people are salt sensitive, i.e. the intake of salt leads to increased the blood pressure. Considering this high percentage, it makes sense for most patients to restrict salt intake (<2,000 mg/day or possibly even lower).[18] Certainly anyone taking a diuretic need to restrict salt intake or the person will increase the salt intake to counteract the diuretic effect. Hence, education on salt intake needs to be done for all patients with hypertension. There has also been much interest in whether specific diets are particularly beneficial in lowering the blood pressure. The Dietary Approaches to Stop Hypertension (DASH) diet has been touted as being particularly beneficial. A recent meta-analysis review of 17 randomized controlled studies reported that the DASH diet, Nordic diet, and Mediterranean diet significantly lowered systolic blood pressure and diastolic blood pressure by 4.26 mm Hg and 2.38 mm Hg, respectively. The authors noted that these diets are rich in fruit, vegetables, whole grains, legumes, seeds, nuts, fish, and dairy and low in meat, sweets, and alcohol.[19] These effects are modest but significant. Diet in combination with weight loss and exercise will lead to even greater decrease in the blood pressure.

Lastly, there has been much interest as to whether specific medications are particularly effective or ineffective in certain ethnic or racial groups. Perhaps this has been best studied in African-Americans. Studies have shown that, in general, African-Americans have less of a response to RAAS inhibitors as compared to others. But these studies have led some to think that these medications are not effective in African-Americans. This is clearly not the case.[20] And although some African-Americans may not respond as well to RAAS inhibition, the utility of RAAS inhibition for cardiac and renal outcomes appears to be seen in African-Americans as well as others. So at this time, one might not want to use RAAS inhibition as a first-line agent in African-Americans but will likely add one of them as a second or third-line medication. Individualized approaches should be done as previously described but less for ethnic or racial reasons. In the future, personalized medicine (may be guided by genomic findings) may lead to insights into which drugs are best for an individual patient.

PRIMARY HYPERALDOSTERONISM AND RENAL ARTERY STENOSIS (BOX 12.3)

Secondary causes of hypertension need to be considered in patients with diabetes mellitus. Of course, any evaluation for a secondary cause of hypertension may includes searching for hyperthyroidism, pheochromocytoma, and hypercortisolism. But the most common causes of

Box 12.3: Secondary causes of hypertension.

- *Reasons to suspect one of the two main secondary causes:*
  - Persistent low or low normal serum potassium
  - Five or more medications needed to control the blood pressure.
- *Primary hyperaldosteronism:*
  - Trial of spironolactone or eplerenone is usually sufficient
  - *Diagnosis*—High serum aldosterone and low renin level. Usually needs to be measured in a controlled setting (stable salt intake, at rest, and stable body position).
- *Renal artery stenosis*—It usually does not need to be diagnosed as medical management is as effective as surgical management.

secondary hypertension in diabetic patients are primary hyperaldosteronism[21] and renal artery stenosis. The most significant sign to be aware of is a low normal or low potassium. This is due to the effect of persistently increased aldosterone causing potassium loss in the urine. Indeed in patients with diabetes it is common to have elevated potassium because most patients are on an ACEI or ARB. In addition some diabetic patients have hyporenin, hypoaldosterone renal tubular acidosis (type 4 RTA) that also leads to elevated serum potassium. The definitive diagnosis of hyperaldosteronism then may be problematic. In primary hyperaldosteronism serum studies should reveal low renin and high aldosterone levels. But random measurements are often not diagnostic as renin and aldosterone are affected by many factors such as salt intake, upright or supine position, diuretics, and by other RAAS inhibitors. So, definitive diagnosis may require carefully controlling conditions and then measuring serum renin and aldosterone levels. In practice, though a trial of an aldosterone antagonist is the best way to determine a role for hyperaldosteronism. Indeed there is a growing interest in using aldosterone antagonists for many patients with diabetes mellitus as studies suggest that aldosterone antagonism significantly improves the cardiac and renal outcomes.

Searching for renal artery stenosis is of less importance as studies have shown that medical management is as effective as surgical management.[22] There is no documented evidence for surgical revascularization to protect the renal function as well. Hence, the main reason to refer a patient for surgical intervention is to decrease the number of medications a person needs to take or rarely to treat uncontrolled hypertension.

FINAL RECOMMENDATIONS

- Aim for blood pressure of 130/80.
- Avoid systolic blood pressure of less than 120 mm Hg.
- Start with the antihypertensive medication that will be most effective to reach blood pressure goal. Although choosing an RAAS inhibitor is reasonable for many patients.
- Choose antihypertensive medications is based on mechanistic rationale (stroke volume, heart rate, or vascular resistance) and for effectiveness, cost, convenience, and comorbidities.
- Most patients will require an RAAS inhibitor at some point.
- Weight loss and exercise as indicated.
- Decrease salt intake (<2,000 mg/day).
- Dietary changes as indicated. Consider using specific diet such as DASH.
- Search for secondary causes of hypertension (primary hyperaldosteronism or renal artery stenosis) if persistent low serum potassium levels and/or on five or more medications needed to control blood pressure.

CONCLUSION

Blood pressure control is of paramount performance in diabetes. The clinician needs to be sure that the measurement of blood pressure is done accurately and often enough to obtain enough information so that optimal treatments can be started. Home blood pressure monitoring is best as long as the patient is well trained. Lifestyle and medication treatment needs to be tailored to the individual patient. There is no one algorithm that fits everyone.

REFERENCES

1. Agarwal R. Home and ambulatory blood pressure monitoring in chronic kidney disease. Curr Opin Nephrol Hypertens. 2009;18(6):507-12.
2. Cohen DL, Huan Y, Townsend RR. Home blood pressure monitoring in CKD. Am J Kidney Dis. 2014;63(5):835-42.
3. Drawz PE, Abdalla M, Rahman M. Blood pressure measurement: clinic, home, ambulatory, and beyond. Am J Kidney Dis. 2012;60(3):449-62.
4. Margolis KL, Asche SE, Bergdall AR, et al. Effect of home blood pressure telemonitoring and pharmacist management on blood pressure control: a cluster randomized clinical trial. JAMA. 2013;310(1):46-56.
5. Bangalore S, Kumar S, Lobach I, et al. Blood pressure targets in subjects with type 2 diabetes mellitus/impaired fasting glucose: observations from traditional and bayesian random-effects meta-analyses of randomized trials. Circulation. 2011;123(24):2799-810.
6. Ettehad D, Emdin CA, Kiran A, et al. Blood pressure lowering for prevention of cardiovascular disease and death: a systematic review and meta-analysis. Lancet. 2016;387(10022):957-67.
7. Grossman E, Messerli FH. Management of blood pressure in patients with diabetes. Am J Hypertens. 2011;24(8):863-75.
8. Volpe M, Tocci G. Redefining blood pressure targets in high-risk patients?: lessons from coronary endpoints in recent randomized clinical trials. Am J Hypertens. 2011;24(10):1060-8.
9. Group AS, Cushman WC, Evans GW, et al. Effects of intensive blood-pressure control in type 2 diabetes mellitus. N Engl J Med. 2010;362(17):1575-85.
10. Cooper-DeHoff RM, Gong Y, Handberg EM, et al. Tight blood pressure control and cardiovascular outcomes among hypertensive patients with diabetes and coronary artery disease. JAMA. 2010;304(1):61-8.
11. Haller H, Ito S, Izzo JL, et al. Olmesartan for the delay or prevention of microalbuminuria in type 2 diabetes. N Engl J Med. 2011;364(10):907-17.
12. Leehey DJ, Zhang JH, Emanuele NV, et al. BP and renal outcomes in diabetic kidney disease: The Veterans Affairs Nephropathy in Diabetes Trial. Clin J Am Soc Nephrol. 2015;10(12):2159-69.
13. Emdin CA, Rahimi K, Neal B, et al. Blood pressure lowering in type 2 diabetes: a systematic review and meta-analysis. JAMA. 2015;313(6):603-15.
14. Do DV, Wang X, Vedula SS, et al. Blood pressure control for diabetic retinopathy. Cochrane Database Syst Rev. 2015;1:CD006127.
15. James PA, Oparil S, Carter BL, et al. 2014 evidence-based guideline for the management of high blood pressure in adults: report from the panel members appointed to the Eighth Joint National Committee (JNC 8). JAMA. 2014;311(5):507-20.
16. Group SR, Wright JT, Williamson JD, et al. A randomized trial of intensive versus standard blood-pressure control. N Engl J Med. 2015;373(22):2103-16.
17. Beckett NS, Peters R, Fletcher AE, et al. Treatment of hypertension in patients 80 years of age or older. N Engl J Med. 2008;358(18):1887-98.
18. Whelton PK, Appel LJ, Sacco RL, et al. Sodium, blood pressure, and cardiovascular disease: further evidence supporting the American Heart Association sodium reduction recommendations. Circulation. 2012;126(24):2880-9.
19. Ndanuko RN, Tapsell LC, Charlton KE, et al. Dietary patterns and blood pressure in adults: a systematic review and meta-analysis of randomized controlled trials. Adv Nutr. 2016;7(1):76-89.
20. Williams SF, Nicholas SB, Vaziri ND, et al. African Americans, hypertension and the renin angiotensin system. World J Cardiol. 2014;6(9):878-89.
21. Umpierrez GE, Cantey P, Smiley D, et al. Primary aldosteronism in diabetic subjects with resistant hypertension. Diabetes Care. 2007;30(7):1699-703.
22. Cooper CJ, Murphy TP, Cutlip DE, et al. Stenting and medical therapy for atherosclerotic renal artery stenosis. N Engl J Med. 2014;370:13-22.

CHAPTER 13

Nonalcoholic Fatty Liver Disease in Diabetes

Karunakaran Indulekha, Ranjit Mohan Anjana, Ranjit Unnikrishnan, Viswanathan Mohan

INTRODUCTION

Nonalcoholic fatty liver disease (NAFLD) is defined as hepatic steatosis and a spectrum of other liver abnormalities and lesions resembling that of alcoholic liver disease, but occurring in individuals not consuming excess alcohol.[1] Although this syndrome was first recognized more than 2 decades ago,[1] its clinical significance has been appreciated only in recent years. A majority of cases of NAFLD are attributed to insulin resistance although other less common causes like drugs, parental nutrition, and inborn errors of metabolism are known to contribute to the pathogenesis.[2] The prevalence of NAFLD in Western nations is around 20–30% and it is now a common problem in Asia as well, owing to the twin epidemics of diabetes and obesity.[3-5] The first report from South Asia by Mohan et al. showed that the prevalence of NAFLD was 32%. This study highlighted the fact that one-third of the general population and half of the type 2 diabetes population of urban India had NAFLD which was significantly associated with diabetes even after adjusting for the confounding effect of several cardiometabolic risk factors.[6] The prevalence of NAFLD among type 1 diabetes subjects has also been reported recently. A South Indian study has shown that 27.7% patients with type 1 diabetes had NAFLD.[7] Owing to lifestyle changes like sedentary behavior and westernized diets, NAFLD has become a global health problem with increasing incidence every year and at younger ages.[8] NAFLD has also been shown to be the most important cause of 'cryptogenic' cirrhosis leading to hepatocellular carcinoma.[9]

CAUSES OF NONALCOHOLIC FATTY LIVER DISEASE

Obesity and dyslipidemia: When intake of calories exceeds the rate of expenditure, obesity ensues. Obese subjects show a high prevalence of NAFLD. In the general population, although the prevalence of NAFLD is 20% and that of nonalcoholic steatohepatitis (NASH) is 3%, the prevalence may go up to 75% in obese subjects.[10] In case of morbidly obese subjects, a 77% prevalence of steatosis has been observed.[11] Increased serum triglycerides, small low-density lipoproteins (LDL), and decreased high-density lipoprotein (HDL) cholesterol levels are common in NAFLD. Hepatic overproduction of very low-density lipoproteins (VLDLs) and defective clearance of circulating lipoproteins have been implicated as the major reasons for dyslipidemia in NAFLD.[12] Visceral fat measured by computed tomography (CT) was found to be significantly associated with NAFLD assessed by liver biopsies and increased visceral adipose tissue area also predicted fibrosis.[13]

- *Type 2 diabetes mellitus:* 50–75% of individuals with type 2 diabetes demonstrate increased fat accumulation in the liver. It has also been proved that NAFLD diagnosed with increased alanine transaminase (ALT) levels predicts the development of diabetes in longitudinal studies.[14] Also diabetes is a well-known risk factor for NASH as hyperglycemic individuals were shown to have a 2.6-fold increased steatohepatitis risk.[15] Evidence also shows that NAFLD patients with type 2 diabetes are at increased risk of progressive forms of liver disease and cirrhosis as compared to patients without diabetes.[16] In patients with NAFLD and type 2 diabetes liver failure may also be a major cause of mortality apart from cardiovascular diseases.[17]
- *Genetics:* Apolipoprotein C3 (APOC3) is a protein component of VLDL which is involved in the regulation of lipid distribution to different tissues and organs. Two gene variants C-482T/T-455C present in the APOC3 gene promoter result in the loss of insulin's inhibitory effect on APOC3.[18] This in turn enhances the levels of plasma of APOC3 and hypertriglyceridemia. In a population of healthy male lean Asian Indians, these gene variations increased the risk of developing insulin resistance and NAFLD.[19] Subjects with these polymorphisms show 30% higher circulating levels of APOC3 and also demonstrate postprandial hypertriglyceridemia as compared to controls.[20] Perilipin-1 is an abundant protein found in adipose tissue that regulates hydrolytic enzymes of tri- and diacylglycerols (DAGs). Frameshift mutations of the *Perilipin-1* gene have been found to be associated with hepatic steatosis, increased triglyceride levels, and type 2 diabetes mellitus.[21] Variants of patatin-like phospholipase domain-containing protein 3 (PNPLA 3) gene abundant in the lipid droplets have been found to be associated with a higher risk of developing NAFLD.[22]

TRENDS IN THE COEXISTENCE OF NONALCOHOLIC FATTY LIVER DISEASE AND DIABETES IN INDIA

Several studies on the Asian Indian population have shown that the prevalence of NAFLD diagnosed by ultrasonography varies from 9% to 35%. Community-based epidemiological data from rural parts of West Bengal show a prevalence of 9%.[23] On the other hand, urban areas like Mumbai report a prevalence of 16.6%.[24] Our study in Chennai reported a prevalence of 32%.[6] A hospital-based report from Cuttack has documented a prevalence of 24.5%.[25]

Nonalcoholic fatty liver disease and type 2 diabetes share a close association. Compared to the general population, NAFLD prevalence is higher in the diabetes and obese subjects since insulin resistance is the central mechanism involved in both the diseases.[26] In an Asian Indian cohort of type 2 diabetes mellitus (T2DM) patients, 87% had NAFLD on liver biopsy.[27] In another report, 88% of patients with T2DM who were non-alcoholics showed fatty liver on ultrasound.[28] In a recent report by Praveenraj et al.[29] in a cohort of morbidly obese subjects with an average body mass index (BMI) of 44 kg/m^2, 65.7% patients had NAFLD, 33.6% had NASH and fibrosis was present in 31.3% subjects. In a report from Mumbai, 49% of T2DM patients had fatty liver among which 65.5%, 12.5%, and 9.35% patients showed mild, moderate, and severe

NAFLD respectively. Further, 21.8% patients recorded fibrosis.[26] In 2013, Kalra et al.[30] assessed the prevalence of NAFLD based on the National Health and Nutrition Examination Survey (NHANES) III criteria of increased aminotransferase levels in a group of 924 subjects from 101 cities. In this study, 56.5% of T2DM subjects had NAFLD and the prevalence was observed to be higher in females (60%) compared to males (54.3%). The NAFLD prevalence was also found to vary from 44% in West India to 72% in North India.[30] In the light of the recent reports on the nationwide prevalence of diabetes and assuming that at least 50% of those with diabetes might be at significant risk of NAFLD, the actual prevalence of NAFLD might be quite large.[31]

PATHOGENESIS OF NONALCOHOLIC FATTY LIVER DISEASE

Two-hit Hypothesis

The pathogenesis and severity of NAFLD are intricately associated with the risk factors of insulin resistance and metabolic syndrome. The association between NAFLD and insulin resistance is complex and the underlying pathological mechanisms are not fully elucidated. The 'two-hit' hypothesis of NAFLD pathogenesis states that the first hit involves fat accumulation in hepatocytes that mediates a variety of metabolic derangements leading to obesity and insulin resistance.[32] This in turn leads to increased free fatty acid (FFA) delivery to the liver which in combination with an impaired fatty acid metabolism culminates in net triglyceride accumulation in the liver. Fat accumulation in the liver has been shown to aggravate insulin resistance by inhibiting the insulin receptor substrate phosphorylation[33] and microsomal cytochrome CYP2E1 increase.[34] These changes lead to a potential vicious cycle wherein insulin resistance causes fat accumulation in the liver and vice versa. Steatosis progresses to steatohepatitis and oxidative stress is believed to be the key second hit in this progression. This involves the peroxidation of the lipids accumulated in the hepatocytes due to reactive oxygen species (ROS) generation and CYP2E1 induction.[35] Other factors involved in disease progression include hepatic inflammation mediated by proinflammatory cytokine release from visceral adipose tissue and reduced secretion of anti-inflammatory cytokines like adiponectin.[36,37]

Subsequent development of fibrosis and cirrhosis involves interactions between lipid accumulated hepatocytes, inflammatory cells, Kupffer cells, and hepatic stellate cells (HSCs). Profibrogenic cytokines like interleukin-10 (IL-10) and transforming growth factor-beta (TGF-beta) are important mediators of fibrogenesis.[38] The hepatic venules can also be occluded by lipid-laden hepatocytes leading to parenchymal collapse and fibrosis.[39]

It has now been proposed that NAFLD is a result of parallel multiple-hits. Insulin resistance leads to increased lipogenesis and FFA uptake. This in turn sensitizes the liver to oxidative damage with activation of HSCs, fibrogenic pathways and adipokine secretion leading to fibrosis.[40]

LIVER INSULIN RESISTANCE AND NONALCOHOLIC FATTY LIVER DISEASE

Fatty acid input to the liver is facilitated by the means of plasma FFA uptake and esterification to triglycerides, whereas fatty acid output is via its oxidation and secretion. When the rate of fatty acid input exceeds fatty acid output, steatosis develops. The close association between insulin resistance and NAFLD can be understood from the fact that liver is also the key producer of causative factors of insulin resistance—fasting serum glucose and VLDL which contains circulating triglycerides.[40] In subjects with NAFLD, insulin's ability to suppress glucose and VLDL production is impaired. Hyperglycemia leads to hyperinsulinemia via stimulating excess insulin secretion. High VLDL levels can also lead to low HDL levels and increased atherogenic small dense LDL levels in addition to increased C-reactive protein (CRP) and coagulation factors.[41] Further, it has been demonstrated that liver-specific knockout of insulin receptor leads to hyperglycemia, insulin resistance, and steatosis, whereas muscle and adipose tissue-specific knockout of insulin receptor resulted in normal glucose levels.[42]

In NAFLD patients, there is also a higher rate of de novo lipogenesis which in turn increases intrahepatic triglyceride accumulation and secretion.[43] Reports also suggest that insulin resistance leads to hepatic triglyceride accumulation by diverting the ingested carbohydrates from muscle glycogen storage toward de novo fatty synthesis. Hepatic de novo lipogenesis is regulated by many enzyme complexes and several nuclear transcription factors including sterol regulatory element-binding proteins (SREBPs)[44] and peroxisome proliferator-activated receptors (PPARs). Insulin and glucose further increase hepatic de novo lipogenesis via activation of the transcription factor SREBP-1c which eventually leads to hepatic steatosis.[45]

On the other hand, impaired oxidation of intrahepatocellular fatty acids in mitochondria is also associated with hepatic steatosis. Data from animal models show that hepatic triglyceride content can be regulated by the activation or inhibition of fatty acid oxidation.[46] Deficiencies in the mitochondrial oxidative enzymes can lead to hepatic steatosis and increasing the expression of fatty acid oxidative enzymes can reduce the triglyceride accumulation.[46,47] NAFLD subjects also demonstrate abnormalities in the structure and function of mitochondria including loss of cristae[48] and paracrystalline inclusions[49] and a reduced activity of mitochondrial respiratory chain.[50]

ADIPOSE TISSUE INSULIN RESISTANCE AND NONALCOHOLIC FATTY LIVER DISEASE

Compared to overweight/obese NAFLD patients, fasting plasma glucose and HOMA-IR were lower and HDL cholesterol levels higher among nonobese NAFLD subjects. Adipocytes are involved in the production of over 60–70% of the FFAs utilized for the synthesis of hepatic triglycerides and VLDL secretion.[51] As adipocytes are tight regulators of energy supply, adipocyte hypertrophy is commonly observed during excessive nutrient supply which initiates a pathogenic crosstalk of adipocytes and macrophages. This leads to chronic release of fatty acids which exert harmful effects on other insulin sensitive tissues like liver, pancreas, and also on the heart and vascular system. The exact mechanism of how adipose tissue insulin resistance affects other tissues is yet to be understood completely. Overproduction of FFAs promotes intramyocellular lipid accumulation and formation of toxic lipid metabolites like ceramide and DAG. These metabolites are important activators of the NF-kB pathway that causes inflammation and insulin resistance. Evidence also points to an important role of FFAs in causing insulin resistance via impaired insulin signaling by stimulating hepatic gluconeogenesis and glycogenolysis.[52] The major risk factors involved in NAFLD pathogenesis are summarized in the Flowchart 13.1.

Flowchart 13.1: Major risk factors in the development of NAFLD.

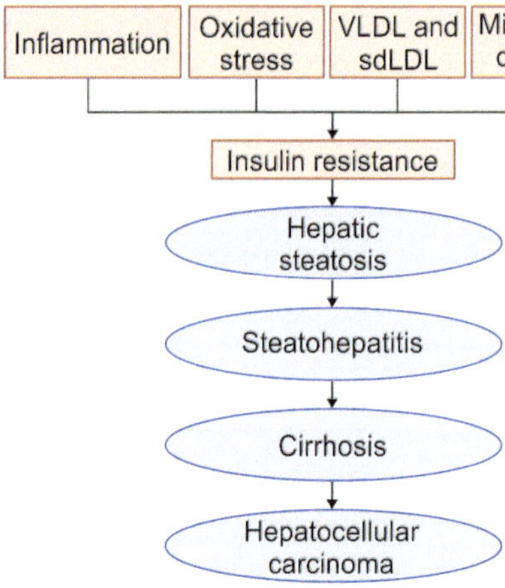

(NAFLD: Nonalcoholic fatty liver disease; sdLDL: Small dense low-density lipoprotein; VLDL: Very low-density lipoprotein)

INFLAMMATION AND OXIDATIVE STRESS LINKING NONALCOHOLIC FATTY LIVER DISEASE AND DIABETES

Oxidative Stress

An imbalance between reactive oxygen and nitrogen species (ROS and RNS) like superoxide, hydroxyl, and hydrogen peroxide and the antioxidant defenses results in oxidative stress.[53] In an Asian Indian cohort, markers of oxidative stress like thiobarbituric acid reactive substances (TBARS) and protein carbonyl content (PCC) levels were significantly elevated and glutathione/glutathione disulfide (GSH/GSSG) ratio was significantly decreased in subjects with diabetes and NAFLD compared to controls.[54] Mitochondria are important sources of ROS as they are the sites of respiratory chain. FFA metabolism occurs via the mitochondrial oxidation and Krebs cycle that produces citrate, a glycolysis inhibitor. During conditions of excess fat storage, FFAs are oxidized in the mitochondria as a compensatory mechanism. Accelerated beta oxidation results in excessive electron flux in the electron transport chain leading to superoxide production and mitochondrial dysfunction.[55] Also mitochondrial deoxyribonucleic acid (DNA) has high susceptibility to oxidative damage owing to the lack of histones and inadequate repair mechanisms which in turn induce somatic mutations and strand breaks. Oxidative damage leads to increased ROS release that can damage other mitochondria and a vicious cycle is created and perpetuated in this manner.[56,57]

Apart from mitochondria, two other organelles, microsomes and peroxisomes, play an important role in fatty acid oxidation and contribute to ROS generation. CYP2E1 is a microsomal enzyme which has been proved to be important for ROS production and therefore liver injury.[58] Another hypothesis states that CYP2E1 induction in fatty liver disease is a means of adaptation to support the inefficient oxidation of fatty acids in the mitochondria or as a consequence of insulin resistance. Superoxide anions and hydrogen peroxide are produced in the endoplasmic reticulum (ER) by the action of cytochrome P450 reductase and monooxygenases. Peroxisomes also serve as rich sources of hydrogen peroxide and are involved in fatty acid oxidation. PPAR-α is the major transcription factor that regulates the expression of the important mitochondrial and peroxisomal beta oxidation enzymes. PPAR-α activation has been shown to be involved in hepatic peroxisomal proliferation and enlargement, a common feature observed in fatty liver patients. The expression of PPAR-α is also increased in experimental murine models of obesity and steatosis.[59]

Inflammation

Adipokines and cytokines secreted by the adipose tissue are the major mediators of inflammation in the liver and adipose tissue. NAFLD is associated with lower serum levels of adiponectin, a predominant anti-inflammatory adipokine independent of conventional cardiovascular risk factors in Asian Indians.[60] Subjects with NAFLD and/or diabetes also had hypoglutathionemia and increased oxidative stress along with hypoadiponectinemia.[61] The degree of liver fibrosis estimated by ultrasound-guided liver biopsy in severe NAFLD cases has been shown to positively correlate with plasma levels of tumor necrosis factor-alpha (TNF-alpha).[62] We have shown that nonspecific inflammatory markers like high-sensitivity C-reactive protein (hsCRP) and leukocyte count increased with increasing severity of NAFLD and were significantly higher in subjects with NAFLD.[63]

Since the Kupffer cells are the resident macrophages in the liver, they are in a unique position to respond to danger signals from the neighboring cells and those reaching the liver through portal circulation. Kupffer cells act via the prominent inflammatory signaling pathways like toll-like receptors (TLRs) and inflammasomes in response to these danger signals. TLRs can recognize a wide array of ligands like saturated fatty acids, endotoxins, and damaged DNA. Signaling via TLRs and inflammasomes results in NF-kB activation and proinflammatory cytokine secretion. TLR inhibition has been shown to suppress liver inflammation and hepatic steatosis and fibrosis.[64] Kupffer cells induce hepatic fibrosis development via inflammasome activation and IL-1 beta secretion.[65] Over a period of time, due to liver injury and organ inflammation, fibrosis of the liver starts to develop. The major characteristic feature of hepatic fibrosis is the activation of HSCs to form a myofibroblastic phenotype and these stellate cells are stimulated by hepatocyte death.[66] HSCs are further activated by ingesting fragments of apoptotic cells and this is evident from the fact that inhibiting apoptosis in the hepatocytes has been shown to suppress hepatic fibrosis.[67] Cytokines like TNF-alpha and IL-1 beta further facilitate the survival and activity of HSC. Stellate cells also express the receptors for TLRs that makes them a potential target for action by endotoxins, fatty acids, and products of dead cells.[68]

DIAGNOSIS, GRADING, AND STAGING OF NONALCOHOLIC FATTY LIVER DISEASE

Nonalcoholic fatty liver disease is diagnosed based on the clinico-pathological criteria of triglyceride accumulation indicated by more than 5% steatotic hepatocytes referred to as hepatocellular steatosis without excess consumption of alcohol (<20 g/day for women and

<30 g/day for men).[69] NAFLD comprises of a spectrum of disorders ranging from simple steatosis to cirrhosis.

Simple steatosis involves the accumulation of fat in the liver and is also called 'pure fatty liver'. The next stage involves *NASH* wherein liver fat accumulation is accompanied by inflammation. *Steatosis accompanied by necroinflammation* (inflammation with necrosis in liver) occurs next followed by *NASH with fibrosis or cirrhosis or both.*[70] Fibrosis occurs as a result of connective tissue formation due to excessive inflammation and cell death. A build-up of connective tissue that obstructs the normal functioning of the liver is called cirrhosis. The final stage in the natural history of NAFLD is the development of *hepatocellular carcinoma* in some cases.

Nonalcoholic fatty liver disease is an asymptomatic disease and diagnosis is based on the incidental observation of abnormal liver enzymes or steatosis on imaging.[71] Although an abnormal liver function test (LFT) with raised ALT, aspartate transaminase (AST), and/or gamma-glutamyl transferase is used for diagnostic purposes, ALT is observed to fall during the progression from fibrosis to cirrhosis. Hence, ALT values are considered to be poor correlates of NAFLD diagnosis.[72] It is of importance to note that the above mentioned histologic features of NAFLD are also evident in nonobese patients and in those with normal liver enzyme levels.[73]

In an attempt to tackle the growing need for standardizing the histological criteria for NASH diagnosis, the first system for grading and staging was introduced in 1999.[74] In this method, grading was done based on the following core pathological features that contribute to the severity of the disease: (i) Steatosis, (ii) Hepatocyte ballooning that involves cellular injury, wherein hepatocytes appear enlarged and swollen, (iii) Lobular inflammation referring to acute as well as chronic infiltration of inflammatory lymphocytes, macrophages, and monocytes within the sinusoids, and (iv) Portal inflammation which is usually chronic and is characterized by the presence of neutrophil infiltration in the portal and periportal regions.

Staging of the disease was done on the basis of the pattern of fibrosis and its evolution. Stage 1 comprises of the involvement of zone 3 perisinusoidal spaces, stage 2 involves portal and/or periportal fibrosis development, and stage 3 incorporates bridging fibrosis and stage 4 involves cirrhosis (Table 13.1). In 2005, another scoring system was developed by NASH Clinical Research Network (CRN), and the National Institute of Diabetes and Digestive and Kidney Diseases (NIDDK) which are most widely used in current practice. The major advantage of the NASH-CRN system is that it assigns a numerical score for grading and also incorporates a NAFLD activity score (NAS) for comparing biopsies in trials before and after treatment. NAS is derived from combining the individual scores for lobular inflammation, hepatocyte ballooning, and steatosis that ranges from 0 to 8 as described in Table 13.1.[75]

However, despite their wide implementation in clinical practice and therapeutic trials there are several shortcomings associated with these scoring systems. For instance, care should be exercised to differentiate hepatocyte ballooning from glycogen rich swollen hepatocytes, a common pattern observed in type 1 diabetes.[75] Since sampling is critical for grading of NASH, there are also several sampling issues associated with diagnosis and grading.[76] Variations in fibrosis and parenchymal injury in different liver regions are quite common. Owing to these variations, there is a fair chance that the actual stage of fibrosis may not be properly assessed from biopsy specimens especially if they are from suboptimal regions.[70] Also, differential diagnosis of NASH and NAFLD with other liver diseases might be complicated due to the fact that liver

Table 13.1: Staging and grading of nonalcoholic steatohepatitis (NASH).

NASH scoring system by Brunt et al.[74]

	Steatosis	*Ballooning*	*Inflammation*	
	1- ≤33% 2- 33–66% 3- ≥66%	(Zonal location and severity)	Lobular 0- Absent 1- <2 2- 2–4 3- >4 foci	Portal 0- Absent 1- Mild 2- Moderate 3- Severe
Grade 1	1–2	Minimal zone 3	1–2	0–1
Grade 2	2–3	Present zone 3	1–2	1–2
Grade 3	2–3	Marked, predominantly zone 3	3	1–2

Fibrosis stages:
1: Zone 3 perisinusoidal fibrosis, focal or extensive
2: Stage 1 with focal or extensive periportal fibrosis
3: Bridging fibrosis
4: Cirrhosis, probable or definite.

Clinical Research Network system for scoring activity and fibrosis in nonalcoholic fatty liver disease*[75]

Steatosis grade (S)	***Lobular inflammation (L)***	***Hepatocyte ballooning (B)***
0: <5%	0: None	0: None
1: 5–33%	1: <2	1: Few ballooned cells
2: 34–66%	2: 2–4	2: Many ballooned cells
3: >66%	3: >4	

Fibrosis stages:
0: None
1: 1a, mild, zone 3 perisinusoidal fibrosis, 1b, moderate, zone 3 perisinusoidal fibrosis, 1c, portal/periportal fibrosis only
2: Zone 3 perisinusoidal fibrosis and portal/periportal fibrosis
3: Bridging fibrosis
4: Cirrhosis, probable or definite.

*Nonalcoholic fatty liver disease activity score: S + L + B (range 0–8).

specimens of hepatitis B infection and primary biliary cirrhosis document the histological features of cirrhosis.[77]

In light of the complicated staging and scoring systems for NAFLD and the inaccuracies associated with these methods, our group has shown that a simple risk score based on waist circumference, age, physical activity, and family history of diabetes could identify individuals at the high-risk of developing NAFLD. This score called the Indian Diabetes Risk Score (IDRS) was originally developed for identifying subjects with type 2 diabetes. Later, it was also shown to be significantly associated with NAFLD even after adjusting for various metabolic risk factors.[78] Hence, it could be highly useful as an initial screening tool in the community-based studies and in the developing countries where imaging and liver enzyme tests are expensive for a major section of the population. Subjects with high IDRS are to be referred for other investigations like imaging and ultrasonography.[79]

MANAGEMENT OF NONALCOHOLIC FATTY LIVER DISEASE

Weight Loss

Weight loss of about 7% has been shown to improve NAFLD in a meta-analysis of randomized control trials. However, it should be noted that this target could be achieved only by less than 50% patients.[80] In order to improve necroinflammation in NAFLD, weight loss of up to 10% has been suggested. The Mediterranean pattern of diet is gaining wide attention as it has emerged as a promising option towards resolution and prevention of metabolic syndrome.[81] Severe caloric restriction on the other hand has proved to be harmful as it decompensates liver function leading to NAFLD aggravation.[82]

Physical Activity

Physical activity has been shown to be effective in improving insulin resistance, dyslipidemia, and metabolic syndrome that constitute the major contributors to NAFLD pathogenesis. The Look Action for Health in Diabetes (LOOK-AHEAD) study is a prospective multicenter study comparing caloric restriction combined with at least 175 minutes of moderate aerobic physical activity per week to standard care in a cohort of subjects with diabetes. The study showed significant hepatic fat reduction after 1 year of intervention and a reduced NAFLD incidence in the patients belonging to the intensive lifestyle modification group.[83] Aerobic and endurance exercises still showed improvements in steatosis even if there was no associated weight loss.[84]

Bariatric Surgery

Although NAFLD per se is not an indication for bariatric surgery, weight loss as a result of bariatric surgery has showed improvements in hepatic steatosis, steatohepatitis, and lipid profile.[85,86] Among the various bariatric procedures, gastric bypass has been documented to produce the maximal sustained weight loss.[87] However, due to lack of long-term outcome data on bariatric surgery as a specific treatment option for NAFLD, it cannot be considered as a first-line treatment option at least at the present time.

Pharmacological Options

The medicines used in the management of NAFLD comprise of the standard medications used in the treatment of associated conditions. Metformin has been shown to have variable outcomes and showed temporary improvement of transaminases without any evidence of histologic data.[88] A convincing effect has been demonstrated by pioglitazone. However, relapse of the disease on stopping pioglitazone was noticed suggesting the need of long-term use of the medicine and given the various side effects of pioglitazone like weight gain, edema, heart failure, and fractures, this is not an attractive option.[89] Statins are another class of drugs that showed some beneficial effect on NAFLD. However, their efficacy is yet to be proven using histological outcomes.[90] Also, drugs that target the antioxidant activity and reduce ER stress like vitamin E,[91] ursodeoxycholic acid[92] have shown promise in treating NASH.

CONCLUSION

Nonalcoholic fatty liver disease is a common condition that affects about 30% of the population. If left unattended, it can lead to significant liver complications and metabolic abnormalities including diabetes, cardiovascular risk, and hepatocellular carcinoma. In this regard, accurate diagnosis, grading, and staging are important in identifying the appropriate treatment plan for NAFLD patients. A multidisciplinary approach involving lifestyle changes targeting at weight loss and improving insulin sensitivity and medications aiming at bringing dyslipidemia and hyperglycemia under control could help in reducing the mortality associated with NAFLD. Public health efforts aimed at curbing overnutrition can also decrease the incidence of NAFLD and its associated complications.

REFERENCES

1. Ludwig J, Viggiano TR, McGill DB, et al. Nonalcoholic steatohepatitis: Mayo Clinic experiences with a hitherto unnamed disease. Mayo Clin Proc. 1980;55(7):434-8.
2. Hübscher SG. Histological assessment of non-alcoholic fatty liver disease. Histopathology. 2006;49(5):450-65.
3. Bellentani S, Saccoccio G, Masutti F, et al. Prevalence of and risk factors for hepatic steatosis in Northern Italy. Ann Intern Med. 2000;132(2):112-7.
4. Bellentani S, Bedogni G, Miglioli L, et al. The epidemiology of fatty liver. Eur J Gastroenterol Hepatol. 2004;16(11):1087-93.
5. Bedogni G, Miglioli L, Masutti F, et al. Prevalence of and risk factors for nonalcoholic fatty liver disease: the Dionysos Nutrition and Liver Study. Hepatology. 2005;42(1):44-52.
6. Mohan V, Farooq S, Deepa M, et al. Prevalence of non-alcoholic fatty liver disease in urban south Indians in relation to different grades of glucose intolerance and metabolic syndrome. Diabetes Res Clin Pract. 2009;84(1):84-91.
7. Vendhan R, Amutha A, Anjana RM, et al. Clinical profile of nonalcoholic fatty liver disease among young patients with type 1 diabetes mellitus seen at a diabetes speciality center in India. Endocr Pract. 2014;20(2):1249-57.
8. Zeng Lu, Tang WJ, Yin JJ, et al. Signal transductions and nonalcoholic fatty liver: a mini-review. Int J Clin Exp Med. 2014;7(7):1624-31.
9. Siriwardana RC, Niriella MA, Dassanayake AS, et al. Clinical characteristics and outcome of hepatocellular carcinoma in alcohol related and cryptogenic cirrhosis: a prospective study. Hepatobiliary Pancreat Dis Int. 2015;14(4):401-5.
10. Bellentani S, Scaglioni F, Marino M, et al. Epidemiology of non-alcoholic fatty liver disease. Dig Dis. 2010;28(1):155-61.
11. Qureshi K, Abrams GA. Prevalence of biopsy-proven non-alcoholic fatty liver disease in severely obese subjects without metabolic syndrome. Clin Obes. 2016;6(2):117-23.
12. Chatrath H, Vuppalanchi R, Chalasani N. Dyslipidemia in patients with nonalcoholic fatty liver disease. Semin Liver Dis. 2012;32(1):22-9.
13. Yu SJ, Kim W, Kim D, et al. Visceral obesity predicts significant fibrosis in patients with nonalcoholic fatty liver disease. Medicine (Baltimore). 2015;94(48):e2159.
14. Vozarova B, Stefan N, Lindsay RS, et al. High alanine aminotransferase is associated with decreased hepatic insulin sensitivity and predicts the development of type 2 diabetes. Diabetes. 2002;51(6):1889-95.
15. Wanless IR, Lentz JS. Fatty liver hepatitis (steatohepatitis) and obesity: an autopsy study with analysis of risk factors. Hepatology. 1990;12(5):1106-10.

16. Angulo P, Keach JC, Batts KP, et al. Independent predictors of liver fibrosis in patients with nonalcoholic steatohepatitis. Hepatology. 1999;30(6):1356-62.
17. Younossi ZM, Gramlich T, Matteoni CA, et al. Nonalcoholic fatty liver disease in patients with type 2 diabetes. Clin Gastroenterol Hepatol. 2004;2(3):262-5.
18. Li WW, Dammerman MM, Smith JD, et al. Common genetic variation in the promoter of the human apoCIII gene abolishes regulation by insulin and may contribute to hypertriglyceridemia. J Clin Invest. 1995;96:2601-605.
19. Petersen KF, Dufour S, Hariri A, et al. Apolipoprotein C3 gene variants in nonalcoholic fatty liver disease. N Engl J Med. 2010;362(12):1082-9.
20. Valenti L, Nobili V, Al-Serri A, et al. The APOC3 T-455C and C-482T promoter region polymorphisms are not associated with the severity of liver damage independently of PNPLA3 I148M genotype in patients with nonalcoholic fatty liver. J Hepatol. 2011;55:1409-14.
21. Gandotra S, Lim K, Girousse A, et al. Human frame shift mutations affecting the carboxyl terminus of perilipin increase lipolysis by failing to sequester the adipose triglyceride lipase (ATGL) coactivator AB-hydrolase-containing 5 (ABHD5). J Biol Chem. 2011;286(40):34998-5006.
22. He S, McPhaul C, Li JZ, et al. A sequence variation (I148M) in PNPLA3 associated with nonalcoholic fatty liver disease disrupts triglyceride hydrolysis. J Biol Chem. 2010;285(9):6706-15.
23. Das K, Das K, Mukherjee PS, et al. Nonobese population in a developing country has a high prevalence of nonalcoholic fatty liver and significant liver disease. Hepatology. 2010;51(5):1593-602.
24. Amarapurkar D, Kamani P, Patel N, et al. Prevalence of non-alcoholic fatty liver disease: population based study. Ann Hepatol. 2007;6(3):161-3.
25. Singh SP, Nayak S, Swain M, et al. Prevalence of nonalcoholic fatty liver disease in coastal eastern India: a preliminary ultrasonographic survey. Trop Gastroenterol. 2004;25(2):76-9.
26. Gupte P, Amarapurkar D, Agal S, et al. Non-alcoholic steatohepatitis in type 2 diabetes mellitus. J Gastroenterol Hepatol. 2004;19:854-8.
27. Prashanth M, Ganesh HK, Vima MV, et al. Prevalence of nonalcoholic fatty liver disease in patients with type 2 diabetes mellitus. J Assoc Physicians India. 2009;57:205-10.
28. Duseja A, Bhansali A, Bhadada S, et al. Nonalcoholic fatty liver disease in patients with recent onset type 2 diabetes mellitus. J Gastroenterol Hepatol. 2004;19:A402.
29. Praveenraj P, Gomes RM, Kumar S, et al. Prevalence and predictors of non-alcoholic fatty liver disease in morbidly obese South Indian patients undergoing bariatric surgery. Obes Surg. 2015;25:2078-87.
30. Kalra S, Vithalani M, Gulati G, et al. Study of prevalence of nonalcoholic fatty liver disease (NAFLD) in type 2 diabetes patients in India (SPRINT). J Assoc Physicians India. 2013;61:448-53.
31. Duseja A, Chawla Y. Nonalcoholic fatty liver disease in India—how much? How soon? Trop Gastroenterol. 2005;26:1-3.
32. Day CP, James OF. Steatohepatitis: a tale of two "hits"? Gastroenterology. 1998;114:842-5.
33. Schattenberg JM, Wang Y, Singh R, et al. Hepatocyte CYP2E1 overexpression and steatohepatitis lead to impaired hepatic insulin signaling. J Biol Chem. 2005;280:9887-94.
34. Chitturi S, Farrell GC. Etiopathogenesis of nonalcoholic steatohepatitis. Semin Liver Dis. 2001;21:27-41.
35. Pessayre D, Fromenty B. NASH: a mitochondrial disease. J. Hepatol. 2005;42:928-40.
36. Diehl AM, Li ZP, Lin HZ, et al. Cytokines and the pathogenesis of non-alcoholic steatohepatitis. Gut. 2005;54:303-6.
37. Bugianesi E, McCullough AJ, Marchesini G. Insulin resistance: a metabolic pathway to chronic liver disease. Hepatology. 2005;42:987-1000.
38. Wanless IR, Shiota K. The pathogenesis of nonalcoholic steatohepatitis and other fatty liver diseases: a four-step model including the role of lipid release and hepatic venular obstruction in the progression to cirrhosis. Semin Liver Dis. 2004;24:99-106.

39. Seppala-Lindroos A, Vehkavaara S, Hakkinen AM, et al. Fat accumulation in the liver is associated with defects in insulin suppression of glucose production and serum free fatty acids independent of obesity in normal men. J Clin Endocrinol Metab. 2002;87:3023-8.
40. Lonardo A, Bellentani S, Ratziu V, et al. Insulin resistance in nonalcoholic steatohepatitis: Necessary but not sufficient—Death of a dogma from analysis of therapeutic studies? Expert Rev Gastroenterol Hepatol. 2011;5:279-89.
41. Adiels M, Westerbacka J, Soro-Paavonen A, et al. Acute suppression of VLDL1 secretion rate by insulin is associated with hepatic fat content and insulin resistance. Diabetologia. 2007;50:2356-65.
42. Biddinger SB, Kahn CR. From mice to men: insights into the insulin resistance syndromes. Annu Rev Physiol. 2006;68:123-58.
43. Musso G, Gambino R, Cassader M. Recent insights into hepatic lipid metabolism in non-alcoholic fatty liver disease (NAFLD). Prog Lipid Res. 2009;48:1-26.
44. Shimomura I, Bashmakov Y, Ikemoto S, et al. Insulin selectively increases SREBP-1c mRNA in the livers of rats with streptozotocin-induced diabetes. Proc Natl Acad Sci U S A. 1999;96:13656-61.
45. Shimomura I, Bashmakov Y, Horton JD. Increased levels of nuclear SREBP-1c associated with fatty livers in two mouse models of diabetes mellitus. J Biol Chem. 1999;274:30028-32.
46. Zhang D, Liu ZX, Choi CS, et al. Mitochondrial dysfunction due to long-chain Acyl-CoA dehydrogenase deficiency causes hepatic steatosis and hepatic insulin resistance. Proc Natl Acad Sci U S A. 2007;104:17075-80.
47. Ibdah JA, Perlegas P, Zhao Y, et al. Mice heterozygous for a defect in mitochondrial trifunctional protein develop hepatic steatosis and insulin resistance. Gastroenterology. 2005;128:1381-90.
48. Sanyal AJ, Campbell-Sargent C, Mirshahi F, et al. Nonalcoholic steatohepatitis: association of insulin resistance and mitochondrial abnormalities. Gastroenterology. 2001;120:1183-92.
49. Caldwell SH, Swerdlow RH, Khan EM, et al. Mitochondrial abnormalities in non-alcoholic steatohepatitis. J Hepatol. 1999;31:430-4.
50. Perez-Carreras M, Del Hoyo P, Martin MA, et al. Defective hepatic mitochondrial respiratory chain in patients with nonalcoholic steatohepatitis. Hepatology. 2003;38(4):999-1007.
51. Cusi K. Nonalcoholic fatty liver disease in type 2 diabetes mellitus. Curr Opin Endocrinol Diabetes Obes. 2009;16:141-9.
52. Cusi K. The role of adipose tissue and lipotoxicity in the pathogenesis of type 2 diabetes. Curr Diab Rep. 2010;10(4):306-15.
53. Murphy MP. How mitochondria produce reactive oxygen species. Biochem J. 2009;417:1-13.
54. Narasimhan S, Gokulakrishnan K, Sampathkumar R, et al. Oxidative stress is independently associated with non-alcoholic fatty liver disease (NAFLD) in subjects with and without type 2 diabetes. Clin Biochem. 2010;43:815-21.
55. Matés JM, Segura JA, Alonso FJ, et al. Intracellular redox status and oxidative stress: implications for cell proliferation, apoptosis, and carcinogenesis. Arch Toxicol. 2008;82:273-99.
56. Bogenhagen DF. Repair of mtDNA in vertebrates. Am J Hum Genet. 1999;64:1276-81.
57. Wallace DC, Fan W. Energetics, epigenetics, mitochondrial genetics. Mitochondrion. 2010;10:12-31.
58. Leclercq IA, Farrell GC, Field J, et al. CYP2E1 and CYP4A as microsomal catalysts of lipid peroxides in murine nonalcoholic steatohepatitis. J Clin Invest. 2001;105:1067-75.
59. Vega RB, Huss JM, Kelly DP. The coactivator PGC-1 cooperates with peroxisome proliferator-activated receptor α in the transcriptional control of nuclear genes encoding mitochondrial fatty acid oxidation enzymes. Mol Cell Biol. 2000;20:1868-76.
60. Gokulakrishnan K, Anjana RM, Indulekha K, et al. Association of hypoadiponectinemia with non-alcoholic fatty liver disease in urban south Indians—(CURES-81). Indian J Med Res. 2010;132:271-7.
61. Sandhya N, Gokulakrishnan K, Ravikumar R, et al. Association of hypoadiponectinemia with hypoglutathionemia in NAFLD subjects with and without type 2 diabetes. Dis Markers. 2010;29:213-21.

62. Lesmana CR, Hasan I, Budihusodo U, et al. Diagnostic value of a group of biochemical markers of liver fibrosis in patients with non-alcoholic steatohepatitis. J Dig Dis. 2009;10:201-6.
63. Zhou YJ, Li YY, Nie YQ, et al. Influence of polygenetic polymorphisms on the susceptibility to non-alcoholic fatty liver disease of Chinese people. J Gastroenterol Hepatol. 2010;25:772-7.
64. Spruss A, Kanuri G, Wagnerberger S, et al. Toll-like receptor 4 is involved in the development of fructose-induced hepatic steatosis in mice. Hepatology. 2009;50:1094-104.
65. Strowig T, Henao-Mejia J, Elinav E, et al. Inflammasomes in health and disease. Nature. 2012;481:278-86.
66. Jiang JX, Mikami K, Venugopal S, et al. Apoptotic body engulfment by hepatic stellate cells promotes their survival by the JAK/STAT and Akt/NF-kappaB-dependent pathways. J Hepatol. 2009;51:139-48.
67. Singh R, Wang Y, Xiang Y, et al. Differential effects of JNK1 and JNK2 inhibition on murine steatohepatitis and insulin resistance. Hepatology. 2009;49:87-96.
68. Witek RP, Stone WC, Karaca FG, et al. Pan-caspase inhibitor VX-166 reduces fibrosis in an animal model of nonalcoholic steatohepatitis. Hepatology. 2009;50:1421-30.
69. Burt AD, Mutton A, Day CP. Diagnosis and interpretation of steatosis and steatohepatitis. Semin Liver Dis. 1998;15:246-58.
70. Brunt EM. Nonalcoholic steatohepatitis: Definition and pathology. Semin Liver Dis. 2001;21:3-16.
71. Mofrad P, Contos MJ, Haque M, et al. Clinical and histologic spectrum of nonalcoholic fatty liver disease associated with normal ALT values. Hepatology. 2003;37:1286-92.
72. McPherson S, Stewart SF, Henderson E, et al. Simple non-invasive fibrosis scoring systems can reliably exclude advanced fibrosis in patients with non-alcoholic fatty liver disease. Gut. 2010;59:1265-9.
73. Kim HJ, Kim HJ, Lee KE, et al. Metabolic significance of nonalcoholic fatty liver disease in nonobese, nondiabetic adults. Arch Intern Med. 2004;164:2169-75.
74. Brunt EM, Janney CG, Di Bisceglie AM, et al. Nonalcoholic steatohepatitis: a proposal for grading and staging the histological lesions. Am J Gastroenterol. 1999;94:2467-74.
75. Kleiner DE, Brunt EM, Van Natta M, et al. Design and validation of a histological scoring system for nonalcoholic fatty liver disease. Hepatology. 2005;41:1313-21.
76. Torbenson M, Chen YY, Brunt E, et al. Glycogenic hepatopathy: an underrecognized hepatic complication of diabetes mellitus. Am J Surg Pathol. 2006;30:508-13.
77. Brunt EM, Ramrakhiani S, Cordes BG, et al. Concurrence of histologic features of steatohepatitis with other forms of chronic liver disease. Mod Pathol. 2003;16:49-56.
78. Brumbaugh DE, Friedman JE. Developmental origins of nonalcoholic fatty liver disease. Pediatr Res. 2014;75:140-7.
79. Araya J, Rodrigo R, Videla LA, et al. Increase in long-chain polyunsaturated fatty acid n-6/n-3 ratio in relation to hepatic steatosis in non-alcoholic fatty liver disease patients. Clin Sci. 2004;106:635-43.
80. Musso G, Cassader M, Rosina F, et al. Impact of current treatments on liver disease, glucose metabolism and cardiovascular risk in non-alcoholic fatty liver disease (NAFLD): A systematic review and meta-analysis of randomised trials. Diabetologia. 2012;55:885-904.
81. Babio N, Toledo E, Estruch R, et al. Mediterranean diets and metabolic syndrome status in the PREDIMED randomized trial. CMAJ. 2014;186:E649-57.
82. Gasteyger C, Larsen TM, Vercruysse F, et al. Effect of a dietary-induced weight loss on liver enzymes in obese subjects. Am J Clin Nutr. 2008;87:1141-7.
83. Lazo M, Solga SF, Horska A, et al. Effect of a 12-month intensive lifestyle intervention on hepatic steatosis in adults with type 2 diabetes. Diabetes Care. 2010;33:2156-63.
84. Albu JB, Heilbronn LK, Kelley DE, et al. Metabolic changes following a 1-year diet and exercise intervention in patients with type 2 diabetes. Diabetes. 2010;59:627-33.
85. Chavez-Tapia NC, Tellez-Avila FI, Barrientos-Gutierrez T, et al. Bariatric surgery for non-alcoholic steatohepatitis in obese patients. Cochrane Database Syst Rev. 2010;1:CD007340.
86. Mummadi RR, Kasturi KS, Chennareddygari S, et al. Effect of bariatric surgery on nonalcoholic fatty liver disease: Systematic review and meta-analysis. Clin Gastroenterol Hepatol. 2008;6:1396-402.

87. Hafeez S, Ahmed MH. Bariatric surgery as potential treatment for nonalcoholic fatty liver disease: A future treatment by choice or by chance? J Obes. 2013;2013:839275.
88. Marchesini G, Brizi M, Bianchi G, et al. Metformin in non-alcoholic steatohepatitis. Lancet. 2001;358:893-4.
89. Stein LL, Dong MH, Loomba R. Insulin sensitizers in nonalcoholic fatty liver disease and steatohepatitis: Current status. Adv Ther. 2009;26:893-907.
90. Nseir W, Mahamid M. Statins in nonalcoholic fatty liver disease and steatohepatitis: Updated review. Curr Atheroscler Rep. 2013;15:305.
91. Shu X, Zhang L, Ji G. Vitamin E therapy in non-alcoholic fatty liver disease. Int J Clin Med. 2014;5:87-92.
92. Chalasani N, Younossi Z, Lavine JE, et al. The diagnosis and management of non-alcoholic fatty liver disease: Practice guideline by the American Association for the Study of Liver Diseases, American College of Gastroenterology, and the American Gastroenterological Association. Am J Gastroenterol. 2012;107:811-26.

CHAPTER 14

Gastrointestinal Complications of Diabetes Mellitus

Parimal Lawate

INTRODUCTION

The gastrointestinal system is affected in diabetes mellitus (DM). The involvement is seen in both type 1 and type 2 diabetes. Involvement is more common in individuals with a longer duration of diabetes. It is believed that autonomic neuropathy related to diabetes is the cause for gastrointestinal involvement and consequent symptoms.

In a large questionnaire-based study done in Australia patients with diabetes had about twice the number of gastrointestinal symptoms as compared to controls.[1]

Figure 14.1 and Table 14.1 show various types of involvement of the gastrointestinal tract in DM.

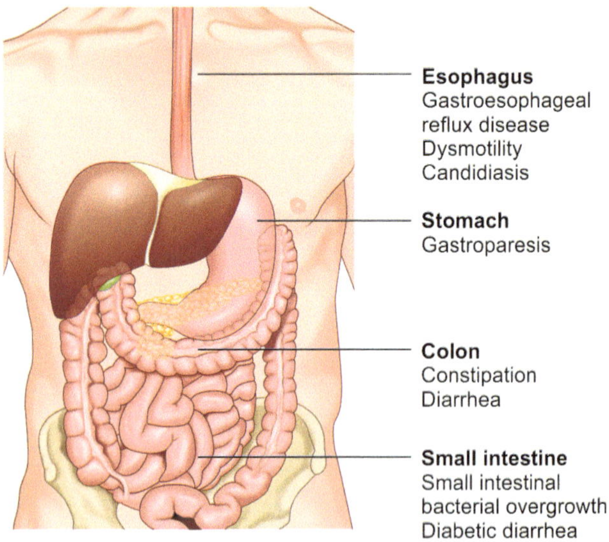

Fig. 14.1: Gastrointestinal involvement in diabetes mellitus.

Table 14.1: Gastrointestinal involvement in diabetes mellitus.

Organ	***Involvement in diabetes***
Esophagus	▪ Candidiasis ▪ Esophageal dysmotility
Stomach	Gastroparesis
Small bowel	Small intestinal bacterial overgrowth
Colon	–
Drug-induced symptoms	Drugs such as metformion, voglibose can lead to various gastrointestinal (GI) symptoms

ESOPHAGEAL INVOLVEMENT

Esophageal Motility Disorder and Gastroesophageal Reflux Disease

The lower third of the esophagus and the lower esophageal sphincter are both under the autonomic control. Studies on esophageal motility disorder have shown reduced esophageal clearance and an increased prevalence of gastroesophageal reflux disease (GERD) in diabetics up to 41%.[2] In this study, there is an increase in erosive esophagitis in patients with neuropathy with this group having more patients with asymptomatic erosive esophagitis.

Esophageal Candidiasis

There is conflicting data on the increased prevalence of esophageal candidiasis in patients with DM. A recent large study of 80,000 patients showed that there DM was not independently associated with esophageal candidiasis.[3]

Symptoms of candida esophagitis include chest pain, chest discomfort, dysphagia, odynophagia, and anorexia.

Diagnosis is on endoscopy which shows characteristic white curd-like precipitates in the esophagus.

Treatment is with oral fluconazole 150 mg per day for 7–10 days.

GASTROPARESIS

Definition

Gastroparesis is defined as delayed gastric emptying in absence of mechanical obstruction.

The cumulative incidence of gastroparesis is 4.8% in type 1 diabetes and 1% in type 2 diabetes. The corresponding figure for nondiabetic people is 0.1% on basis of data from Olmsted County.[4]

A high index of suspicion is needed to diagnose this condition as the symptom profile can mimic many other gastrointestinal disorders such as functional dyspepsia, irritable bowel syndrome, and lactose intolerance. The importance of diagnosing this condition is twofolds, it not only affects the quality of life in these patients with consequent nutritional deficiency but it also compounds difficulties in managing hyperglycemia. Glucose levels may swing between hyperglycemia and hypoglycemia. The pattern of antidiabetic medication especially insulin may have to be modified in patients with diabetic gastroparesis.

In a recently reported study,[5] (from Olmsted County, the cumulative proportions developing gastroparesis over a 10-year time period were 5.2% in type 1 DM and 0.2% in type 2 DM). This was in contrast to 0.2% observed in controls.

Gastric Physiology in Relevance to Gastroparesis

The gastric physiology in relevance to gastroparesis is described in the Figure 14.2.

Pathophysiology of Gastroparesis

Gastric neuropathy and gastric cajalopathy are supposed to be associated with gastroparesis. Full thickness biopsies from the stomach show that interstitial cells of Cajal (ICC) are depleted (<5/HPF). Gastric enteric neurons show reduced numbers and an immune infiltration of macrophages around these (Flowchart 14.1).

Approach to Diagnosis

- Suspicion of gastroparesis
- Documentation of absence of outlet obstruction in the stomach
- Documentation of slow gastric emptying
- Treatment with dietary and pharmacologic measures
- Newer forms of treatment (Flowchart 14.2).

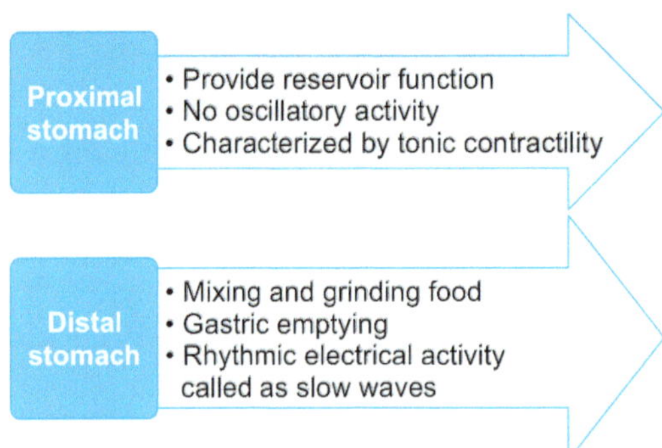

Fig. 14.2: Gastric physiology in relevance to gastroparesis.

Flowchart 14.1: Pathophysiology of gastroparesis.

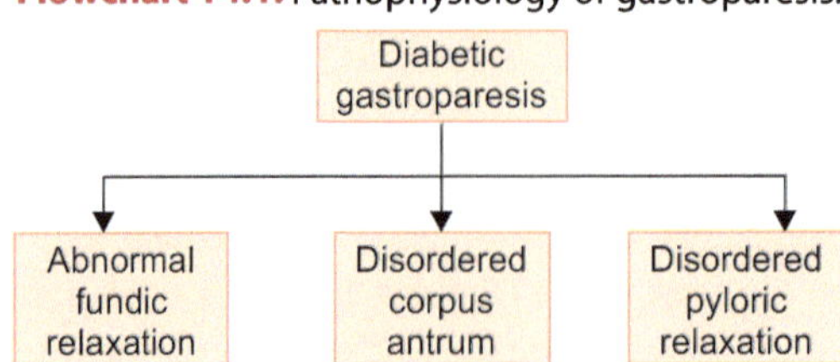

Flowchart 14.2: Diagnosis of gastroparesis.

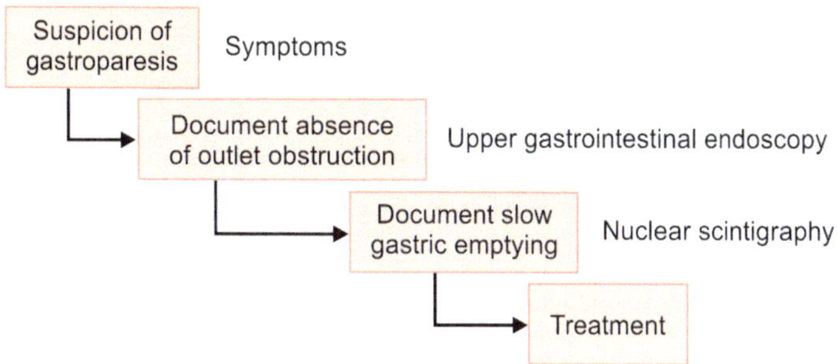

Suspicion of Diabetic Gastroparesis

Diabetic gastroparesis often occurs with about 10 years of pre-existing diabetes. Diabetic gastroparesis presents with abdominal pain, fullness, early satiety, vomiting, and poor glycemic control in some patients. Effortless regurgitation of gastric contents has also been described. Poor control of glycemia in patients who were otherwise well controlled should also raise the suspicion of gastroparesis. Physical examination is normal.

Establishing the Absence of Mechanical Obstruction

An upper gastrointestinal endoscopy is now considered as the test of choice for first-line evaluation in patients with suspected diabetic gastroparesis. The aim is to rule out a mechanical obstruction as a cause for symptoms. The endoscope is advanced till deep in the duodenum. Often food residue of food eaten over 12 hours is visualized in the stomach. Phytobezoars can rarely be found (Figs. 14.3A to D).

Documentation of Slow Gastric Emptying

This can be done with the help of scintigraphic documentation of gastric emptying in (Table 14.2).

Treatment of Gastroparesis

Diet in Gastroparesis

Dietary restrictions of diabetes need to be continued. Patients with fullness can have frequent feeds with antidiabetics timed accordingly. High fiber in the diet may have to be avoided as this can lead to formation of phytobezoars. High fat diet should be avoided as this slows gastric emptying further and can aggravate symptoms (Fig. 14.4).

Prokinetics

Prokinetics are drugs which promote motility in the gastrointestinal tract. The drugs promote motility by various mechanisms as shown in the Tables 14.3 and 14.4. The drugs have to be preferably given about 0.5 hour before meals to be effective. Availability of prokinetics varies within countries.

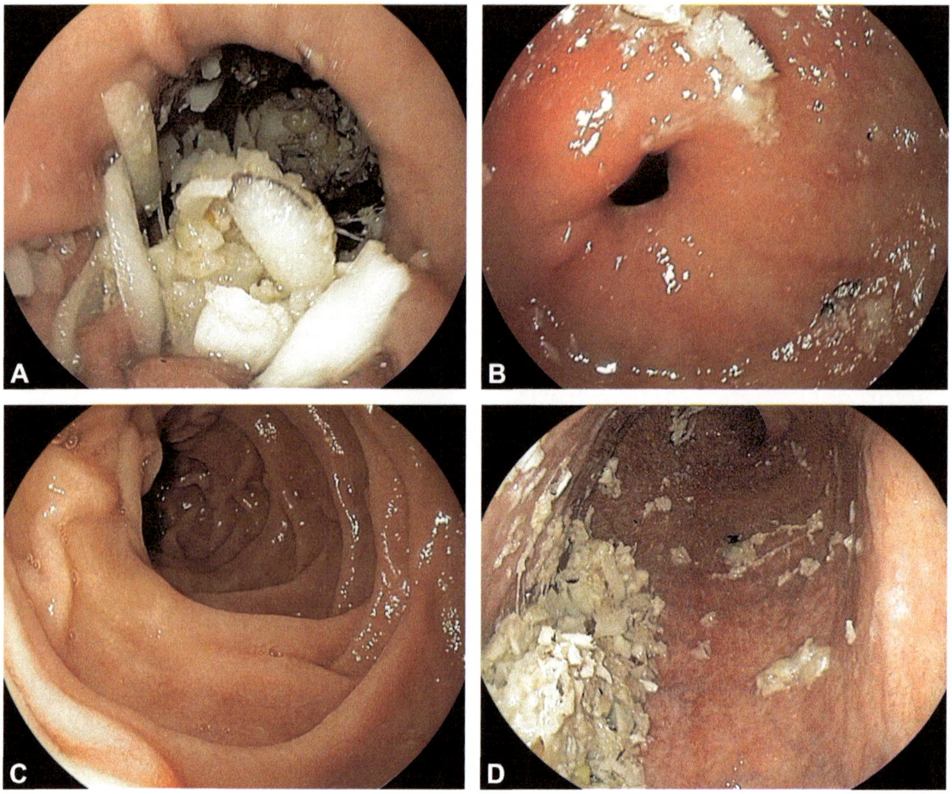

Figs. 14.3A to D: Endoscopy in a patient with diabetic gastroparesis showing solid food residue in the stomach despite and overnight fast and in absence of pyloric narrowing.

Table 14.2: Scintigraphic documentation of gastric emptying.

Method	*Principle*	*Comments*
Radionuclide gastric emptying scintigraphy	Technetium 99m sulfur colloid radiolabeled meal	▪ Gold standard test ▪ Assess solid and liquid emptying ▪ Radiation exposure
Barium studies	Assesses emptying of barium from the stomach	▪ May rule out obstruction ▪ Not very physiological ▪ Rarely used
Breath tests	Nonradioactive isotope carbon 13 is used to label octanoate, or acetate or Spirulina platensis which is bound to a solid meal	▪ Noninvasive ▪ Needs normal small bowel absorption, liver function
Wireless motility capsule	Ingestible capsule ingested with a 250 calories energy bar, measures pH, temperature, and pressure	Capsule gastric residence time has good correlation with radionuclide emptying
Electrogastrography	Noninvasive measurement of myoelectrical activity	Diagnosis of gastric dysrhythmias

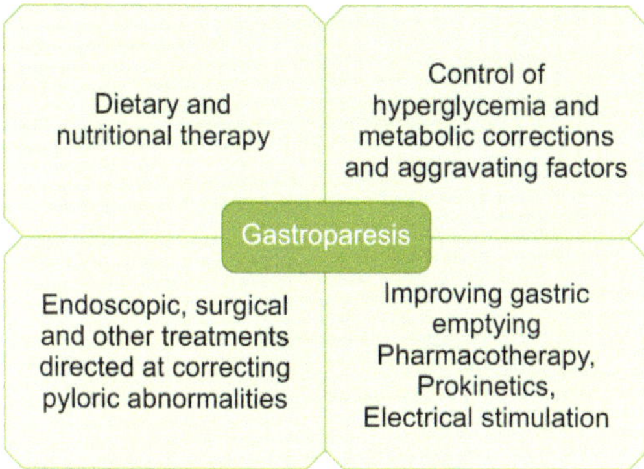

Fig. 14.4: Diet in gastroparesis.

Table 14.3: Various drugs promote motility by different mechanisms.

Category	*Prototype*	*Mechanism of action*
Muscarinic agonist	Bethanechol	Increased gastrointestinal (GI) motility
Anticholinesterase	Neostigmine	▪ Increased GI motility ▪ Inhibit acetylcholine degradation
Dopamine D2 blockers	▪ Metoclopramide ▪ Domperidone ▪ Itopride	Blocks inhibitory D2 receptor
5-HT4 agonists	▪ Cisapride ▪ Tegaserod ▪ Prucalopride ▪ Mosapride	Activate excitatory 5-HT4 receptors
Motilin receptor agonists	▪ Erythromycin ▪ Azithromycin	Activate neural and smooth muscle motilin receptors
Novel molecules acting through muscarinic receptors	Acotiamide	Acts on muscarinic receptors and increases local acetylcholine by increasing release and preventing reuptake from the presynaptic neuron
Ghrelin agonists	Relamorelin	Improved gastric emptying

Table 14.4: Different drugs having various side effects.

Agent	*Route*	*Dose*	*Side effects*
Domperidone	Oral	10 mg thrice	▪ Gynecomastia ▪ Free of extrapyramidal
Metoclopramide	▪ Oral ▪ Intravenous	10 mg for both routes	▪ Extrapyramidal ▪ Drowsiness
Levosulpiride	▪ Oral ▪ Intravenous	25 mg oral thrice	Drowsiness Extrapyramidal syndromes
Mosapride	Oral	5 mg thrice	No significant

Contd...

Contd...

Agent	Route	Dose	Side effects
Erythromycin	▪ Oral ▪ Intravenous	500 mg thrice 3 mg/kg/ 24 hour	▪ Diarrhea ▪ Dyspepsia ▪ Thrombophlebitis
Azithromycin	▪ Oral ▪ Intravenous	500 mg	Diarrhea
Acotiamide	Oral	100 mg thrice daily	Nil significant
Relmorelin	Subcutaneous	10 mcg twice daily	Headache Worsening diabetes in some patients

Table 14.5: Treatments directed at the pylorus.

Modality	Comments
Botulinum toxin	Neurotoxic protein which binds to presynaptic cholinergic receptors and inhibits acetylcholine release, ending of muscle relaxation
Transpyloric stent placement	▪ Done in a few patients with symptomatic relief ▪ May help to decide which patients are likely to benefit from pyloromyotomy
Surgical pyloroplasty	Improvement in gastric emptying time with symptomatic improvement and decreased use of prokinetics
Endoscopic pyloromyotomy	Similar to per-oral endoscopic myotomy (POEM) for achalasia. Recently reported with benefit

Source: Anthony Lembo, Michel Camilleri, Richard McCallum. Relamorelin Reduces Vomiting Frequency and Severity and Accelerates Gastric Emptying in Adults with Diabetic Gastroparesis. Gastroenterology. 2016;151(1):87-96.

TREATMENTS DIRECTED AT THE PYLORUS

The treatments directed at the pylorus are given in Table 14.5.

REFERENCES

1. Bytzer P, Talley NJ, Leemon M, et al. Prevalence of gastrointestinal symptoms associated with diabetes mellitus: a population-based survey of 15,000 adults. Arch Intern Med. 2001;161(16):1989-96.
2. Wang X, Pitchumoni CS, Chandrarana K, et al. Increased prevalence of symptoms of gastroesophageal reflux diseases in type 2 diabetics with neuropathy. World J Gastroenterol. 2008;14:709-12.
3. Takahashi Y, Nagata N, Shimbo T, et al. Long-term trends in esophageal candidiasis prevalence and associated risk factors with or without HIV infection: Lessons from an endoscopic study of 80,219 patients. PLoS One. 2015;10:e0133589.
4. Choung RS, Locke GR, Schleck C, et al. Cumulative incidence of gastroparesis in people with type 1 and 2 diabetes and in the general population. Am J Gastroenterol. 2008;103:S309.
5. Choung RS, Locke GR, Schleck CD, et al. Risk of gastroparesis in subjects with type 1 and 2 diabetes in the general population. Am J Gastroenterol. 2012;107(1):82-8.

CHAPTER 15

Diabetes and Pregnancy

Jennifer A Wyckoff, Florence M Brown

INTRODUCTION

The purpose of this chapter is to provide clinicians with an understanding of the challenges of managing diabetes and prediabetes before, during, and immediately after pregnancy. Care for all women should begin preconception by assessing alcohol use, prescription medications, general nutrition, obesity, and smoking. Obesity alone is a risk factor for poor outcomes. For women with overt diabetes, preconception care (PC) is crucial to prevent congenital malformations (CMs) by achieving adequate blood glucose control through optimization of diabetes, self-management skills including medical nutrition therapy (MNT) and basal/bolus insulin administration. An assessment of the maternal health status includes screening for complications of diabetes, and evaluation of concurrent conditions to reduce maternal and fetal risks and improve pregnancy and neonatal outcomes.

Many women with obesity, polycystic ovarian syndrome (PCOS), or prediabetes develop gestational diabetes mellitus (GDM) during pregnancy. The definition and epidemiology of GDM will be discussed along with controversies in the diagnosis of GDM, its treatment with oral medications versus insulin, and which glycemic targets to use for treatment goals.

During pregnancy and through delivery, frequent visits are required to address progressive changes in insulin resistance, monitor for diabetes and pregnancy complications, and fetal well being. Immediately postpartum, abrupt changes to insulin requirements require close monitoring. At later postpartum visits, contraception options should be discussed and a final assessment of maternal health status should be made. Women should set personal goals around having a healthy lifestyle and focus on diabetes self-care despite the challenges of motherhood they should be reminded of the importance of PC for future pregnancies.

HISTORICAL PERSPECTIVE

Prior to the introduction of insulin in 1922, pregnancy outcomes in women with diabetes were abysmal. Type 1 diabetes (DM1) was universally fatal outside of pregnancy, and pregnancy only accelerated the course of the disease. Pregnancies complicated by type 2 diabetes (DM2) were plagued with nearly 50% maternal mortality as well as high rates of intrauterine fetal demise (IUFD) and CMs.[1]

In 1949, Priscilla White at the Joslin Diabetes Center published her experience with insulin treatment in 439 pregnant women with mostly DM1.[1] She reported a fetal mortality of 18%. She described 34 IUFD associated with either diabetic ketoacidosis (DKA) or vascular disease and 44 neonatal deaths associated with either CM or preterm delivery (PTD). These outcomes were considered substantially superior to the standard of care at the time.

For decades, women with diabetes were advised against pregnancies due to poor maternal and fetal outcomes. While maternal and fetal outcomes have dramatically improved, the rates of IUFD, CM, and PTD remain substantially higher for women with diabetes as compared to the normal population.[2-6]

DEFINITIONS

Hyperglycemia in pregnancy is categorized as either GDM or preexisting diabetes mellitus (PEDM). GDM is defined as hyperglycemia that is less severe than overt diabetes that first present in pregnancy.[7] PEDM is any form of diabetes present prior to conception or identified in pregnancy by usual diagnostic criteria for diabetes.

This means that PEDM encompasses all forms of diabetes including the classic autoimmune-mediated complete insulin deficiency of DM1, the genetically diverse syndromes of hyperglycemia and insulin resistance called DM2, and an increasingly recognized group of unique diabetes phenotypes.[8] An in-depth review of types of diabetes is beyond the scope of this chapter, and the reader is referred to American Diabetes Association's (ADAs) guidelines on classification.[8] However, recognition of the correct diagnosis underlying PEDM and GDM is important as it will change the treatment decisions.

Recognizing which women are at risk for DKA by identifying those patients with PEDM who have latent autoimmune diabetes of the adult or ketosis prone DM2 is important. Perhaps even more important in preventing DKA is to recognize that possibility of the development of DM1 in a younger, thinner, and often Caucasian woman with other autoimmune disease whose has just been diagnosed with GDM. Diabetes can be a part of other genetic syndromes (like myotonic dystrophy or Wolfram's syndrome) or a manifestation of endocrinopathies (like Cushing's syndrome) as well.

Most atypical genetic forms of diabetes are rare and many individuals with one of these atypical forms are misdiagnosed as having either DM1 or DM2. Therefore, there is relatively sparse literature on the prenatal management of these forms of diabetes, though it is probable that these women have unique needs. For example, the management of cystic fibrosis-related diabetes during pregnancy is unique in the need for an altered approach to MNT and the confusion over appropriate prenatal vitamin supplementation. The literature is very limited.[9]

An interesting recent revelation is the contribution of maturity onset diabetes of the young (MODY) in a subset of GDM.[10,11] MODY is classically characterized by antibody-negative diabetes in young, lean individuals without metabolic syndrome. MODY is a group of monogenic, autosomal dominant forms of diabetes due to mutations in genes important in beta cell development or insulin production.[12] In the Atlantic Diabetes in Pregnancy Cohort, GCK-

MODY (MODY2) was found in 1.1/1,000 women with GDM.[10] The Hyperglycemia and Adverse Pregnancy Outcome (HAPO) study found that GCK genotype was associated with high fasting glucose.[11] The optimal screening strategy for GCK-MODY in GDM has not been established, nor has ideal treatment.

EPIDEMIOLOGY

As the prevalence of obesity and DM2 has dramatically increased globally, so it has the prevalence of both PEDM and GDM. Interestingly, there has also been a rise in the prevalence of DM1.[13,14] In the US, recent estimates suggest that 1.3–1.8% of pregnancies are complicated by PEDM.[15,16]

In a recent retrospective analysis of the Truven Health MarketScan® database from 2005–2011, Jovanovic and colleagues reviewed 839,792 pregnancies in North America and found that 7.9% were associated with diabetes: 0.1% with type 1 diabetes mellitus (T1DM); 1.2% with type 2 diabetes mellitus (T2DM); 6.3% with GDM; and 0.2% with GDM that progressed to DM2.[16]

One of the most alarming aspects of GDM is the 50–100% increase in its prevalence over recent 10–15 year periods.[17-19] GDM prevalence increases with maternal age, number of children, lower socioeconomic status as defined by Special Supplemental Nutrition Program for Women, Infants, and Children (WIC) use, and decreases with higher education. Prevalence varied by maternal race/ethnicity with Asian/Pacific Islanders and Hispanics having the highest prevalence estimates (16.3% and 12.1%, respectively). Non-Hispanic whites had the lowest prevalence estimate (6.8%).[20] Notably, age is an important risk factor for GDM as women ages more than or equal to 30 years have prevalence of GDM approaching 8% (Figs. 15.1 and 15.2).[19]

The rising prevalence of GDM parallels the rising prevalence of overweight and obesity. In a meta-analysis, the odds ratio (OR) of developing GDM for overweight, moderately obese,

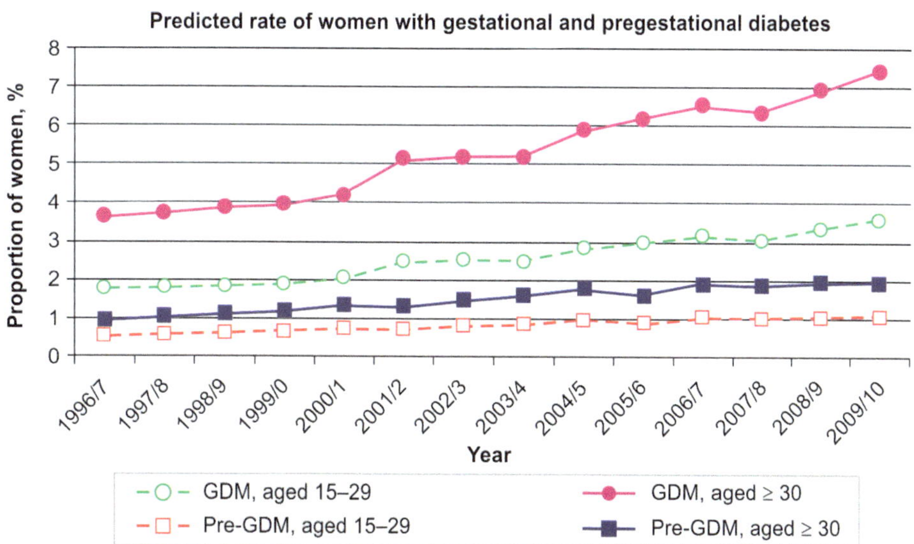

Fig. 15.1: Trends in incidence.[19]
Source: Reprinted with permission from American Diabetes Association.

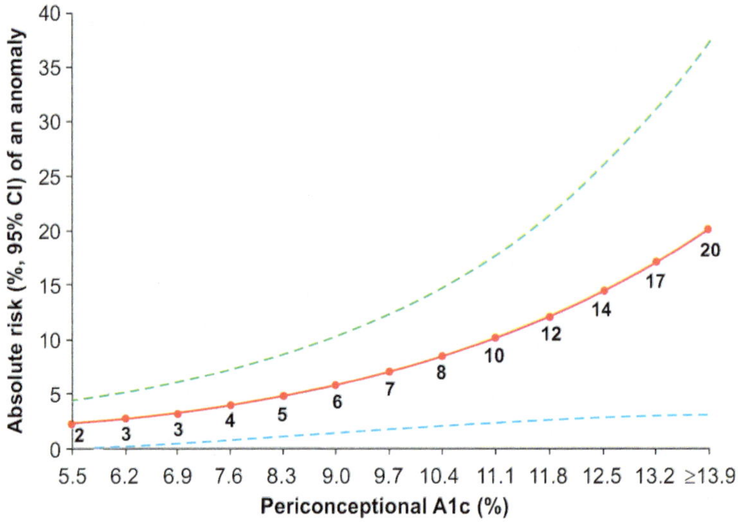

Fig. 15.2: Risk of major or minor anomaly according to periconception A1c.
*Data are presented as an absolute risk (solid line and blue values) ± 95% CIs (dashed lines).
(CIs: confidence intervals; SDs: standard deviations).
Source: Reprinted with permission from American Diabetes Association.

and morbidly obese women were 1.97 [95% confidence interval (CI) 1.77–2.19], 3.01 (95% CI 2.34–3.87), and 5.55 (95% CI 4.27–7.21), respectively. For every 1 kg/m^2 increase in body mass index (BMI), the prevalence of GDM increased by 0.92% (95% CI 0.73–1.10).[21]

GLUCOSE METABOLISM IN PREGNANCY

During pregnancy, there is a normal increase in insulin resistance in the late 2nd and 3rd trimesters which favors fuel delivery to the fetus. The physiology of this is not well understood. A number of placental hormones have been implicated including cortisol, human placental lactogen, progesterone, prolactin, placental growth hormone, tumor necrosis factor-α, and leptin.[22] Studies demonstrate that increasing levels of placental cytokines may contribute to low-grade systemic inflammation which also induces maternal insulin resistance.[23] Other studies suggest a role for placental growth hormone as a mediator of the insulin resistance of normal pregnancy by inducing postreceptor insulin signaling changes as demonstrated in a transgenic mouse model.[24]

Women who develop GDM have either baseline *preconception* insulin resistance or reduced insulin secretion or both. Normally, insulin secretion increases during pregnancy to compensate for the normal physiologic increase in insulin resistance. However, in women with GDM, the reduced baseline insulin secretory capacity is unable to overcome the combined underlying (baseline preconception) and gestational insulin resistance, so a state of carbohydrate intolerance results. The details of the studies demonstrating changes in insulin secretion, insulin resistance, and insulin signaling are beyond the scope of this chapter but are discussed thoroughly by Catalano.[25] In PEDM, this is manifest as a progressive increase in insulin requirements from around 16 weeks gestation until around 36 weeks gestation followed by a rapid decrease in insulin resistance and insulin requirements at the time of delivery.[26]

THE PRECONCEPTION PERIOD

The Woman at Risk for Type 2 Diabetes

Achieving good pregnancy outcomes starts preconception. Overweight and obese women and those with PCOS have increased risk of many pregnancy complications, including GDM.[27,28] Overweight and obese women have increased prevalence of hypertensive disorders, cesarean delivery, macrosomia and shoulder dystocia as well as severe birth-asphyxia-related complications.[29,30] Ideally women who are overweight and obese with/without known impaired glucose metabolism should be referred for MNT with a goal of 5–10% weight loss prior to pregnancy, per Institute of Medicine (IOM) 2009 recommendations.[31] It is the position of the Academy of Nutrition and Dietetics: Obesity, Reproduction, and Pregnancy Outcomes that 'behavioral counseling to improve dietary intake and physical activity should be provided to overweight and obese women, beginning in the preconception period and continuing throughout pregnancy for at least 12–18 months postpartum.'[27] Glucose metabolism should be evaluated prior to pregnancy to screen for PEDM or impaired fasting glucose or impaired glucose tolerance. For women with a previous history of GDM, the risk of GDM in subsequent pregnancies is approximately 50% in primiparous women whose GDM was treated with diet alone. The risk of recurrence is less in those women who lost weight between the first and the subsequent pregnancy, supporting preconception lifestyle management for women with prior GDM as well.[32]

Fertility and Contraception

One of the most important aspects of PC is contraception. Many women with obesity, PCOS, or diabetes believe that they have decreased fertility. While for some this is true, most women with diabetes are able to become pregnant without undue difficulty. This misconception about fertility and the lack of patient education regarding the risks of diabetes and pregnancy result in less than half of women with PEDM getting PC.[33-35] A contraceptive plan is an essential component of the general care for all women especially those with any form of PEDM.

Both PCOS and obesity have been shown to decrease fertility, and are common in women with DM2.[36] Studies looking at fertility in women with DM1 are somewhat lacking. Women with DM1 have an increased risk of premature ovarian failure and there are population studies suggesting a subtle decrease in the fertility rate.[37]

Preconception Care for Preexisting Diabetes and Medical Nutrition Therapy

In women with PEDM, the most effective way of substantially reducing poor pregnancy outcomes is preconception counseling and intense and comprehensive diabetes care.[33,38-44] PC is best delivered by a multidisciplinary team including a maternal fetal medicine specialist, an endocrinologist, a certified diabetes educator, and a dietitian.[45,46] It is imperative that all women with PEDM who are considering pregnancy get PC to reduce the risk of CM.[47]

The hemoglobin A1c (HbA1c) at the time of conception is strongly associated with poor maternal and fetal outcomes, most notably the occurrence of CM.[48-52] In a 2001 meta-analysis of PC, the relative risk of CM was 0.42 (95% CI 0.22–0.60) in those pregnancies that received PC.[53] While the prevention of CM is thought to be the primary benefit of PC, PC has also been shown to reduce the risk of PTD.[33]

Table 15.1 provides a checklist for comprehensive preconception counseling and care for the woman with PEDM. One essential component is a diabetes education assessment and comprehensive diabetes education including MNT.[46] This is the ideal time for this intervention for some patients as the desire to ensure a healthy pregnancy is often a powerful motivator for most women.

Medical Nutrition Therapy

For women with PEDM starting preconception and women with GDM, dietary recommendations call for a diet that is rich in nonstarchy vegetables, whole grains, and lean proteins (including beans) and healthy (poly and monounsaturated) fats, avoiding simple sugars, processed grains, and saturated and trans fats. The optimal daily nutrition of macronutrient breakdown is not well studied. Typically, diets lower in carbohydrates have been recommended with the goal of reducing glycemic excursions.[54,55] A typical macronutrient breakdown is carbohydrates 40–45%, fats 30–40%, and proteins 15–20% of total calories. The total daily carbohydrate is approximately 175 g divided over three meals and three snacks. However, the relative contribution of carbohydrates versus fats has been called into question in recent small studies in pregnant patients with GDM. While both a lower complex carbohydrate/higher fat 'conventional' diet and a higher complex carbohydrate diet/lower fat diet effectively controlled glycemia, free fatty acids were higher with the 'conventional diet'.[56] In a very small study, the higher complex carbohydrate/lower fat diet may also reduce maternal insulin resistance.[57] Follow-up visits with the dietitian are helpful to review the quality of the diet and to liberalize complex carbohydrates, if glycemic targets are met.

Prenatal vitamin supplements should be started 3 months prior to conception. Both the National Institute for Health and Care Excellence (NICE) and the Endocrine Society recommend the high dose of folic acid (5 mg) for women with PEDM.[46,47] The ADA recommends a moderate intake of 600 μg per day of folic acid through supplementation or fortified food sources for women with PEDM during the periconception and prenatal period.[58] A vitamin B_{12} level should be checked when high doses of folic acid are prescribed, as high doses of folic acid may mask B_{12} deficiency.

The National Institute for Health and Care Excellence recommends that women with GDM take regular exercise 'such as walking for 30 minutes after a meal' to improve blood glucose control.[46]

Preconception Monitoring and Treatment Goals

Fasting preconception blood glucose targets of 80–110 mg/dL (4.4–6.1 mmol/L) are recommended.[59] 2 hours postprandial targets of less than 155 mg/dL (less than 8.6 mmol/L) are

Table 15.1: Checklist for preconception care.

Preconception care checklist ***Initial visit to MFM or endocrinologist***	
Counsel	Detailed explanation of maternal and fetal risks and risk reduction
	Natural history of insulin resistance in pregnancy
	Clear understanding of time commitment and expectations
	Smoking cessation (if applicable)
	Hypoglycemia safety
Establish	Contraception plan
Set	Clear glycemic goals
Order	Referrals to comprehensive team: Maternal fetal medicine, endocrinology, diabetes education, and MNT
	Baseline A1c, TSH, lipids, CBC, creatinine, AST, ALT, and uric acid
	Baseline evaluation of either urine protein excretion or albumin/creatinine ratio
	Comprehensive eye examination
	Routine pap smear, if indicated
	Baseline ECG and exercise echocardiogram in select patients
Prescribe	Prenatal vitamin
First follow-up visit	
Counsel	Follow-up questions for initial visit counseling
Confirm	Contraception plan
	Clear glycemic goals
Review	Test results
Optimize	Glycemic management
	Treatment and medications for comorbid conditions and complications
Offer	Genetic counseling
Consider	Nephrology consult, if urine albumin/creatinine ratio > 300 or GFR < 60
Reinforce	Comprehensive diabetes education including testing, hypoglycemia safety, prevention of DKA, and sick day rules
Subsequent visits	
Order	A1c every 1–2 months
	Discontinue contraception once therapy for comorbid conditions and complications is optimized and glycemic goals are met

(ALT: alanine transaminase; AST: aspartate transaminase; CBC: complete blood count; DKA: diabetic ketoacidosis; ECG: electrocardiogram; GFR: glomerular filtration rate; MNT: medical nutrition therapy; TSH: thyroid-stimulating hormone)

recommended, though we prefer this target at 1 hour as chosen in a randomized controlled trial of insulin aspart versus regular human insulin.[60] Data support the recommendation to optimize glycemic control prior to conception with A1c less than 6.5% (48 mmol/mol) associated with the lowest risk of congenital anomalies. This target may need to be relaxed for patients with

Table 15.2: Glycemic goals for GDM and PEDM.

	ADA for GDM[217]	***ADA for PEDM***[215]	***ACOG for PEDM***[45]	***ENDO for GDM and PEDM***[48]	***NICE for GDM and PEDM***[47]
A1c		6–6.5% (42–48 mmol/L)	<6% (<42 mmol/L)	<6.5% (<48 mmol/L)	–
Fasting	<95 mg/dL (5.3 mmol/L)	<95 mg/dL (5 mmol/L)	<95 mg/dL (5.3 mmol/L)	<95 mg/dL (5.3 mmol/L)	<95 mg/dL (5.3 mmol/L)
1 hour postprandial	<140 mg/dL (7.8 mmol/L)	<140 mg/dL (7.8 mmol/L)	<140 mg/dL (7.8 mmol/L)	<140 mg/dL (7.8 mmol/L)	<140 mg/dL (7.8 mmol/L)
2 hours postprandial	<120 mg/dL (6.6 mmol/L)	<120 mg/dL (6.6 mmol/L)	<120 mg/dL (6.6 mmol/L)	<120 mg/dL (6.6 mmol/L)	<115 mg/dL (6.4 mmol/L)

(ACOG: American College of Obstetricians and Gynecologists; ADA: American Diabetes Association; GDM: gestational diabetes mellitus; NICE: National Institute for Health and Care Excellence; PEDM: preexisting diabetes mellitus)

hypoglycemia unawareness.[50] In general, it is recommend to have blood glucose and A1c levels as close to normal as possible without undue hypoglycemia (Table 15.2).[47]

Glycemic Management for Preexisting Diabetes

Insulin is the standard of care for women with PEDM. Increase in insulin resistance renders oral hypoglycemic agents for DM2 inadequate to the task of controlling blood glucose during pregnancy. As glycemic control is of paramount importance at conception and in the 1st trimester, titration of the insulin regimen to achieve ideal control prior to pregnancy is essential. Women with DM2 who are achieving preconception glycemic goals with diet alone should be aware that they will most likely require insulin therapy during their pregnancy. The safety of noninsulin injectable agents is not established. During PC, all oral or noninsulin injectable hypoglycemic agents with the possible exception of metformin should be discontinued, and insulin should be started.[47] Multiple daily injections (MDIs) in a basal bolus pattern or an insulin pump are the recommended formats for insulin delivery.[47] An insulin pump can be used to provide excellent glycemic control.[61,62] There is some evidence that continuous glucose monitoring system (CGMS) may improve glycemic control during pregnancy, and an argument can also be made for it reducing of severe hypoglycemia and the risk of injury in the setting of severe hypoglycemia.[63,64] However, the benefit of these technologies over MDI in pregnancy is not clearly established.[65,66] A recent study demonstrated that patients with type 1 diabetes may benefit from continuous glucose monitoring.[67]

Lispro is superior when compared to regular insulin in pregnancy for achieving postprandial targets.[68,69] Both lispro and aspart[70] have been studied in pregnancy, and are Food and Drug Administration (FDA) approved for use in pregnancy.[47] Glulisine is not.[15,16,47]

Neutral protamine Hagedorn (NPH) has traditionally been the choice for long-acting insulin. However, detemir is now FDA approved for pregnancy, and has been shown to cause less nocturnal hypoglycemia.[71] Glargine is not FDA approved, but some retrospective cohort and case-controlled studies do support its use in pregnancy.[47,72-74] However, there are no randomized controlled trials (RCTs) of glargine in pregnancy and glargine

Table 15.3: Maternal and fetal risks.

Fetal and neonatal risks	***Maternal risks***	***Pregnancy complications***
Congenital malformations	Myocardial infarction/ postpartum cardiomyopathy	Cesarean section
Miscarriage	Hypoglycemia	Preterm delivery
IUFD	DKA and hyperglycemia	
IUGR	Hypertension/PIH/preeclampsia	
Macrosomia	Progression of retinopathy	
Shoulder dystocia	Progression of nephropathy	
Perinatal and neonatal mortality		
Respiratory problems		
Neonatal hypoglycemia		
Hyperbilirubinemia		

(DKA: diabetic ketoacidosis; IUGR: intrauterine growth retardation; IUFR: intrauterine fetal demise; PIH: pregnancy-induced hypertension)

has increased affinity for the insulin-like growth factor-1 (IGF-1) receptor which plays an important role in fetal development.[75] Metformin may be continued preconception, if it is deemed beneficial in the specific case. There is data surrounding the use of metformin at conception and in the 1st trimester in women with PCOS, and as an adjunct therapy for DM2 in pregnancy. Unfortunately, many of these studies are small and are not RCTs. It is outside the scope of this chapter to review all this data in detail, but several recent systematic reviews are recommended.[76,77] In women with PCOS, metformin treatment in the 1st trimester did not improve outcomes of pre-eclampsia, preterm delivery, or gestational diabetes.[78] The risk of overweight in offspring was increased.[79] A 9-year follow-up study of a randomized control trial of metformin versus insulin in the treatment of GDM demonstrated greater measures of obesity in the offspring, including weight, arm and waist circumferences, waist:height ratios, BMI and triceps skinfold thickness, and abdominal fat volume with MRI.[80] Metformin may affect mitochondrial oxidative metabolism and gene expression.[81]

Counseling for Maternal and Fetal Risks

An important component of PC is a discussion of the maternal and fetal risks associated with PEDM and pregnancy (Table 15.3).

Perinatal and neonatal mortality: Perinatal mortality rate (PMR) for the infant of a diabetic mother (IDM) remains substantially higher than that for the general population.[82] One study reported a PMR in DM2 of 39.1/1,000 live births as compared to 12.5/1,000 live births in the general population.[4] Half of this increased mortality was due to the presence of CM.[4] A worrisome trend is that PMR due to PEDM may be increasing due to increased rates of PEDM, older maternal age, more complicated diabetes, and obesity.[3,82]

Congenital malformations: Infants of diabetic mothers have an increased risk of CM.[42,48,50,53,83-87] There is substantial evidence that maternal hyperglycemia causes CM, and tight glycemic control preconception can prevent many of these CM. An A1c of 6% is associated with a rate of CM of 2–3% which is similar to that of normal pregnancies.[44] An A1c of 10% is associated with a rate of CM of 20–25%.[88] Congenital heart defects and central nervous system defects are two of the most common. A retrospective study from the Mayo Clinic found that 7.9% of their patients with PEDM had a congenital heart defect.[85] This is consistent with other studies which have reported rates between 5.6% and 15%.[16,85] Caudal regression in which the lower part of the spinal cord fails to form resulting in denervation of the bowel, bladder, and legs is pathognomonic of PEDM. In Jovanovic's recent retrospective review of 839,792 pregnancies in the Truven database, 66,041 of which were complicated by some form of diabetes, the rates of major CMs were 11.4% for DM1, 10.9% for DM2, 6.9% for GDM, and 9.5% for GDM which progressed to DM2 by the end of pregnancy.[16] This was compared to a rate of 5.9% for pregnancies not complicated by DM.

Miscarriage: Preexisting diabetes mellitus has been associated with a higher rate of miscarriage or spontaneous abortion (SAB). Estimated rates vary from 13.5% to 25%,[16,83,89,90] with some studies suggesting a higher rate in women with DM2.[16] Several factors may contribute to this higher rate of SAB including severe CM, poor glycemic control, and DKA. In women with DM2, another reason for the increased SAB rate may be the presence of PCOS as a comorbid state. A higher SAB rate is observed in women with PCOS.[91,92] PC and tight glycemic control have been shown to reduce this rate in women with PEDM.[93]

Intrauterine fetal demise: Intrauterine fetal demise occurs at about double the rate in pregnancies complicated by PEDM compared to normal pregnancies.[16,82] Severe CM, poor glycemic control, and DKA may be contributing factors. Poor glycemic control is thought to contribute to fetal cardiac hypertrophy which may contribute to a fifth of the cases of IUFD in IDM.[94] A recent study of DKA in pregnancy found that fetal demise occurred in 15.6% pregnancy cases. Maternal ICU admission and higher serum osmolality were risk factors for fetal demise.[95]

Diabetic ketoacidosis and hyperglycemia: Diabetic ketoacidosis has been reported to occur in 0.5–10% of pregnancies complicated by PEDM.[96,97] While the majority of cases are in women with T1DM, it has also been reported in women with ketosis-prone DM2 and those diagnosed with GDM.[97] A unique presentation of DKA in pregnancy is euglycemic diabetic ketoacidosis.[98] A high index of suspicion for DKA should be present when any pregnant woman with any form of diabetes presents with hyperglycemia and symptoms consistent with DKA. It is important to test for ketonemia in this setting.[46] The fetal mortality rate associated with maternal DKA has been reported as low as 10% and as high as 90%.[97,99-101] In a decade of observation at University of Tennessee Women's Hospital, DKA occurred in 1.2% of women with PEDM and had a fetal death rate of 27%.[97] Continuous fetal heart rate monitoring typically shows recurrent late decelerations.[44] These decelerations typically resolve with treatment of DKA.[97]

Large for gestational age/macrosomia: Macrosomia is defined as a fetal weight more than 4,000 g. Large for gestational age (LGA) is defined as a weight above the 90th percentile for gestational age. In Jovanovic's review of the Truven database, 11% of infants born to mothers with DM1 and 6.6% of those born to mothers with DM2 had macrosomia. Risk factors for macrosomia include higher A1c at conception, and higher postprandial glucose levels in the 3rd trimester, maternal obesity, previous delivery of a macrosomic infant, and family history of macrosomia.[102]

Macrosomic infants are at higher risk for birth injuries including shoulder dystocia, Erb's palsy, and death.

Neonatal hypoglycemia: 7.8% of IDM experience neonatal hypoglycemia.[103] If untreated, neonatal hypoglycemia can result in seizures and long-term neurologic damage.

Cesarean section: Women with PEDM are up to a 4.5 times more likely to undergo cesarean section (C-section) than women without PEDM.[6,16,18,104] In Jovanovic's recent study, 52.5% of women with DM1 and 48.5% of women with DM2 underwent C-section compared to 27.4% of women without PEDM.[16]

Intrauterine growth retardation: While in modern practice, we frequently see LGA, IDM, pregnancies complicated by preeclampsia, nephropathy, smoking, or vascular disease may demonstrate intrauterine growth retardation (IUGR) and small for gestational age (SGA) infants.[105]

Preterm labor and delivery: Women with PEDM have an increased risk of PTD.[106] In part this is due to an increased rate of early deliveries from induction or C-section due to preeclampsia. However, there is also an increased risk of preterm labor (PTL) and polyhydramnios.[44] In a prospective multicenter observational study, Sibai noted that 38% of women with PEDM had a PTD compared with only 13.9% of women without PEDM.[106] One study found that factors associated with PTL in PEDM include polyhydramnios and poor glycemic control, and that factors associated with indicated PTD included preeclampsia, worsening retinopathy or nephropathy, and poor glycemic control.[107] Jovanovic's recent study found that 15.5% of mothers with DM1 and 12.5% of mothers with DM2 had PTD compared to 6.1% of the normal population.[16]

Long-term neurologic outcomes in offspring: In one study, IDM achieved similar grades in primary school to a matched cohort, though there was a negative association between maternal A1c and the children's grades.[108] In another similar study, attention and motor performance appeared to be negatively associated with maternal A1c.[109]

Risk of diabetes mellitus in infant of a diabetic mother: The genetics of DM1 and DM2 differ. Most genes associated with DM1 are involved in immune regulation, and are associated with a variety of other autoimmune diseases. IDM have a 3.5% cumulative risk of developing DM1. Interestingly, the risk is 7.6% if the infant's father has DM1.[110]

Understanding the risk of parental transmission of DM2 is more complicated. The risk of a child of a parent with DM2, developing DM2 can vary between about 15% and about 50% depending on the age of the parent's diagnosis, the gender of the affected parent, whether the mother had diabetes during her pregnancy, and what genes are involved.

There are dozens of disparate genes associated with various forms of DM2. This is further complicated by the observation that prenatal exposure to maternal hyperglycemia and/or being an LGA or macrosomic infant increases the risk of metabolic syndrome, obesity, and DM2 later in life.[111] One of the first observations of this was Dabalea's description of discordant sibships in the Pima Native American population.[112,113] Even the offspring of women with DM1 seem to have a higher risk of DM2 presumably due to the intrauterine exposure to hyperglycemia.[114] The risk of DM2 in IDM may also vary with the gender of the affected parent, but not all studies have found this.[115,116]

Hypertension, nephropathy, and preeclampsia: There is a complex relationship between hypertension, nephropathy, and preeclampsia confounded by varying criteria used to define these diagnoses. Pregnancy demands an increase in glomerular filtration rate (GFR), and the urine albumin excretion rate increase normally in all pregnancies.[117] Fortunately, for most patients including those with diabetes, this returns to baseline after the pregnancy. Several studies have shown that in women with diabetes and normal renal function, including those with microalbuminuria, pregnancy does not increase the risk of developing or progressing renal disease.[118-120] However, between 40% and 65% of women with moderate to severe renal impairment will have progression of renal disease during pregnancy.[121,122] In one study of women with serum creatinine > 2.0 mg/dL, seven out of 20 progressed to require dialysis.[122]

Chronic hypertension, microalbuminuria, chronic kidney disease, and PEDM are all risk factors for preeclampsia.[6,104,105,123,124] The level of glycemic control during a pregnancy also impacts the rate of preeclampsia.[125,126] In general, the more severe the kidney disease, the higher the risks of progressive renal disease, preeclampsia, PTD, and perinatal mortality.[127]

In one study, preeclampsia occurred in 18.1% of pregnancies with PEDM.[6] In Jovanovic's retrospective claims analysis, hypertension complicating pregnancy was not separated out into subcategories, so the rate of preeclampsia versus chronic hypertension could not be ascertained.[16] However, it was clear from that analysis that hypertension of some form complicated about half of pregnancies with PEDM.

Progression of retinopathy: Diabetic retinopathy can progress rapidly during pregnancy and the peripartum period.[119,120,128-130] Therefore, a comprehensive preconception ophthalmologic examination is a part of appropriate PC.[47] The risk of women with PEDM and no baseline retinopathy, developing retinopathy during pregnancy is about 10%.[128,129] Roughly 20% of those with nonproliferative diabetic retinopathy will progress, and about 55% of those with proliferative retinopathy. Women found to have active proliferative retinopathy on their preconception examination should consider delaying pregnancy until the retinopathy has been treated and stabilized.[47] An eye examination is recommended every trimester to assess for progression. If unstable proliferative retinopathy develops, an assisted vaginal delivery or a C-section may be considered. Other risk factors for progression of retinopathy include poor glycemic control, duration of diabetes, smoking, and rapid improvement in glycemic control.[119,120,128,130]

Myocardial infarction/postpartum cardiomyopathy: Myocardial infarction (MI), congestive heart failure, and postpartum cardiomyopathy are fortunately rare events in pregnancy. However, PEDM is a risk factor for cardiac complications during pregnancy.[16] Maternal and fetal mortality associated with MI during pregnancy are high (11% and 9%, respectively).[131] Screening for coronary artery disease (CAD) is recommended by some for older women with PEDM of long duration and multiple risk factors.[47]

Preconception Management of Comorbid Conditions

Table 15.2 outlines the examinations and tests recommended in the evaluation and screening for diabetes comorbidities and complications.

Preconception management of overweight and obesity is an emerging problem. One study of a regional health system in Alabama found that in 1999, almost 25% of women presenting for their first prenatal visit are over 200 pounds and 4.9% were over 300 pounds. Maternal obesity is associated with not only GDM but also preeclampsia, C-section, obstructive sleep apnea, and complications at the time of labor and delivery.[132] Furthermore, weight gain during pregnancy exceeding recommended guidelines is reported in roughly 59% of overweight women and 56% of obese women.[132] While there are recommendations to refer women with overweight and obesity to a dietitian and to encourage healthy lifestyle and attainment of a healthy body weight,[46,132] a 2015 Cochrane review of preconception interventions for obesity found no studies eligible for review.[133]

For women with chronic hypertension, angiotensin converting enzyme (ACE) inhibitors and angiotensin receptor blockers (ARBs) should be discontinued[47,134,135] and if necessary replaced by antihypertensive medication considered safe in pregnancy such as nifedipine or labetalol. The 8th Joint National Committee (JNC8) recommends blood pressure (BP) goals of systolic BP less than 140 mm Hg and diastolic BP less than 90 mm Hg in nonpregnant patients with diabetes.[136] Nephrology consult should be obtained for women with a urine microalbumin more than 300 or a decreased GFR.

Statin, niacin, and fibric acid medications should be discontinued prior to conception.[47,58] However, it is important to be aware of the rare but serious cases of hypertriglyceridemia-induced pancreatitis during pregnancy seen in women with familial hypertriglyceridemia.[137,138] Women at risk for this should receive specialized MNT and omega-3 fatty acids to prevent pancreatitis.[139]

A careful review of all medications is an important part of PC. For example, many women with DM2 have PCOS. One common treatment for PCOS is spironolactone. This should be stopped prior to conception.

Thyroid disorders are common in women with diabetes. Women on thyroid hormone replacement should be advised that once pregnancy is confirmed, the thyroid hormone dose will need to be increased by 25%. This may be done conveniently by adding two additional tablets to the usual dose each week.[140]

PREGNANCY

Screening for Diabetes during Pregnancy

There is a uniform agreement that PEDM should be identified and treated as soon as possible in pregnancy.[141] However, there is no uniform agreement on whom and how to screen for overt diabetes and for lesser degrees of impaired glucose metabolism. The American College of Obstetricians and Gynecologists (ACOG) recommends screening high-risk women including those with prior history of GDM, glucose intolerance, or BMI greater than 30 using the two-step method to rule out overt diabetes.[142] The International Association of Diabetes and Pregnancy Study Groups (IADPSG) recommendations called for screening of some or all women early in pregnancy subject to differences in prevalence of diabetes in local populations.[143] The diagnosis of overt (preexisting) diabetes is made with a fasting glucose $\geq$ 126, or random glucose [or 2 hours after 75 g oral glucose tolerance test (OGTT)] $\geq$ 200 mg/dL (11.1 mmol/L), or A1c $\geq$ 6.5.[144] Underscoring the concern that intermediate levels of glycemia, less than overt diabetes may impart greater risks of adverse outcomes,[145] IADPSG also recommended that 1st trimester fasting glucose $\geq$ 92 mg/dL (5.1 mmol/L) be consistent with the diagnosis of GDM.[143] However, more recently the fasting glucose has been shown to decline in pregnancy so that 1st trimester fasting glucose less than 110 mg/dL (6.1 mmol/L) is less predictive of GDM later in pregnancy. While 1st trimester fasting glucose 92 to less than 110 mg/dL (5.1–6.1 mmol/L) is also associated with higher risk of GDM, the incidence may not be sufficient to warrant early detection of GDM.[146] Zhu and Yang et al. recommend identifying women with fasting glucose 110–125 mg/dL (6.10–6.99 mmol/L) for early intervention, as 66.2% will develop GDM later in pregnancy. They suggest this as a practical approach as there is no RCT outcome data to support early intervention in this intermediate range of glucose.

Early pregnancy A1c ≥ 5.9 is associated with worse outcomes including increased risk of CM, preeclampsia, shoulder dystocia, and perinatal death. It identified all the patients in the cohort who had overt diabetes.[147] Women with A1c ≥ 5.9 represented only 2.9% of the total cohort. However, among women with A1c ≥ 5.9 early in pregnancy, 74% had GDM [diagnosed by IADPSG/World Health Organization (WHO) criteria either early or later in pregnancy] or overt diabetes (10.4% of this group). As noted earlier, the sensitivity of diagnosing women with overt diabetes was 100%. However, the sensitivity was not as good at diagnosing GDM, as 12% of women with A1c less than 5.9 were diagnosed with GDM earlier than 20 weeks and 13% were diagnosed later than 20 weeks, underscoring the need for either a one step or two step screen at 24–28 weeks in women with an initial A1c less than 5.9.

In summary, at this time, the authors are not aware of data to support the ACOG recommendation for the use of the two-step method early in pregnancy to identify women with overt diabetes or at high-risk of developing GDM. As the purpose of a screening test is to identify a disease or risk factor for a disease in large numbers of apparently healthy individuals, there is no point in offering a 1 hour 50 g glucose loading test (GLT) to a group of women who are already at high-risk for a disease. These women should undergo a diagnostic 2 hour 75 g OGTT. Alternatively, we and others find a threshold A1c of 5.9 to be a compelling early pregnancy diagnostic test. Fasting glucose ≥ 126 identifies women with overt diabetes and glucose ≥ 110 mg identifies those who are at very high-risk of developing GDM for early intervention.[148]

All women without PEDM or the early diagnosis of overt diabetes or GDM should be screened for GDM at 24–28 weeks gestation with either the one step or two-step method. Selective screening for historical risk factors may not be efficient, as only 10% of women meet the low-risk characteristics that would not require laboratory screening.[149] Women who are at high-risk for GDM but had a negative test early in pregnancy should undergo a diagnostic test skipping the screening test.

Diagnosis of Gestational Diabetes

In 1964, O'Sullivan and Mahan published data which defined GDM based on whole blood glucose levels that were two standard deviations (SDs) above the mean for normal and correlated it with a future maternal risk of diabetes of 50% over the next 20 years.[150] Neonatal and pregnancy outcomes were not evaluated. Subsequently, the National Diabetes Data Group (NDDG) adjusted these criteria by taking into account changes from whole blood to plasma measurements.[151] The Carpenter and Coustan criteria adjusted for changes in the measurement of glucose from the nonspecific Somogyi-Nelson to the glucose oxidase method.[152] An initial 50 g GLT screening test, if positive, was followed by a diagnostic 3 hours 100 g OGTT, comprising a two-step method.

For decades, there was lack of consensus among healthcare providers and institutions across the world regarding these and other criteria because there was insufficient data to determine which criteria best predicted adverse neonatal and pregnancy outcomes. For this reason, the observational HAPO study was designed to investigate the impact of maternal glycemia which is less severe than overt diabetes, on the risk of adverse neonatal and pregnancy outcomes.[153] The HAPO study demonstrated a linear increase in the risk of primary outcomes including > 90th percentile for infant birth weight (LGA) and cord C-peptide, clinically diagnosed neonatal hypoglycemia, and the need for cesarean delivery with increasing degrees of hyperglycemia at all time points, as assessed by a fasting 75 g 2 hours OGTT at fasting, 1 and 2 hours. The secondary outcomes of preeclampsia, PTD (<37 weeks gestation), and shoulder dystocia or birth injury also increased with increasing glycemia.[147] Neonatal skinfold thicknesses more than 90% exhibited a linear relationship with increasing glycemia.[154] RCTs on treatment of GDM demonstrated reductions in adverse pregnancy and neonatal outcomes with treatment, although neither of these studies uses the exact GDM thresholds proposed by the IADPSG.[143,155,156]

As a result of the aforementioned studies, IADPSG convened a consensus conference to arrive at diagnostic targets for the 75 g 2 hours OGTT. The challenge for the group entailed how and at what values to establish dichotomous targets for the fasting, 1 hour and 2 hour values, when the risk of adverse outcomes is continuous and linear. An OR of 1.75 times the mean was selected for the outcomes of increased neonatal body fat, LGA, and cord C-peptide greater than the 90th percentile to arrive at the recommended diagnostic criteria for GDM. While mean values for fasting plasma glucose, 1 hour and 2 hours OGTT plasma glucose concentrations were 4.5 mmol/L (81 mg/dL), 7.4 mmol/L (133 mg/dL), and 6.2 mmol/L (112 mg/dL), respectively. The plasma glucose levels corresponding to or above an OR of 1.75 were fasting plasma glucose ≥ 5.1 mmol/L (92 mg/dL), 1 hour plasma glucose ≥10 mmol/L (180 mg/dL), and 2 hours plasma glucose ≥ 8.5 mmol/L (153 mg/dL). GDM was diagnosed if one or more values were met but were less than overt diabetes criteria.[143] Because of the linear relationship of glucose levels with higher frequencies of adverse outcomes, the choice of IADPSG thresholds was necessarily arbitrary and underscores the underlying controversy about these thresholds. The higher risk of adverse outcomes when one or more glucose values are equal to or above the IADPSG thresholds is shown in the Table 15.4.

Table 15.4: Frequency of outcomes when all glucose values are below threshold or any one or more is equal to or above threshold[+]

Outcome	***FPG, 1-hr and 2-hr OGTT values all < threshold***	***FPG and /or 1-hr and/or 2-hr OGTT values ≥ threshold***
Birthweight > 90th percentile	8.3%	16.2%**
Cord C-peptide > 90th percentile	6.7%	17.5%**
Percent body fat > 90th percentile	8.5%	16.6%**
Preeclampsia	4.5%	9.1%**
Preterm delivery (< 37 weeks)	6.4%	9.4%**
Primary cesarean section	16.8%	24.4%**

Contd...

Contd...

Outcome	FPG, 1-hr and 2-hr OGTT values all < threshold	FPG and /or 1-hr and/or 2-hr OGTT values ≥ threshold
Shoulder dystocia and/or bith injury	1.3%	1.8%*
Clinical neonatal hypoglycemia	1.9%	2.7%*
Hyperbilirubinemia	8.0%	10.0%**
Intensive neonatal care	7.8%	9.1%*

(FPG: fasting plasma glucose; HAPO: Hyperglycemia and Adverse Pregnancy Outcome; IADPSG: International Association of Diabetes and Pregnancy Study Groups; OGTT: oral glucose tolerance test)
+Threshold values: FPG ≥ 5.1 mmol/L (92 mg/dL), 1-hr PG ≥ 10.0 mmol/L (180 mg/dL), 2-hr ≥ 8.5 mmol/L (153 mg/dL)
*Difference between groups significant at p < 0.01
**Difference between groups significant at p < 0.001
Source: Reprinted with permission from American Diabetes Association.

The American Diabetes Association endorsed the IADPSG guidelines in 2011 stating that 'these diagnostic criteria changes are being made in the context of worrisome worldwide increases in obesity and diabetes rates with the intent of optimizing gestational outcomes for women and their babies.'[157] The Endocrine Society adopted them in 2013.[47] The WHO adopted them in 2013 based on a simulation study that demonstrated some advantages of the IADPSG criteria compared with the previous WHO criteria with lower numbers needed to screen to prevent adverse outcomes and in the interest of moving toward a universal standard recommendation for the diagnosis of GDM.[158] However, in 2011, a committee opinion of the ACOG continued to recommend the two-step method, expressing concern that approximately 18% of women would be diagnosed with GDM based on IADPSG guidelines.[159] An National Institutes of Health (NIH) Consensus Conference concurred.[160] An ACOG practice bulletin in 2013 reaffirmed their position recommending a 1 hour 50 g screening test at 24–28 weeks for women with risk factors and if the screen is abnormal, the diagnosis of GDM should be based on the 3 hours 100 g (OGTT).[142] The ACOG bulletin lists two separate criteria for the diagnosis of GDM: (1) The NDDG, and (2) Carpenter and Coustan (C + C) criteria, shown here in Table 15.5.[142] The ADA softened their position, acknowledging the GDM screening and diagnosis controversy, in their 2015 practice guidelines, and opted to recommend either the one step IADPSG or the two-step method (either NDDG or C + C criteria) preferred by ACOG.[144] Outside the United States (US), the International Federation of Gynecology and Obstetrics (FIGO) supports the use of the IADPSG criteria.[161] Other varieties of responses to the IADPSG recommendations from the other nations also demonstrate the complexity and controversy especially given concerns around access to health care and costs.[162]

For those advocating the use of the two-step method the question remains whether to use the NDDG criteria or C + C criteria. In a secondary analysis of a RCT of Landon 2009,[156] use of C + C criteria compared with NDDG criteria increases the number of women diagnosed with GDM by 30–50% but similar benefit of treatment was derived in both groups.[156] The p value for interaction was not significant for any neonatal outcomes suggesting that those diagnosed by C + C criteria benefit equally from treatment compared with those diagnosed by the NDDG criteria. With the exception of shoulder dystocia, the number needed to treat to prevent a single outcome of cesarean delivery, pregnancy-induced hypertension, shoulder dystocia, LGA, and

Table 15.5: Criteria for diagnosis of GDM.

	O'Sullivan[150]	NDDG[151]	Carpenter and Coustan[152]	IADPSG[143]	Adapted from IADPSG, WHO,[158] and Endocrine Society[47]	NICE
	1964	1979	1982	2010	2013	2015
	Whole blood	Plasma				
	Two step: 50 g glucose load test—One abnormal value 100 g—Two abnormal values			75 g—One abnormal value		
Fasting (mg/dL)	90	105	95	92	92–125	101
1 hour	165	190	180	180	180	–
2 hours	145	165	155	153	153–199	145
3 hours	125	145	140	–	–	–
Endorsed by	O'Sullivan whole blood[144]	ACOG[142] ADA[223]	ACOG[142] ADA[223]	ADA[213]	WHO[158]	NICE[45]

(ACOG: American College of Obstetricians and Gynecologists; ADA: American Diabetes Association; GDM: gestational diabetes mellitus; IADPSG: International Association of Diabetes and Pregnancy Study Groups; NDDG: National Diabetes Data Group; NICE: National Institute for Health and Care Excellence; WHO: World Health Organization)
Source: American Diabetes Association (ADA). (2017). Diabetes Care. [online] Available from www.care.diabetesjournals.org/cgi/content/full/dc09-1848/DC1. [Accessed February, 2018].

macrosomia was small (20 or less for the overall group) and similar for both C + C and NDDG criteria.[163] At many institutions, there is disagreement over the method of diagnosing GDM (Table 15.5). The Joslin Diabetes Center has adapted its guidelines to accommodate these differences, opting for either the one step IADPSG method or the two-step method with Carpenter and Coustan criteria (Flowchart 15.1).[152]

Several outcome studies compare the use of IADPSG criteria versus other criteria. Meek et al. evaluated UK NICE criteria versus IADPSG criteria found that women who 'fell through the net,' testing NICE negative but IADPSG positive (n = 387), had a higher risk of having a LGA infant [birth weight > 90th percentile for gestational age; adjusted OR (95% CI) 3.12 (2.44, 3.98)], cesarean delivery [1.44 (1.15, 1.81)], and polyhydramnios [6.90 (3.94,12.08)] compared with women with negative screening results and no OGTT (n = 21,695).[164]

Wei et al. evaluated a 75 g OGTT diagnostic test using NDDG criteria versus IADPSG criteria, and found a 125% increase in women diagnosed with GDM by IADPSG criteria (8.4% vs. 18.9% of cohort). The group with GDM based on IADPSG that was untreated had the highest rates of macrosomia and cesarean delivery compared with three different groups with normal glucose tolerance, treated GDM by NDDG criteria, and treated GDM by IADPSG.[165]

In a retrospective cohort study, Feldman and colleagues evaluated whether change from the two-step method using Carpenter–Coustan criteria (two step) to the one-step approach to GDM screening and diagnosis using the IADPSG criteria (one step) was associated with improved

Flowchart 15.1: Joslin guidelines for gestational diabetes mellitus (GDM) diagnosis.

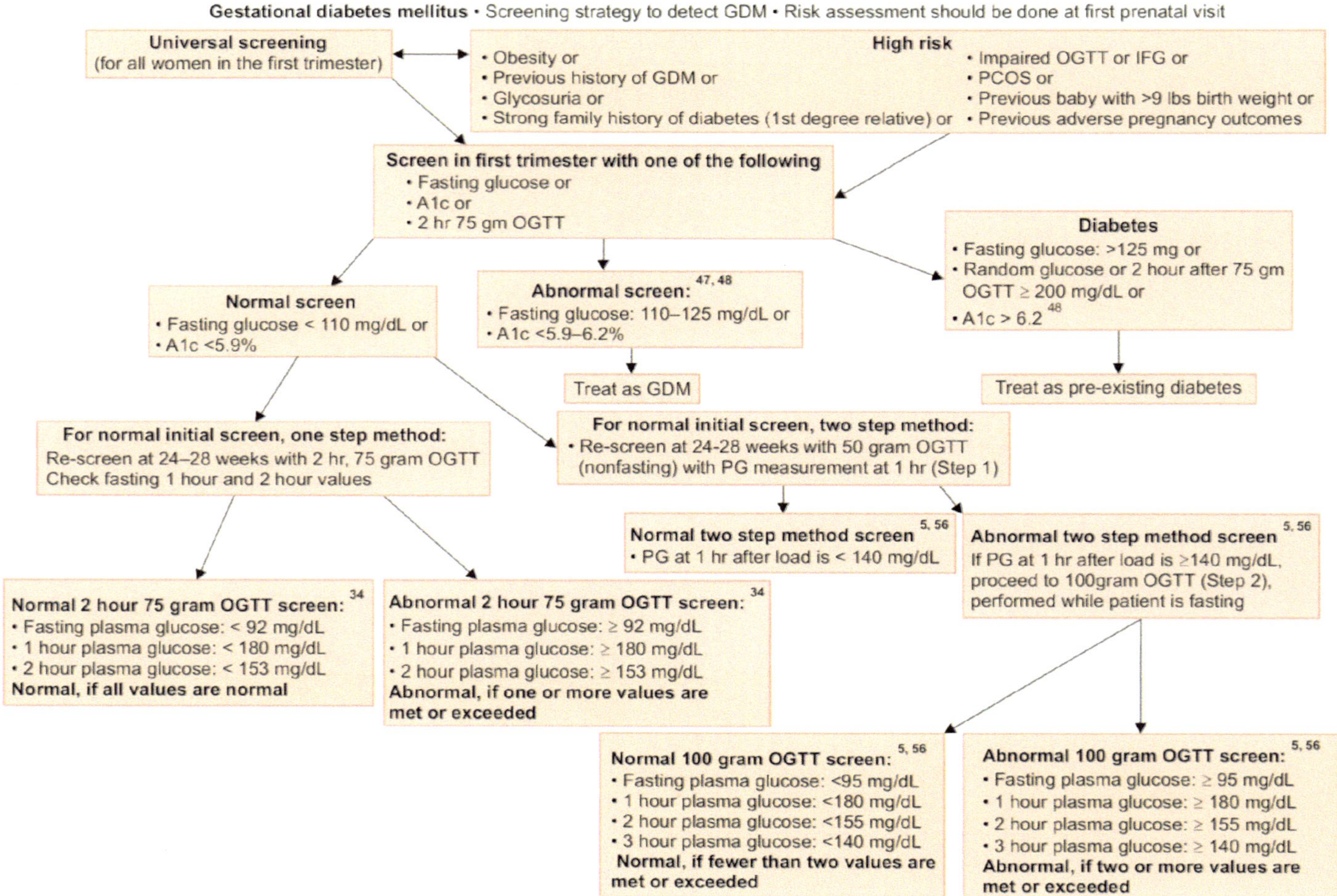

(IFG: impaired fasting glucose; PCOS: polycystic ovary syndrome; OGTT: oral glucose tolerance test)

Source: Reprinted with permission from Joslin Diabetes Center.

maternal and perinatal outcomes.[166] The diagnosis of GDM increased over the study period from 17% (two step) to 27% (one step). There was no significant difference in the rates of the primary outcome of LGA neonates (10% and 9%, respectively) or any other secondary perinatal measure between the two groups. However, the primary cesarean delivery rate significantly increased from 16% (two step) to 20% (one step). The authors point out that routine early screening for PEDM did not occur in the two-step group and that more patients were diagnosed with overt diabetes in the one-step group (4% compared with 15%, P 0.001). They did not exclude these women because they considered that the two-step group likely also had some patients with undiagnosed overt diabetes. They also reported a significantly increased use of glyburide in the after patients which is noteworthy given the effect of glyburide on neonatal outcomes (see section on treatment of GDM).[166]

Long-term Risks and Outcomes of Gestational Diabetes Mellitus in Offspring

The effect of fetal exposure to increasing maternal glycemia independent of maternal prepregnancy BMI on later childhood adiposity has been the subject of many studies and systematic analyses. These studies suggest an association of GDM with childhood obesity, although this may be less influential than maternal preconception BMI.[167] In longer follow-up studies, childhood Z-scores are increased at 7 years in association with increasing maternal fasting glucose at 24–28 weeks gestation, after adjustment for confounders including maternal prepregnancy BMI.[168] A longitudinal study of 421 mother-daughter pairs at Kaiser Permanente Northern California evaluated maternal pregnancy glucose values and the association with adiposity outcomes measured annually: (1) More than or equal to 85th age-specific percentile for BMI; (2) Percent body fat; and (3) Waist-to-height ratio. Girls who were exposed to maternal GDM or hyperglycemia in utero were at higher risk of childhood adiposity; risk increases if the mother was overweight or obese.[169]

In a follow-up study of children (ages 5–10 years) of women previously enrolled in a multicenter trial of treatment versus no treatment of mild GDM,[156] height, weight, blood pressure, waist circumference, fasting glucose, fasting insulin, triglycerides, and high-density lipoprotein (HDL) cholesterol were measured.[170] No reduction in childhood obesity or metabolic dysfunction in the offspring of treated women was found. However, sex-specific differences were noted in female offspring of women treated for mild GDM having lower fasting glucose and log HOMA-IR (P for interaction = 0.002 and 0.02, respectively) than the untreated group.[170] A recent review looks at the complexities of the debate between use of the one-step and two-step for diagnosing GDM, including differences in prevalence of diagnosis, effects of outcomes, and medical costs.[171]

Treatment of Gestational Diabetes Mellitus and Preexisting Diabetes Mellitus

Medical Nutrition Therapy, Monitoring, and Goals

Medical nutrition therapy in conjunction with self-monitoring of blood glucose (SMBG) are mainstays of the treatment of GDM and PEDM (see PC—MNT earlier). Food records and SMBG records are required to assess the effectiveness of MNT. Carbohydrate counting skills are taught for a consistent carb intake. Food records and SMBG records should be reviewed weekly by a combination of electronic, phone, and face to face visits. During pregnancy, the caloric intake should be increased by about 300 kcal above basal requirements.[43]

The IOM also recommends specific goals for weight gain during pregnancy based on preconception or first prenatal visit BMI (Table 15.6) A recent RCT provides a compelling argument for lifestyle intervention in early gestation in women at high-risk of GDM (prior history of GDM or obesity). Moderate lifestyle intervention resulted in a 39% reduction in the incidence of GDM.[172] However, another RCT did not demonstrate significant improved in neonatal or pregnancy outcomes with lifestyle intervention in pregnancy in a moderate risk (overweight and obese) cohort.[173]

Ensuring an A1c in the target range is the primary goal of PEDM. To achieve this, patients need to perform SMBG: Fasting, before meals, and 1 or 2 hours postprandial.[47] Postprandial monitoring of blood glucose results in better outcomes than preprandial monitoring.[174] Various guidelines, ACOG, ADA, Endocrine Society, and FIGO recommends target glucose fasting is less than 95 mg/dL (5.3 mmol/L), 1 hour less than 140 mg/dL (7.8 mmol/L), or 2 hours less than 120 mg/dL (6.6 mmol/L) (Table 15.2).[47,54,58,142] These goals were reinforced by a systematic review commissioned by the Endocrine Society.[175] Yet, the ADA also targets lower 1 hour peak postprandial blood glucose of less than 130 mg/dL for women with PEDM.[47,58]

Normative data should be considered when formulating therapeutic goals. The HAPO study demonstrated mean fasting glucose of 81 mg/dL ± 7 mg/dL (4.5 mmol/L ± 0.39 mmol/L) between 24 weeks and 32 weeks.[153] Ambulatory continuous glucose monitoring of interstitial fluid in nondiabetic pregnancies demonstrates that the mean of peak postprandial glucose concentration approximates 110 ± 16 mg/dL (6.1 ± 0.9 mmol/L) and that there is substantial intra- and inter subject variation of the time to the peak glucose excursion after starting the meal (range 45–120 min).[176] It should be noted that the aforementioned target fasting and

Table 15.6: IOM weight gain. New recommendations for total and rate of weight gain during pregnancy by prepregnancy BMI.

Prepregnancy BMI	***Total weight gain***		***Rates of weight gain* 2nd and 3rd trimesters***	
	Range in kg	***Range in lbs***	***Mean (range) in kg/week***	***Mean (range) in lbs/week***
Underweight (<18.5 kg/m^2)	12.5–18	28–40	0.51 (0.44–0.58)	1 (1–1.3)
Normal weight (18.5–24.9 kg/m^2)	11.5–16	25–35	0.42 (0.35–0.50)	1 (0.8–1)
Overweight (25.0–29.9 kg/m^2)	7–11.5	15–25	0.28 (0.23–0.33)	0.6 (0.5–0.7)
Obese (≥30.0 kg/m^2)	5–9	11–20	0.22 (0.17–0.27)	0.5 (0.4–0.6)

(BMI: body mass index; IOM: Institute of Medicine)

*Calculations assume a 0.5–2 kg (1.1–4.4 lbs) weight gain in the 1st trimester (based on Siega-Riz et al. 1994; Abrams et al. 1995; Carmichael et al. 1997).

Source: The National Academies Press (NAP). (2009). Weight gain during pregnancy: reexamining the guidelines. [online] Available from www.nap.edu/catalog/12584/weight-gain-during-pregnancy-reexamining-the-guidelines. [Accessed February, 2018].

1 hour targets above are approximately two SD above normal. Lower targets may need to be considered, especially in the setting of fetal abdominal circumference more than or equal to 75%, when data suggest that mean blood glucose for fasting (80 mg/dL, 4.5 mmol/L) and 1 hour after meals (110 mg/dL, 6.1 mmol/L) should be targeted.[177]

We have found that weekly glucose log reviews with ideally twice monthly face to face visits and monthly A1c checks achieves target glucose and A1c goals for most patients.

Oral Hypoglycemic Treatment of Gestational Diabetes Mellitus

Insulin has been the mainstay for the medical treatment of GDM, if diet and exercise are insufficient in achieving glycemic targets. It continues to be the standard of care endorsed by ACOG, ADA, Endocrine Society, and FIGO.[47,142,144,161] However, in the last 15 years, glyburide has been increasingly used to treat GDM in the US,[178] and metformin has been steadily gaining acceptance in other countries.

Two different initial RCTs one comparing glyburide versus insulin and the other metformin versus insulin demonstrated favorable pregnancy and neonatal outcomes to support their use.[179,180] Presently, neither glyburide nor metformin are approved by the FDA for use in pregnancy. In 2000, Langer et al. described a RCT of 404 singleton pregnancies with GDM treated with either glyburide or insulin.[179] 4% of subjects in the glyburide arm were not able to achieve glycemic goals and were started on insulin. The primary outcome variable was level of glycemic control based on home SMBG and A1c. With treatment, the mean SMBG [105 mg/dL ± 16 mg/dL (5.8 mmol/L ± 0.9) vs. 105 mg/dL ± 18 mg/dL (5.8 mmol/L ± 1; P = 0.99] and A1c (5.5 ± 0.7 vs. 5.4 ± 0.6; P = 0.12) did not differ between the treatment and control groups, respectively. No differences were noted in neonatal outcomes. This study led to glyburide's increasing use in pregnancy with every calendar year from a US commercial insurance database.[178] In 2001, 7.4% of women with GDM who required medication for glycemic control were treated with glyburide compared with 92.6% treated with insulin. By 2011, 65% of women with GDM requiring medication were treated with glyburide and 35% of women were treated with insulin.[178] It is more convenient and cheaper than insulin. In a cost analysis, Goetzl et al. found that the average cost savings per patient treated with glyburide instead of insulin was US$165.84.[181] However, since then numerous retrospective and prospective clinical trials demonstrate higher glyburide failure rates of approximately 20%.[182] Concerns have been raised from a pharmacologic study of glyburide that showed it crosses the placenta with an average glyburide umbilical cord to maternal plasma concentration ratio at the time of delivery of 0.7 ± 0.4. This study differs from Langer 2000 in which cord glyburide level were undetectable in a less sensitive assay. Also while fasting blood glucose levels were normal, peak postprandial blood glucose levels were elevated following a mixed meal tolerance test in GDM women on their stable glyburide dose compared with normal pregnant women having 167 ± 33 mg/dL versus 122 ± 16 mg/dL (9.3 mmol/L ± 1.8 vs. 6.8 mmol/L ± 0.5).[183] Two recent meta-analyses of RCTs demonstrate worse outcomes with glyburide compared to insulin. Both demonstrate at least a doubling of the risk of macrosomia and neonatal hypoglycemia with glyburide.[184,185]

The Metformin in Gestational Diabetes Trial (MiG Trial) was an RCT of metformin versus insulin.[180] Subjects were randomized to receive metformin (<2.5 g/day) or insulin. Women with blood glucose that were not controlled with metformin alone (46% of the metformin group) also received insulin. The composite primary endpoint included neonatal hypoglycemia, respiratory distress, the need for phototherapy, birth trauma, Apgar score less than 7 at 5 minutes, preterm birth, and admission and duration of admission to neonatal intensive care unit (NICU). No significant difference was seen in the composite primary endpoint rates between the women receiving metformin versus insulin (32.0% vs. 32.2%, P = 0.95). However, the prevalence of severe neonatal hypoglycemia was lower in the metformin group than the insulin group (3.3% vs. 8.1%, P = 0.008), but preterm birth (<37 weeks) was more prevalent in women taking metformin compared to insulin (12.1% vs. 7.6%, P = 0.04). There was no difference in secondary outcomes including neonatal factors such as gestational age at birth, birth weight percentile, umbilical cord serum insulin concentration, and maternal factors such as glycemic control at various times during pregnancy, hypertension, postpartum, oral glucose tolerance testing results, and BMI. There was no significant difference in glycemic control between the two groups as measured by A1c at weeks 36–37 (5.6% ± 0.5% in the metformin group vs. 5.7% ± 0.6% in the insulin group, P = 0.25) nor fasting SMBG at randomization until delivery (93.6 ± 10.8 mg/dL in the metformin group vs. 91.8 ± 12.6 mg/dL in the insulin group) 1 week after randomization (100.8 ± 16.2 mg/dL in the metformin group vs. 99.0 ± 18 mg/dL in the insulin group, P = 0.33).[180] However, there was a significant difference in 2 hours postprandial glucose from randomization until delivery (111.6 ± 10.8 mg/dL in the metformin group vs. 115.2 ± 16.2 mg/dL in the insulin group, P = 0.003) and at 1 week after randomization (117 ± 16.2 mg/dL in the metformin group vs. 120.6 ± 18 mg/dL in the insulin group, P = 0.006) which implies that women treated with metformin reached postprandial glucose goals earlier than women treated with insulin.[126] Pharmacokinetic studies demonstrate that metformin crosses the placenta achieving therapeutic concentrations that are similar to maternal levels.[186] This level of fetal exposure to metformin poses a long-term concern for infant health. In the Metformin in Gestational Diabetes the Offspring Follow-Up (MiG TOFU) study, children 2 years of age whose mothers had participated in the MiG study had higher mid-upper arm circumferences in the metformin compared to insulin group. There was no significant difference in total fat mass and percentage body fat assessed by bioimpedance and dual-energy X-ray absorptiometry.[187] Blood pressure and neurodevelopment did not differ in the offspring of the two groups.[188] Long-term safety data are not available.

All groups (ACOG, ADA, Endocrine Society, FIGO, and UK NICE) endorse the use of insulin to treat GDM.[46,47,142,144,161] All groups except ADA also endorse the use of the oral hypoglycemic agents, glyburide/glibenclamide and metformin to treat GDM. ADA cites concern over lack of long-term safety data with the oral agents. We agree with the position of the ADA as both drugs cross the placenta. The increasing use of glyburide/glibenclamide in the US is particularly concerning, as its use is associated with a doubling of macrosomia and neonatal hypoglycemia. We recommend the earlier groups reconsider their endorsement of glyburide for the treatment of GDM.

Glycemic Management in Preexisting Diabetes Mellitus

In the first 9 weeks of pregnancy there is an initial increase in insulin requirements followed by a decline in insulin requirements between weeks 9 and weeks 16.[26] While tight control is crucial during early pregnancy to reduce the risk of miscarriage and CM, maternal hypoglycemia must be considered. Maternal hypoglycemia does not seem to be associated with CM or other adverse fetal outcome.[42,44,189] However, maternal hypoglycemia can be dangerous.[190,191] Severe hypoglycemia is most likely to occur in the 1st trimester.[192] Previous history of severe hypoglycemia, A1c less than 6.5%, long duration of diabetes, and presence of hypoglycemic unawareness have been identified as risk factors.[191,192] Careful patient and family education on the detection, treatment, and prevention of hypoglycemia is important. Specific attention should be paid to safe driving practices including testing blood glucose prior to driving. The use of CGM should be considered.

Prenatal Care

Women with overt diabetes diagnosed in pregnancy and those with PEDM who have not had PC should be scheduled for diabetes education, nutrition, and medical consultation at the earliest possible time. The first visit should include the counseling and assessment recommended for PC.

Frequency of visits depends on a variety of factors including gestational age, patient adherence, glycemic control, and complications. Optimally, glucose logs should be reviewed twice a week for those not meeting glycemic goals and weekly to once every other week for those meeting goals. Visits should occur approximately every 1–2 weeks in the 1st and 2nd trimesters and then weekly after 28–30 weeks gestation.[44] Given the steady increase in insulin resistance that occurs in the second half of pregnancy, these frequent insulin adjustments are necessary to maintain tight control.

A sudden drop in insulin requirement greater than 15% later in pregnancy is associated with markers of placental insufficiency, increased risk for preeclampsia, earlier delivery, and NICU admission.[193]

Baby aspirin 81 mg daily as recommended from 12 weeks to 36 weeks help to reduce the risk for preeclampsia in patients with PEDM.[194]

An ultrasound (USG) at early in gestation is recommended to accurately date the pregnancy and demonstrate fetal viability.[44,46] An USG at 18–20 weeks is performed to assess growth and for CM.[44] Fetal echocardiography is routinely performed around 22 weeks to screen further for congenital heart defects and for fetal cardiac hypertrophy. In a retrospective study from the Mayo Clinic, routine anatomic surveys picked up only a third of congenital cardiac anomalies.[80] This highlights the importance of fetal echocardiogram in the routine care of preexisting diabetes. Following this, USG may be done every 4 weeks after 28 weeks gestation to assess fetal growth and amniotic fluid.[46]

Fetal movement counting, nonstress tests, biophysical profiles, and contraction stress tests are performed weekly usually starting at 32–34 weeks of gestation. The timing of initiation of testing may vary in pregnancies complicated by more high-risk conditions. As pregnancy progresses, twice weekly testing is often initiated.[44]

It is important to remember to advise women around 34–36 weeks gestation about the management of their diabetes during and after labor and delivery, breastfeeding, and contraception.

Medical Management of Comorbidities

Blood pressure measurements at every visit are essential to detect the development of hypertensive disorders in pregnancy. Women with known renal dysfunction prior to conception should have regular assessments during pregnancy of their renal function with creatinine and a urine protein assessment.[46] Women with nephrotic range of proteinuria are at increased risk for thrombotic events, and prophylaxis should be considered.[46] Refer to the ACOG guidelines for an in-depth review of hypertensive disorders in pregnancy.[195] ACOG has recently changed their position on the use of oral agents glyburide and metformin in pregnancy and now considers insulin the preferred treatment.[196]

Type 1 diabetes mellitus (and to a lesser extent T2DM) are associated with an increased risk of thyroid abnormalities.[197] We recommend screening women with PEDM without known thyroid disease and no previous screening with a thyroid-stimulating hormone (TSH). NICE supports this recommendation for women with DM1.[46] Women with known hypothyroidism who are on levothyroxine will require an increase of about 25% in their dose at the onset of pregnancy and continued monitoring throughout pregnancy with levothyroxine dose adjustments to achieve target TSH levels.[140]

Labor and Delivery

Women with diabetes should give birth in hospitals with NICUs, and written policies for the prevention, detection, and management of neonatal hypoglycemia.[46]

Maternal hyperglycemia during labor and delivery increases the risk of neonatal hypoglycemia. A continuous intravenous infusion of regular insulin titrated hourly is recommended during labor and delivery.[44] Alternatively, patients who manage their diabetes with an insulin pump may continue their basal rates during labor as long as it is considered safe to do so. Guidelines agree that glucose control during labor and delivery should be tight, but specific targets vary from less than 110 mg/dL to less than 126 mg/dL (6.1–7 mmol/L).[44,47]

When steroids are required for fetal lung maturation, either subcutaneous insulin doses will need to be adjusted or an insulin drip protocol should be employed. DKA has been reported in this setting and increased monitoring should be in place to prevent this.[44] Mathiesen found that up to a 40–45% increase in insulin doses was required to maintain good glucose control.[198] Betamimetic medicines for tocolysis should be avoided in women with diabetes because of an increased risk for hyperglycemia and DKA.[46]

Continuous fetal monitoring during labor and delivery is recommended.

Vaginal delivery is preferred with C-section reserved for nonreassuring fetal heart rate, failure to progress, breech presentation, and macrosomia more than 4,500 g.[44] Induction of labor in pregnancies complicated by macrosomia does not reduce birth injuries and may increase the rate of C-section.[44]

Complications and comorbidities often seen in pregnancy complicated by diabetes may need to be considered when deciding the route of delivery. Preeclampsia is a common concern. Proliferative diabetic retinopathy is another circumstance where C-section or assisted vaginal delivery may be considered.

THE POSTPARTUM PERIOD

Medical Management

Insulin requirements drop rapidly at delivery.[44] For patients who required insulin prior to pregnancy, approximately one-half of the prepregnancy insulin dose should be started after delivery. In one retrospective study of women with DM1 there was a 34% reduction in total daily insulin requirement in the postpartum period from preconception levels.[199] Women should be counseled to expect an increase in their insulin dose to around prepregnancy doses in the first few weeks postpartum. For women who were treated with oral hypoglycemic agents prepregnancy, one must first determine if they are planning on breastfeeding. Not all oral hypoglycemic are considered safe in pregnancy (see below).

For women with diabetes, special attention should be paid to wound healing as there is a 2.5-fold increase in wound complications.[200]

For women with hypothyroidism, the levothyroxine dose should be decreased to the prepregnancy dose. Women with DM1 should be screened with a TSH for postpartum thyroiditis at 3 and 6 months.[47]

Breastfeeding

Diabetes is not a contraindication to breastfeeding and we strongly encourage 6 months of exclusive breastfeeding and continued breastfeeding for 1 year for mothers with either GDM or PEDM.[47] In one very small study of women with DM2 who were breastfeeding no glyburide or glipizide was detected in breast milk and no infant hypoglycemia was reported.[193] Metformin is excreted in breast milk, mean estimated infant dose as a percentage of the mothers weight adjusted dose has been reported between 2% and 0.65%.[202,203] Based on this limited data, glyburide and metformin may be used during breastfeeding.[46,47] A recent study has demonstrated a relationship between longer duration of breastfeeding and lower risk of DM2 in the mom when tested 2 years after delivery.[204] Breastfeeding reduces the risk of obesity in all children.[205-208] Maternal overweight or obesity may have a strong positive effect on the risk of infant overweight at 2 years of age that may be reduced by breastfeeding. Studies of longer duration of follow-up such as 5–10 years suggest GDM as an independent risk factor for childhood overweight and obesity that may be reduced by breastfeeding.[209]

Hypoglycemia can occur overnight in insulin-requiring women who are breastfeeding. Small snacks before breastfeeding or an adjustment in basal insulin may be needed. One small study comparing women with DM1 who were or were not breastfeeding showed a reduced total daily insulin dose and increased hypoglycemia in women who were breastfeeding.[208] Another retrospective study of women with DM1 found no difference in total daily insulin requirement between women who were breastfeeding and those who were not.[199]

Screening and Long-term Follow-up of Gestational Diabetes Mellitus

The elevated blood glucose associated with GDM usually resolve after delivery. We advise monitoring blood glucoses prebreakfast and 2 hours post meals for the first 24 hours after

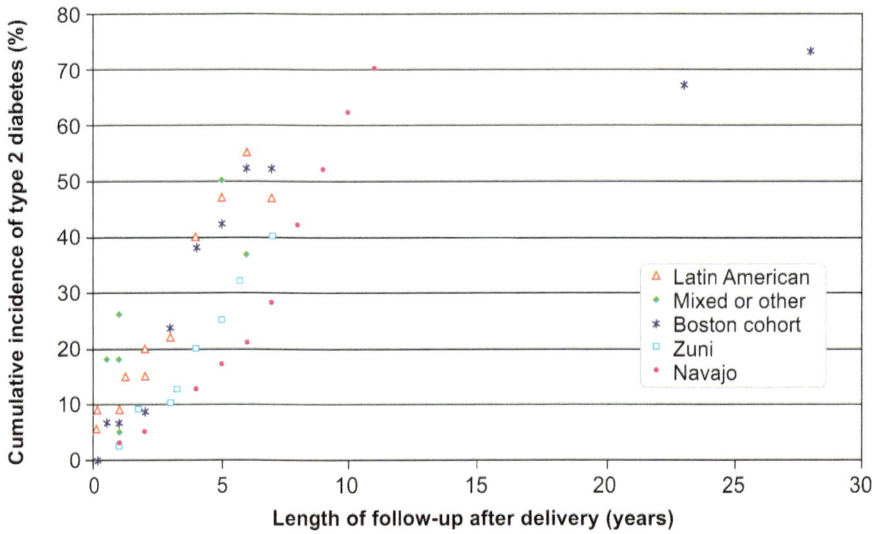

Fig. 15.3: Cathy Kim image

Source: Reprinted with permission from American Diabetes Association.

delivery and discontinuing SMBG, if they are normal. Some women may have underlying abnormal glucose metabolism or overt diabetes that may have been undiagnosed prior to pregnancy. In this case, hyperglycemia may not resolve. In addition, women with GDM are at high-risk of developing T2DM. The cumulative risk is approximately 50% over the next 7–10 years (Fig. 15.3).[210] A systematic review and meta-analysis demonstrates that factors that increase the risk of progression to DM2 include BMI, family history of diabetes, nonwhite ethnicity, advanced maternal age, early diagnosis of GDM, elevated fasting glucose, increased HbA1c, and need for insulin. Multiparity, hypertensive disorders in pregnancy, and PTD were also associated with future diabetes.[211] Women who had GDM should receive regular screening for diabetes. This is usually done in 6 weeks after delivery and at yearly medical visits. The ADA recommends a 75 g 2 hours OGTT postpartum at 6 weeks, 1 year, and every 3 years alternating with a fasting plasma glucose yearly.[54]

Lifestyle management with moderate weight loss has been shown to reduce the risk of DM2 in high-risk persons.[212-215] Targeting a weight that is 7% less than the preconception weight for women who have elevated BMI (≥25 for non-Asians and ≥23 for Asians),[216] or targeting the preconception weight for women with normal BMI, by optimizing diet and physical activity reduces the risk of diabetes. This is variably true in women with a history of GDM.[217,218] Adherence to lifestyle management is challenging in the GDM group as they may have reduced commitment to changing behaviors given the demands of motherhood. How to better engage these women in healthy lifestyle education and implementation is a priority for future research.[219-221]

Economic and Societal Impacts of Gestational and Preexisting Diabetes Mellitus

There is relatively little data on the economic impact of diabetes and pregnancy. However, in a systematic literature review from 2013, it is clear that PTL and delivery and other complications especially diabetes are major cost drivers in pregnancy care.[214] In one study which analyzed pregnancies from 2004 to 2011, the mean total medical cost for a pregnancy was $14,355 for patients without diabetes compared to $27,531 for patients with DM1 and $22,739 for patients with DM2.[16] Estimates for women treated with an insulin pump are considerably higher.[222,223]

There is really no data on the total economic and societal impact of diabetes in pregnancy. Data on the direct costs of care associated with the epidemic of gestational and preexisting diabetes seen in recent years is limited. There is no data on the economic losses related to complicated labor and delivery and recovery for women affected by diabetes and their families. Furthermore and ominously, it is not known what the extent of the personal and financial impact to families nor the larger societal and economic implications of the increase in the number of children affected by CMs or PTD resulting from the epidemic of diabetes and pregnancy will be.

REFERENCES

1. White P. Pregnancy complicating diabetes. Am J Med. 1949;7(5):609-16.
2. Hadden DR, McCance DR. Advances in management of Type 1 diabetes and pregnancy. Curr Opin Obstet Gynecol. 1999;11(6):557-62.
3. Clausen TD, Mathiesen E, Ekbom P, et al. Poor pregnancy outcome in women with Type 2 diabetes. Diabetes Care. 2005;28(2):323-8.
4. Cundy T, Gamble G, Townend K, et al. Perinatal mortality in Type 2 diabetes mellitus. Diabet Med. 2000;17(1):33-9.
5. Cundy T, Slee F, Gamble G, et al. Hypertensive disorders of pregnancy in women with Type 1 and Type 2 diabetes. Diabet Med. 2002;19(6):482-9.
6. Jensen DM, Damm P, Moelsted-Pedersen L, et al. Outcomes in Type 1 diabetic pregnancies: A nationwide, population-based study. Diabetes Care. 2004;27(12):2819-23.
7. Buchanan TA, Xiang A, Kjos SL, et al. What is gestational diabetes? Diabetes Care. 2007;30(Suppl 2):S105-11.
8. American Diabetes Association. Diagnosis and classification of diabetes mellitus. Diabetes Care. 2010;33(Suppl 1):S62-69.
9. Moran A, Brunzell C, Cohen RC, et al. Clinical care guidelines for cystic fibrosis-related diabetes: A position statement of the American Diabetes Association and a clinical practice guideline of the Cystic Fibrosis Foundation, endorsed by the Pediatric Endocrine Society. Diabetes Care. 2010;33(12):2697-708.
10. Chakera AJ, Spyer G, Vincent N, et al. The 0.1% of the population with glucokinase monogenic diabetes can be recognized by clinical characteristics in pregnancy: The Atlantic Diabetes in Pregnancy Cohort. Diabetes Care. 2014;37(5):1230-6.
11. Freathy RM, Hayes MG, Urbanek M, et al. Hyperglycemia and Adverse Pregnancy Outcome (HAPO) Study: common genetic variants in GCK and TCF7l2 are associated with fasting and postchallenge glucose levels in pregnancy and with the new consensus definition of gestational diabetes mellitus from the International Association of Diabetes and Pregnancy Study Groups. Diabetes. 2010;59(10):2682-9.
12. Tuomi T, Miettinen PJ, Hakaste L, et al. Atypical forms of diabetes. In: De Groot LJ, Beck-Peccoz P, Chrousos G, Dungan K, Grossman A, Hershman JM (Eds). Endotext. South Dartmouth: MDText.com; 2000.
13. Maahs DM, West NA, Lawrence JM, et al. Epidemiology of Type 1 diabetes. Endocrinol Metab Clin North Am. 2010;39(3):481-97.
14. Guariguata L, Whiting DR, Hambleton I, et al. Global estimates of diabetes prevalence for 2013 and projections for 2035. Diabetes Res Clin Pract. 2014;103(2):137-49.

15. Lawrence JM, Contreras R, Chen W, et al. Trends in the prevalence of preexisting diabetes and gestational diabetes mellitus among a racially/ethnically diverse population of pregnant women, 1999–2005. Diabetes Care. 2008;31(5):899-904.
16. Jovanovič L, Liang Y, Weng W, et al. Trends in the incidence of diabetes, its clinical sequelae, and associated costs in pregnancy. Diabetes Metab Res Rev. 2015;31(7):707-16.
17. Bardenheier BH, Imperatore G, Gilboa SM, et al. Trends in gestational diabetes among hospital deliveries in 19 U.S. States, 2000–2010. Am J Prev Med. 2015;49(1):12-9.
18. Feig DS, Razzaq A, Sykora K, et al. Trends in deliveries, prenatal care, and obstetrical complications in women with pregestational diabetes: A population-based study in Ontario, Canada, 1996-2001. Diabetes Care. 2006;29(2):232-5.
19. Feig DS, Hwee J, Shah BR, et al. Trends in incidence of diabetes in pregnancy and serious perinatal outcomes: a large, population-based study in Ontario, Canada, 1996-2010. Diabetes Care. 2014;37(6):1590-6.
20. DeSisto CL, Kim SY, Sharma AJ. Prevalence estimates of gestational diabetes mellitus in the United States, Pregnancy Risk Assessment Monitoring System (PRAMS), 2007-2010. Prev Chronic Dis. 2014;11:E104.
21. Torloni MR, Betrán AP, Horta BL, et al. Prepregnancy BMI and the risk of gestational diabetes: a systematic review of the literature with meta-analysis. Obes Rev. 2009;10(2):194-203.
22. Ryan EA. Hormones and insulin resistance during pregnancy. Lancet. 2003;362(9398):1777-8.
23. Hauguel-de Mouzon S, Guerre-Millo M. The placenta cytokine network and inflammatory signals. Placenta. 2006;27(8):794-8.
24. Barbour LA, Shao J, Qiao L, et al. Human placental growth hormone increases expression of the p85 regulatory unit of phosphatidylinositol 3-kinase and triggers severe insulin resistance in skeletal muscle. Endocrinology. 2004;145(3):1144-50.
25. Catalano PM. Trying to understand gestational diabetes. Diabet Med. 2014;31(3):273-81.
26. García-Patterson A, Gich I, Amini SB, et al. Insulin requirements throughout pregnancy in women with type 1 diabetes mellitus: three changes of direction. Diabetologia. 2010;53(3):446-51.
27. Stang J, Huffman LG. Position of the Academy of Nutrition and Dietetics: Obesity, Reproduction, and Pregnancy Outcomes. J Acad Nutr Diet. 2016;116(4):677-91.
28. Goodman NF, Cobin RH, Futterweit W, et al. American Association of Clinical Endocrinologists, American College of Endocrinology, and Androgen Excess and PCOS Society disease state clinical review: guide to the best practices in the evaluation and treatment of polycystic ovary syndrome—Part 2. Endocr Pract. 2015;21(12):1415-26.
29. Owens LA, O'Sullivan EP, Kirwan B, et al. Atlantic dip: The impact of obesity on pregnancy outcome in glucose-tolerant women. Diabetes Care. 2010;33(3):577-9.
30. Persson M, Johansson S, Villamor E, et al. Maternal overweight and obesity and risks of severe birth-asphyxia-related complications in term infants: a population-based cohort study in Sweden. PLoS Med. 2014;11(5):e1001648.
31. Rasmussen KM, Yaktine AL. Weight Gain During Pregnancy: Reexamining the Guidelines. Washington DC: National Academy of Sciences; 2009.
32. Kruse AR, Darling MS, Hansen MK, et al. Recurrence of gestational diabetes in primiparous women. Acta Obstet Gynecol Scand. 2015;94(12):1367-72.
33. Temple RC, Aldridge VJ, Murphy HR. Prepregnancy care and pregnancy outcomes in women with Type 1 diabetes. Diabetes Care. 2006;29(8):1744-9.
34. Kim C, Ferrara A, McEwen LN, et al. Preconception care in managed care: The translating research into action for diabetes study. Am J Obstet Gynecol. 2005;192(1):227-32.
35. Varughese GI, Chowdhury SR, Warner DP, et al. Preconception care of women attending adult general diabetes clinics—are we doing enough? Diabetes Res Clin Pract. 2007;76(1):142-5.

36. Linné Y. Effects of obesity on women's reproduction and complications during pregnancy. Obes Rev. 2004;5(3):137-43.
37. Jonasson JM, Brismar K, Sparen P, et al. Fertility in women with Type 1 diabetes: A population-based cohort study in Sweden. Diabetes Care. 2007;30(9):2271-6.
38. Dunne FP, Brydon P, Smith T, et al. Pre-conception diabetes care in insulin-dependent diabetes mellitus. QJM. 1999;92(3):175-6.
39. McElvy S, Miodovnik M, Rosenn B, et al. A focused preconceptional and early pregnancy program in women with Type 1 diabetes reduces perinatal mortality and malformation rates to general population levels. J Matern Fetal Med. 2000;9(1):14-20.
40. Suhonen L, Hiilesmaa V, Teramo K. Glycaemic control during early pregnancy and fetal malformations in women with Type I diabetes mellitus. Diabetologia. 2000;43(1):79-82.
41. Pregnancy outcomes in the Diabetes Control and Complications Trial. Am J Obstet Gynecol. 1996;174(4):1343-53.
42. Kitzmiller JL, Gavin LA, Gin GD, et al. Preconception care of diabetes: Glycemic control prevents congenital anomalies. JAMA. 1991;265(6):731-6.
43. Willhoite MB, Bennert HW, Palomaki GE, et al. The impact of preconception counseling on pregnancy outcomes. The experience of the Maine Diabetes in Pregnancy Program. Diabetes Care. 1993;16(2):450-5.
44. ACOG Committee on Practice Bulletins. ACOG practice bulletin. Clinical management guidelines for obstetrician-gynecologists. Number 60, March 2005. Pregestational diabetes mellitus. Obstet Gynecol. 2005;105(3):675-85.
45. Correa A, Bardenheier B, Elixhauser A, et al. Trends in prevalence of diabetes among delivery hospitalizations, United States, 1993–2009. Matern Child Health J. 2014;19(3):635-42.
46. National Institute for Health and Care Excellence (NICE). (2015). Diabetes in pregnancy: management from preconception to the postnatal period. [online] Available from www.nice.org.uk/guidance/ng3/chapter/1-Recommendations#antenatal-care-for-women-with-diabetes-2. [Accessed February, 2018].
47. Blumer I, Hadar E, Hadden DR, et al. Diabetes and pregnancy: An Endocrine Society Clinical Practice Guideline. J Clin Endocrinol Metab. 2013;98(11):4227-49.
48. Miller E, Hare JW, Cloherty JP, et al. Elevated maternal hemoglobin A1c in early pregnancy and major congenital anomalies in infants of diabetic mothers. N Engl J Med. 1981;304(22):1331-4.
49. Galindo A, Burguillo AG, Azriel S, et al. Outcome of fetuses in women with pregestational diabetes mellitus. J Perinat Med. 2006;34(4):323-31.
50. Guerin A, Nisenbaum R, Ray JG. Use of maternal GHb concentration to estimate the risk of congenital anomalies in the offspring of women with prepregnancy diabetes. Diabetes Care. 2007;30(7):1920-5.
51. Nielsen GL, Moller M, Sorensen HT. HbA1c in early diabetic pregnancy and pregnancy outcomes: A Danish population-based cohort study of 573 pregnancies in women with type 1 diabetes. Diabetes Care. 2006;29(12):2612-6.
52. Greene MF, Hare JW, Cloherty JP, et al. First-trimester hemoglobin A and risk for major malformation and spontaneous abortion in diabetic pregnancy. Teratology. 1989;39(3):225-31.
53. Ray JG, O'Brien TE, Chan WS. Preconception care and the risk of congenital anomalies in the offspring of women with diabetes mellitus: a meta-analysis. QJM. 2001;94(8):435-44.
54. Metzger BE, Buchanan TA, Coustan DR, et al. Summary and recommendations of the Fifth International Workshop-Conference on gestational diabetes mellitus. Diabetes Care. 2007;30(Suppl 2):S251-60.
55. Han S, Crowther CA, Middleton P, et al. Different types of dietary advice for women with gestational diabetes mellitus. Cochrane Database Syst Rev. 2013;(3):CD009725.
56. Hernandez TL, Van Pelt RE, Anderson MA, et al. A higher-complex carbohydrate diet in gestational diabetes mellitus achieves glucose targets and lowers postprandial lipids: a randomized crossover study. Diabetes Care. 2014;37(5):1254-62.

57. Hernandez TL, Van Pelt RE, Anderson MA, et al. Women with gestational diabetes mellitus randomized to a higher-complex carbohydrate/low-fat diet manifest lower adipose tissue insulin resistance, inflammation, glucose, and free fatty acids: a pilot study. Diabetes Care. 2016;39(1):39-42.
58. Kitzmiller JL, Block JM, Brown FM, et al. Managing preexisting diabetes for pregnancy: summary of evidence and consensus recommendations for care. Diabetes Care. 2008;31(5):1060-79.
59. American Diabetes Association. Preconception care of women with diabetes. Diabetes Care. 2004;27(Suppl 1):S76-8.
60. Mathiesen ER, Kinsley B, Amiel SA, et al. Maternal glycemic control and hypoglycemia in type 1 diabetic pregnancy: A randomized trial of insulin aspart versus human insulin in 322 pregnant women. 2007;30(4):771-6.
61. Cyganek K, Hebda-Szydlo A, Katra B, et al. Glycemic control and selected pregnancy outcomes in type 1 diabetes women on continuous subcutaneous insulin infusion and multiple daily injections: the significance of pregnancy planning. Diabetes Technol Therap. 2010;12(1):41-7.
62. Talaviya PA, Saboo BD, Joshi SR, et al. Pregnancy outcome and glycemic control in women with type 1 diabetes: a retrospective comparison between CSII and MDI treatment. Diabetes Metab Syndr. 2013;7(2):68-71.
63. Polsky S, Giordano D, Voelmle MK, et al. Using technology to advance type 1 diabetes care among women during the reproductive years and in pregnancy. Postgrad Med. 2016;128(4):418-26.
64. Secher AL, Stage E, Ringholm L, et al. Real-time continuous glucose monitoring as a tool to prevent severe hypoglycaemia in selected pregnant women with Type 1 diabetes - an observational study. Diabet Med. 2014;31(3):352-6.
65. Mukhopadhyay A, Farrell T, Fraser RB, et al. Continuous subcutaneous insulin infusion vs intensive conventional insulin therapy in pregnant diabetic women: a systematic review and meta-analysis of randomized, controlled trials. Am J Obstet Gynecol. 2007;197(5):447-56.
66. Ranasinghe PD, Maruthur NM, Nicholson WK, et al. Comparative effectiveness of continuous subcutaneous insulin infusion using insulin analogs and multiple daily injections in pregnant women with diabetes mellitus: a systematic review and meta-analysis. J Womens Health (Larchmt). 2015;24(3):237-49.
67. Feig DS, Donovan LE, Corcoy R, et al. Continuous glucose monitoring in pregnant women with type 1 diabetes (CONCEPTT): a multicentre international randomised controlled trial. Lancet. 2017;390(10110):2347-59.
68. Di Cianni G, Volpe L, Ghio A, et al. Maternal metabolic control and perinatal outcome in women with gestational diabetes mellitus treated with lispro or aspart insulin: comparison with regular insulin. Diabetes Care. 2007;30(4):e11.
69. Mecacci F, Carignani L, Cioni R, et al. Maternal metabolic control and perinatal outcome in women with gestational diabetes treated with regular or lispro insulin: comparison with non-diabetic pregnant women. Eur J Obstet Gynecol Reprod Biol. 2003;111(1):19-24.
70. Hod M, Damm P, Kaaja R, et al. Fetal and perinatal outcomes in type 1 diabetes pregnancy: a randomized study comparing insulin aspart with human insulin in 322 subjects. Am J Obstet Gynecol. 2008;198(2):186.e1-7.
71. Bartley PC, Bogoev M, Larsen J, et al. Long-term efficacy and safety of insulin detemir compared to neutral protamine Hagedorn insulin in patients with Type 1 diabetes using a treat-to-target basal-bolus regimen with insulin aspart at meals: a 2-year, randomized, controlled trial. Diabetic Med. 2008;25(4):442-9.
72. Price N, Bartlett C, Gillmer MD. Use of insulin glargine during pregnancy: a case-control pilot study. BJOG. 2007;114(4):453-7.
73. Fang YM, MacKeen D, Egan JF, et al. Insulin glargine compared with Neutral Protamine Hagedorn insulin in the treatment of pregnant diabetics. J Matern Fetal Neonatal Med. 2009;22(3):249-53.

74. Di Cianni G, Torlone E, Lencioni C, et al. Perinatal outcomes associated with the use of glargine during pregnancy. Diabetic Med. 2008;25(8):993-6.
75. Tennagels N, Werner U. The metabolic and mitogenic properties of basal insulin analogues. Arch Physiol Biochem. 2013;119(1):1-14.
76. Kollmann M, Martins WP, Lima ML, et al. Strategies for improving outcome of assisted reproduction in women with polycystic ovary syndrome: systematic review and meta-analysis. Ultrasound Obstet Gynecol. 2016:48(6):709-18.
77. Lautatzis ME, Goulis DG, Vrontakis M. Efficacy and safety of metformin during pregnancy in women with gestational diabetes mellitus or polycystic ovary syndrome: a systematic review. Metabolism. 2013;62(11):1522-34.
78. Vanky E, Stridsklev S, Heimstad R, et al. Metformin versus placebo from first trimester to delivery in polycystic ovary syndrome: a randomized, controlled multicenter study. J Clin Endocrinol Metab. 2010;95(12):E448-55.
79. Engen Hanem LG, Stridsklev S, Júlíusson PB, et al. Metformin use in PCOS pregnancies increases the risk of offspring overweight at 4 years of age; follow-up of two RCTs. J Clin Endocrinol Metab. 2018. [Epub ahead of print]
80. Rowan JA, Rush EC, Plank LD, et al. Metformin in gestational diabetes: the offspring follow-up (MiG TOFU): body composition and metabolic outcomes at 7-9 years of age. BMJ Open Diabetes Res Care. 2018;6(1):e000456.
81. Lindsay RS, Loeken MR. Metformin use in pregnancy: promises and uncertainties. Diabetologia. 2017;60(9):1612-9.
82. Vitoratos N, Vrachnis N, Valsamakis G, et al. Perinatal mortality in diabetic pregnancy. Ann New York Acad Sci. 2010;1205(1):94-8.
83. Pearson DW, Kernaghan D, Lee R, et al. The relationship between pre-pregnancy care and early pregnancy loss, major congenital anomaly or perinatal death in type I diabetes mellitus. BJOG. 2007;114(1):104-7.
84. Kucera J. Rate and type of congenital anomalies among offspring of diabetic women. J Reprod Med. 1971;7(2):73-82.
85. Nassr AA, El-Nashar SA, Shazly SA, et al. Expected probability of congenital heart disease and clinical utility of fetal echocardiography in pregnancies with pre-gestational diabetes. Eur J Obstet Gynecol Reprod Biol. 2016;201:121-5.
86. Rosenn BM, Combs CA, Khoury J, et al. Glycemic thresholds for spontaneous abortion and congenital malformations in insulin-dependent diabetes mellitus. Obstet Gynecol. 1994;84(4):515-20.
87. Farrell T, Neale L, Cundy T. Congenital anomalies in the offspring of women with Type 1, Type 2 and gestational diabetes. Diabetic Med. 2002;19(4):322-6.
88. Kitzmiller JL, Buchanan TA, Siri K, et al. Pre-conception care of diabetes, congenital malformations, and spontaneous abortions. Diabetes Care. 1996;19(5):514-41.
89. Lorenzen T, Pociot F, Johannesen J, et al. A population-based survey of frequencies of self-reported spontaneous and induced abortions in Danish women with Type 1 diabetes mellitus. Diabetic Med. 1999;16(6):472-6.
90. Casson IF, Clarke CA, Howard CV, et al. Outcomes of pregnancy in insulin dependent diabetic women: results of a five year population cohort study. BMJ. 1997;315(7103):275-8.
91. Rees DA, Jenkins-Jones S, Morgan CL. Contemporary reproductive outcomes for patients with polycystic ovary syndrome: a retrospective observational study. J Clin Endocrinol Metab. 2016;101(4):1664-72.
92. Jakubowicz DJ, Iuorno MJ, Jakubowicz S, et al. Effects of metformin on early pregnancy loss in the polycystic ovary syndrome. J Clin Endocrinol Metab. 2002;87(2):524-9.
93. Dicker DD, Feldberg D, Samuel N, et al. Spontaneous abortion in patients with insulin-dependent diabetes mellitus: the effect of preconceptional diabetic control. Am J Obstet Gynecol. 1988;158(5):1161-4.

94. Russell NE, Holloway P, Quinn S, et al. Cardiomyopathy and cardiomegaly in stillborn infants of diabetic mothers. Pediatr Dev Pathol. 2008;11(1):10-4.
95. Morrison FJ, Movassaghian M, Seely EW, et al. Fetal outcomes after diabetic ketoacidosis during pregnancy. Diabetes Care. 2017;40(7):e77-9.
96. Dalfrà MG, Burlina S, Sartore G, et al. Ketoacidosis in diabetic pregnancy. J Matern Fetal Neonatal Med. 2016;29(17):2889-95.
97. Schneider MB, Umpierrez GE, Ramsey RD, et al. Pregnancy complicated by diabetic ketoacidosis: maternal and fetal outcomes. Diabetes Care. 2003;26(3):958-9.
98. Guo RX, Yang LZ, Li LX, et al. Diabetic ketoacidosis in pregnancy tends to occur at lower blood glucose levels: Case-control study and a case report of euglycemic diabetic ketoacidosis in pregnancy. J Obstet Gynaecol Res. 2008;34(3):324-30.
99. Veciana MDe. Diabetes ketoacidosis in pregnancy. Semin Perinatol. 2013;37(4):267-73.
100. Kamalakannan D, Baskar V, Barton DM, et al. Diabetic ketoacidosis in pregnancy. Postgrad Med J. 2003;79(934):454-7.
101. Montoro MN, Myers VP, Mestman JH, et al. Outcome of pregnancy in diabetic ketoacidosis. Am J Perinatol. 1993;10(1):17-20.
102. Combs CA, Gunderson E, Kitzmiller JL, et al. Relationship of fetal macrosomia to maternal postprandial glucose control during pregnancy. Diabetes Care. 1992;15(10):1251-7.
103. Weintrob N, Karp M, Hod M. Short- and long-range complications in offspring of diabetic mothers. J Diabetes Complications. 1996;10(5):294-301.
104. Evers IM, de Valk HW, Visser GH. Risk of complications of pregnancy in women with type 1 diabetes: nationwide prospective study in the Netherlands. BMJ. 2004;328(7445):915.
105. Ekbom P, Damm P, Feldt-Rasmussen B, et al. Pregnancy outcome in type 1 diabetic women with microalbuminuria. Diabetes Care. 2001;24(10):1739-44.
106. Sibai BM, Caritis SN, Hauth JC, et al. Preterm delivery in women with pregestational diabetes mellitus or chronic hypertension relative to women with uncomplicated pregnancies. Am J Obstet Gynecol. 2000;183(6):1520-4.
107. Lepercq J, Coste J, Theau A, et al. Factors associated with preterm delivery in women with type 1 diabetes: a cohort study. Diabetes Care. 2004;27(12):2824-8.
108. Knorr S, Clausen TD, Vlachová Z, et al. Academic achievement in primary school in offspring born to mothers with type 1 diabetes (the EPICOM study): a register-based prospective cohort study. Diabetes Care. 2015;38(7):1238-44.
109. Ornoy AA, Ratzon N, Greenbaum C, et al. School-age children born to diabetic mothers and to mothers with gestational diabetes exhibit a high rate of inattention and fine and gross motor impairment. J Pediatr Endocrinol. 2001;14 (Suppl 1):681-9.
110. Tuomilehto J, Podar T, Tuomilehto-Wolf E, et al. Evidence for importance of gender and birth cohort for risk of IDDM in offspring of IDDM parents. Diabetologia. 1995;38(8):975-82.
111. Boney CM, Verma A, Tucker R, et al. Metabolic syndrome in childhood: association with birth weight, maternal obesity, and gestational diabetes mellitus. Pediatrics. 2005;115(3):e290-6.
112. Dabelea D, Hanson RL, Lindsay RS, et al. Intrauterine exposure to diabetes conveys risks for type 2 diabetes and obesity: a study of discordant sibships. Diabetes. 2000;49(12):2208-11.
113. Dabelea DD, Pettitt DJ. Intrauterine diabetic environment confers risks for type 2 diabetes mellitus and obesity in the offspring, in addition to genetic susceptibility. J Pediatr Endocrinol. 2001;14(8):1085-91.
114. Clausen TD, Mathiesen ER, Hansen T, et al. High prevalence of type 2 diabetes and pre-diabetes in adult offspring of women with gestational diabetes mellitus or type 1 diabetes. Diabetes Care. 2008;31(2):340-6.
115. Wang C, Yatsuya H, Tamakoshi K, et al. Association between parental history of diabetes and the incidence of type 2 diabetes mellitus differs according to the sex of the parent and offspring's body weight: A finding from a Japanese worksite-based cohort study. Prev Med. 2015;81:49-53.

116. Meigs JB, Cupples LA, Wilson PW. Parental transmission of type 2 diabetes: The Framingham Offspring Study. Diabetes. 2000;49(12):2201-7.
117. McCance DR, Traub AI, Harley JM, et al. Urinary albumin excretion in diabetic pregnancy. Diabetologia. 1989;32(4):236-9.
118. Rossing K, Jacobsen P, Hommel E, et al. Pregnancy and progression of diabetic nephropathy. Diabetologia. 2002;45(1):36-41.
119. Diabetes Control and Complications Trial Research Group. Effect of pregnancy on microvascular complications in the diabetes control and complications trial. The Diabetes Control and Complications Trial Research Group. Diabetes Care. 2000;23(8):1084-91.
120. Vérier-Mine O, Chaturvedi N, Webb D, et al. Is pregnancy a risk factor for microvascular complications? The EURODIAB Prospective Complications Study. Diabetic Med. 2005;22(11):1503-9.
121. Jones DC, Hayslett JP. Outcome of pregnancy in women with moderate or severe renal insufficiency. N Engl J Med. 1996;335(4):226-32.
122. Gordon M, Landon MB, Samuels P, et al. Perinatal outcome and long-term follow-up associated with modern management of diabetic nephropathy. Obstet Gynecol. 1996;87(3):401-9.
123. Duckitt K, Harrington D. Risk factors for pre-eclampsia at antenatal booking: systematic review of controlled studies. BMJ. 2005;330(7491):565.
124. Reece EA, Leguizamon G, Homko C. Pregnancy performance and outcomes associated with diabetic nephropathy. Am J Perinatol. 1998;15(7):413-21.
125. Hiilesmaa V, Suhonen L, Teramo K. Glycaemic control is associated with pre-eclampsia but not with pregnancy-induced hypertension in women with Type I diabetes mellitus. Diabetologia. 2000;43(12):1534-9.
126. Cohen AL, Wenger JB, James-Todd T, et al. The association of circulating angiogenic factors and HbA1c with the risk of preeclampsia in women with preexisting diabetes. Hypertens Pregnancy. 2014;33(1):81-92.
127. Williams D, Davison J. Chronic kidney disease in pregnancy. BMJ. 2008;336(7637):211-5.
128. Chew EY, Mills JL, Metzger BE, et al. Metabolic control and progression of retinopathy. The Diabetes in Early Pregnancy Study. National Institute of Child Health and Human Development Diabetes in Early Pregnancy Study. Diabetes Care. 1995;18(5):631-7.
129. Rahman W, Rahman FZ, Yassin S, et al. Progression of retinopathy during pregnancy in type 1 diabetes mellitus. Clin Exp Ophthalmol. 2007;35(3):231-6.
130. Temple RC, Aldridge VA, Sampson MJ, et al. Impact of pregnancy on the progression of diabetic retinopathy in Type 1 diabetes. Diabetic Med. 2001;18(7):573-7.
131. Roth A, Elkayam U. Acute myocardial infarction associated with pregnancy. Ann Intern Med. 1996;125(9):751-62.
132. Downs DS. Obesity in special populations: pregnancy. Prim Care. 2016;43(1):109-20.
133. Opray N, Grivell RM, Deussen AR, et al. Directed preconception health programs and interventions for improving pregnancy outcomes for women who are overweight or obese. Cochrane Database Syst Rev. 2015;(7):CD010932.
134. Cooper WO, Hernandez-Diaz S, Arbogast PG, et al. Major congenital malformations after first-trimester exposure to ACE inhibitors. N Engl J Med. 2006;354(23):2443-51.
136. Bos-Thompson MA, Hillaire-Buys D, Muller F, et al. Fetal toxic effects of angiotensin II receptor antagonists: case report and follow-up after birth. Ann Pharmacother. 2005;39(1):157-61.
136. James PA, Oparil S, Carter BL, et al. 2014 evidence-based guideline for the management of high blood pressure in adults: Report from the panel members appointed to the eighth Joint National Committee (JNC 8). JAMA. 2014;311(5):507-20.
137. Russi G. Severe dyslipidemia in pregnancy: The role of therapeutic apheresis. Transfus Apher Sci. 2015;53(3):283-7.

138. Safi FF, Toumeh A, Abuissa Qadan M, et al. Management of familial hypertriglyceridemia-induced pancreatitis during pregnancy with therapeutic plasma exchange: a case report and review of literature. Am J Ther. 2014;21(5):e134-6.
139. Nakao J, Ohba T, Takaishi K, et al. Omega-3 fatty acids for the treatment of hypertriglyceridemia during the second trimester. Nutrition. 2015;31(2):409-12.
140. Alexander EK, Marqusee E, Lawrence J, et al. Timing and magnitude of increases in levothyroxine requirements during pregnancy in women with hypothyroidism. N Engl J Med. 2004;351(3):241-9.
141. Ainuddin JA, Karim N, Zaheer S, et al. Metformin treatment in type 2 diabetes in pregnancy: an active controlled, parallel-group, randomized, open label study in patients with type 2 diabetes in pregnancy. J Diabetes Res. 2015;2015(11):325851.
142. Committee on Practice Bulletins—Obstetrics. Practice Bulletin No. 137: Gestational diabetes mellitus. Obstet Gynecol. 2013;122(2 Pt 1):406-16.
143. International Association of Diabetes and Pregnancy Study Groups Consensus Panel, Metzger BE, Gabbe SG, et al. International Association of Diabetes and Pregnancy Study Groups recommendations on the diagnosis and classification of hyperglycemia in pregnancy. Diabetes Care. 2010;33(3):676-82.
144. International Association of Diabetes and Pregnancy Study Groups. Classification and diagnosis of diabetes. Diabetes Care. 2014;38(Supp 1):S8-16.
145. Riskin-Mashiah S, Younes G, Damti A, et al. First-trimester fasting hyperglycemia and adverse pregnancy outcomes. Diabetes Care. 2009;32(9):1639-43.
146. Zhu WW, Yang HX, Wei YM, et al. Evaluation of the value of fasting plasma glucose in the first prenatal visit to diagnose gestational diabetes mellitus in China. Diabetes Care. 2013;36(3):586-90.
147. Hughes RC, Moore MP, Gullam JE, et al. An early pregnancy HbA1c ≥5.9% (41 mmol/mol) is optimal for detecting diabetes and identifies women at increased risk of adverse pregnancy outcomes. Diabetes Care. 2014;37(11):2953-9.
148. McIntyre HD, Sacks DA, Barbour LA, et al. Issues with the diagnosis and classification of hyperglycemia in early pregnancy. Diabetes Care. 2016;39(1):53-4.
149. Danilenko-Dixon DR, Van Winter JT, Nelson RL, et al. Universal versus selective gestational diabetes screening: Application of 1997 American Diabetes Association recommendations. Am J Obstet Gynecol. 1999;181(4):798-802.
150. O'Sullivan JB, Mahan CM. Criteria for the oral glucose tolerance test in pregnancy. Diabetes. 1964;13:278-85.
151. Classification and diagnosis of diabetes mellitus and other categories of glucose intolerance. National Diabetes Data Group. Diabetes. 1979;28(12):1039-57.
152. Carpenter MW, Coustan DR. Criteria for screening tests for gestational diabetes. Am J Obstet Gynecol. 1982;144(7):768-73.
153. HAPO Study Cooperative Research Group, Metzger BE, Lowe LP, et al. Hyperglycemia and adverse pregnancy outcomes. N Engl J Med. 2008;358(19):1991-2002.
154. HAPO Study Cooperative Research Group. Hyperglycemia and Adverse Pregnancy Outcome (HAPO) Study: associations with neonatal anthropometrics. Diabetes. 2009;58(2):453-9.
155. Crowther CA, Hiller JE, Moss JR, et al. Effect of treatment of gestational diabetes mellitus on pregnancy outcomes. N Engl J Med. 2005;352(24):2477-86.
156. Landon MB, Spong CY, Thom E, et al. A multicenter, randomized trial of treatment for mild gestational diabetes. N Engl J Med. 2009;361(14):1339-48.
157. Basevi V, Di Mario S, Morciano C, et al. Comment on: American Diabetes Association. Standards of medical care in diabetes—2011. Diabetes Care 2011;34(Suppl. 1):S11-S61. Diabetes Care. 2011;34(5):e53.

158. World Health Organization (WHO). (2013). Diagnostic criteria and classification of hyperglycaemia first detected in pregnancy. [online] Available from www.apps.who.int/iris/bitstream/10665/85975/1/WHO_NMH_MND_13.2_eng.pdf. [Accessed February, 2018].
159. Committee opinion no. 504: Screening and diagnosis of gestational diabetes mellitus. Obstet Gynecol. 2011;118(3):751-3.
160. National Institutes of Health (NIH). (2013). NIH Development Conference: Diagnosing Gestational Diabetes Mellitus. [online] Available from www.consensus.nih.gov/2013/gdmabstracts.htm. [Accessed February, 2018].
161. Hod M, Kapur A, Sacks DA, et al. The International Federation of Gynecology and Obstetrics (FIGO) Initiative on gestational diabetes mellitus: A pragmatic guide for diagnosis, management, and care. Int J Gynaecol Obstet. 2015;131 Suppl 3:S173-211.
162. Wong VW. Diagnosis of gestational diabetes mellitus: Where are we at? Int J Diabetes Clin Diagn. 2014;1(4):104.
163. Harper LM. Carpenter-Coustan compared with National Diabetes Data Group criteria for diagnosing gestational diabetes. Obstet Gynecol. 2016;127(5):893-8.
164. Meek CL, Lewis HB, Patient C, et al. Diagnosis of gestational diabetes mellitus: falling through the net. Diabetologia. 2015;58(9):2003-12.
165. Wei YY. International Association of Diabetes and Pregnancy Study Group criteria is suitable for gestational diabetes mellitus diagnosis: further evidence from China. Chinese Med J. 2014;127(20):3553-6.
166. Feldman R. Gestational diabetes screening: The International Association of the Diabetes and Pregnancy Study Groups compared with Carpenter-Coustan screening. Obstet Gynecol. 2016;127(1):10-7.
167. Kim SY, England JL, Sharma JA, et al. Gestational diabetes mellitus and risk of childhood overweight and obesity in offspring: a systematic review. Exp Diabetes Res. 2011;2011:541308.
168. Zhu Y, Olsen SF, Mendola P, et al. Growth and obesity through the first 7 years of life in association with levels of maternal glycemia during pregnancy: a prospective cohort study. Am J Clin Nutr. 2016;103(3):794-800.
169. Kubo A, Ferrara A, Windham GC, et al. Maternal hyperglycemia during pregnancy predicts adiposity of the offspring. Diabetes Care. 2014;37(11):2996-3002.
170. Landon MB, Rice MM, Varner MW, et al. Mild gestational diabetes mellitus and long-term child health. Diabetes Care. 2015;38(3):445-52.
171. Brown FM, Wyckoff J. Application of One-Step IADPSG Versus Two-Step Diagnostic Criteria for Gestational Diabetes in the Real World: Impact on Health Services, Clinical Care, and Outcomes. Curr Diabetes Rep. 2017;17(10):85.
172. Koivusalo SB, Rönö K, Klemetti MM, et al. Gestational diabetes mellitus can be prevented by lifestyle intervention: The Finnish Gestational Diabetes Prevention Study (RADIEL): a randomized controlled trial. Diabetes Care. 2016;39(1):24-30.
173. Dodd JM, Turnbull D, McPhee AJ, et al. Antenatal lifestyle advice for women who are overweight or obese: LIMIT randomised trial. BMJ. 2014;348:g1285.
174. de Veciana M, Major CA, Morgan MA, et al. Postprandial versus preprandial blood glucose monitoring in women with gestational diabetes mellitus requiring insulin therapy. N Engl J Med. 1995;333(19):1237-41.
175. Prutsky GJ, Domecq JP, Wang Z, et al. Glucose targets in pregnant women with diabetes: a systematic review and meta-analysis. J Clin Endocrinol Metab. 2013;98(11):4319-24.
176. Yogev Y, Ben-Haroush A, Chen R, et al. Diurnal glycemic profile in obese and normal weight nondiabetic pregnant women. Am J Obstet Gynecol. 2004;191(3):949-53.

177. Kjos SL, Schaefer-Graf UM. Modified therapy for gestational diabetes using high-risk and low-risk fetal abdominal circumference growth to select strict versus relaxed maternal glycemic targets. Diabetes Care. 2007;30(Suppl 2):S200-5.
178. Castillo WC, Boggess K, Stürmer T, et al. Trends in glyburide compared with insulin use for gestational diabetes treatment in the United States, 2000–2011. Obstet Gynecol. 2014;123(6):1177-84.
179. Langer O, Conway DL, Berkus MD, et al. A comparison of glyburide and insulin in women with gestational diabetes mellitus. N Engl J Med. 2000;343(16):1134-8.
180. Rowan JA, Hague WM, Gao W, et al. Metformin versus insulin for the treatment of gestational diabetes. N Engl J Med. 2008;358(19):2003-15.
181. Goetzl LL, Wilkins I. Glyburide compared to insulin for the treatment of gestational diabetes mellitus: a cost analysis. J Perinatol. 2002;22(5):403-6.
182. Buschur E, Brown F, Wyckoff J. Using oral agents to manage gestational diabetes: what have we learned? Curr Diabetes Rep. 2015;15(2):1-8.
183. Hebert MF, Ma X, Naraharisetti SB, et al. Are we optimizing gestational diabetes treatment with glyburide? The pharmacologic basis for better clinical practice. Clin Pharmacol Ther. 2009;85(6):607-14.
184. Zeng YC, Li MJ, Chen Y, et al. The use of glyburide in the management of gestational diabetes mellitus: a meta-analysis. Adv Med Sci. 2014;59(1):95-101.
185. Balsells M, García-Patterson A, Solà I, et al. Glibenclamide, metformin, and insulin for the treatment of gestational diabetes: a systematic review and meta-analysis. BMJ. 2015;350:h102.
186. Vanky E, Zahlsen K, Spigset O, et al. Placental passage of metformin in women with polycystic ovary syndrome. Fertil Steril. 2005;83(5):1575-8.
187. Rowan JA, Rush EC, Obolonkin V, et al. Metformin in gestational diabetes: The Offspring Follow-Up (MiG TOFU): Body composition at 2 years of age. Diabetes Care. 2011;34(10):2279-84.
188. Wouldes TA, Battin M, Coat S, et al. Neurodevelopmental outcome at 2 years in offspring of women randomised to metformin or insulin treatment for gestational diabetes. Arch Dis Child Fetal Neonatal Ed. 2016. [Epub ahead of print]
189. Steel JM, Johnstone FD, Hepburn DA, et al. Can prepregnancy care of diabetic women reduce the risk of abnormal babies? BMJ. 1990;301(6760):1070-4.
190. Rosenn BM, Miodovnik M, Holcberg G, et al. Hypoglycemia: The price of intensive insulin therapy for pregnant women with insulin-dependent diabetes mellitus. Obstet Gynecol. 1995;85(3):417-22.
191. Evers IM, ter Braak EW, de Valk HW, et al. Risk indicators predictive for severe hypoglycemia during the first trimester of type 1 diabetic pregnancy. Diabetes Care. 2002;25(3):554-9.
192. Nielsen LR, Pedersen-Bjergaard U, Thorsteinsson B, et al. Hypoglycemia in pregnant women with type 1 diabetes: predictors and role of metabolic control. Diabetes Care. 2008;31(1):9-14.
193. Padmanabhan S, McLean M, Cheung NW. Falling insulin requirements are associated with adverse obstetric outcomes in women with preexisting diabetes. Diabetes Care. 2014;37(10):2685-92.
194. US Preventive Services Task Force. (2014). Low-Dose Aspirin Use for the Prevention of Morbidity and Mortality From Preeclampsia: Preventive Medication. [online] Available from www.uspreventiveservicestaskforce.org/Page/Document/RecommendationStatementFinal/low-dose-aspirin-use-for-the-prevention-of-morbidity-and-mortality-from-preeclampsia-preventive-medication. [Accessed February, 2018].
195. American College of Obstetricians and Gynecologists (ACOG). (2013). Hypertension in pregnancy. [online] Available from www.acog.org/Clinical-Guidance-and-Publications/Task-Force-and-Work-Group-Reports/Hypertension-in-Pregnancy. [Accessed February, 2018].
196. Committee on Practice Bulletins—Obstetrics. ACOG Practice Bulletin No. 190: Gestational Diabetes Mellitus. Obstet Gynecol. 2018;131(2):e49-64.
197. Umpierrez GE, Latif KA, Murphy MB, et al. Thyroid dysfunction in patients with type 1 diabetes: a longitudinal study. Diabetes Care. 2003;26(4):1181-5.

198. Mathiesen ER, Christensen AB, Hellmuth E, et al. Insulin dose during glucocorticoid treatment for fetal lung maturation in diabetic pregnancy: test of an algorithm [correction of analgoritm]. Acta Obstet Gynecol Scand. 2002;81(9):835-9.
199. Roeder H. Changes in postpartum insulin requirements for patients with well-controlled type 1 diabetes. Am J Perinatol. 2016;33(7):683-7.
200. Takoudes TC, Weitzen S, Slocum J, et al. Risk of cesarean wound complications in diabetic gestations. Am J Obstet Gynecol. 2004;191(3):958-63.
201. Feig DS, Briggs GG, Kraemer JM, et al. Transfer of glyburide and glipizide into breast milk. Diabetes Care. 2005;28(8):1851-5.
202. Hale T, Kristensen J, Hackett L, et al. Transfer of metformin into human milk. Diabetologia. 2002;45(11):1509-14.
203. Gardiner SJ, Kirkpatrick CM, Begg EJ, et al. Transfer of metformin into human milk. Clin Pharmacol Ther. 2003;73(1):71-7.
204. Gunderson EP, Hurston SR, Ning X, et al. Lactation and progression to type 2 diabetes mellitus after gestational diabetes mellitus: a prospective cohort study. Ann Intern Med. 2015;163(12):889-98.
205. Yan J, Liu L, Zhu Y, et al. The association between breastfeeding and childhood obesity: a meta-analysis. BMC Public Health. 2014;14:1267.
206. Bider-Canfield Z, Martinez MP, Wang X, et al. Maternal obesity, gestational diabetes, breastfeeding and childhood overweight at age 2 years. Pediatr Obes. 2017;12(2):171-8.
207. Briggs G. Excretion of metformin into breast milk and the effect on nursing infants. Obstet Gynecol. 2005;105(6):1437-41.
208. Riviello C, Mello G, Jovanovic L. Breastfeeding and the basal insulin requirement in Type 1 diabetic women. Endocr Pract. 2009;15(3):187-93.
209. Zhao YL, Ma RM, Lao TT, et al. Maternal gestational diabetes mellitus and overweight and obesity in offspring: a study in Chinese children. J Dev Orig Health Dis. 2015;6(6):479-84.
210. Kim C, Newton KM, Knopp RH. Gestational diabetes and the incidence of type 2 diabetes: a systematic review. Diabetes Care. 2002;25(10):1862-8.
211. Rayanagoudar G, Hashi AA, Zamora J, et al. Quantification of the type 2 diabetes risk in women with gestational diabetes: a systematic review and meta-analysis of 95,750 women. Diabetologia. 2016;59(7):1403-11.
212. Diabetes Prevention Program Research Group. Reduction in the incidence of type 2 diabetes with lifestyle intervention or metformin. N Engl J Med. 2002;346(6):393-403.
213. Tuomilehto J, Lindström J, Eriksson JG, et al. Prevention of type 2 diabetes mellitus by changes in lifestyle among subjects with impaired glucose tolerance. N Engl J Med. 2001;344(18):1343-50.
214. Pan XR, Li GW, Hu YH, et al. Effects of diet and exercise in preventing NIDDM in people with impaired glucose tolerance. The Da Qing IGT and Diabetes Study. Diabetes Care. 1997;20(4):537-44.
215. Ramachandran A, Snehalatha C, Mary S, et al. The Indian Diabetes Prevention Programme shows that lifestyle modification and metformin prevent type 2 diabetes in Asian Indian subjects with impaired glucose tolerance (IDPP-1). Diabetologia. 2006;49(2):289-97.
216. Hsu WC, Araneta MR, Kanaya AM, et al. BMI cut points to identify at-risk Asian Americans for type 2 diabetes screening. Diabetes Care. 2015;38(1):150-8.
217. Ratner RE, Christophi CA, Metzger BE, et al. Prevention of diabetes in women with a history of gestational diabetes: effects of metformin and lifestyle interventions. J Clin Endocrinol Metab. 2008;93(12):4774-9.
218. Guo J, Chen JL, Whittemore R, et al. Postpartum lifestyle interventions to prevent type 2 diabetes among women with history of gestational diabetes: a systematic review of randomized clinical trials. J Womens Health (Larchmt). 2016;25(1):38-49.
219. Ferrera A, Ehrlich SF. Strategies for diabetes prevention before and after pregnancy in women with GDM. Curr Diabetes Rev. 2011;7(2):75-83.

220. Peacock AS, Bogossian F, McIntyre HD, et al. A review of interventions to prevent Type 2 diabetes after gestational diabetes. Women Birth. 2014;27(4):e7-15.
221. Bennett WL, Ennen CS, Carrese JA, et al. Barriers to and facilitators of postpartum follow-up care in women with recent gestational diabetes mellitus: a qualitative study. J Womens Health (Larchmt). 2011;20(2):239-45.
222. Huynh L, McCoy M, Law A, et al. Systematic literature review of the costs of pregnancy in the US. Pharmacoeconomics. 2013;31(11):1005-30.
223. American Diabetes Association. Management of diabetes in pregnancy: Standards of medical care in diabetes. Diabetes Care. 2018;41(Suppl 1):S137-43.

CHAPTER 16

Skin Lesions in Diabetes

Arturo R Rolla

INTRODUCTION

Diabetes mellitus (DM) frequently causes changes and lesions in the skin, often completely asymptomatic, but they are important at times for the diagnosis of diabetes, its complications and pathogenesis. We could classify them in several groups (Box 16.1):

Box 16.1: Skin lesions in diabetes.

- Dermopathies usually associated with diabetes mellitus (DM)
- Complications of treatments
- Lesions due to metabolic alterations
- Skin infections more common in DM
- Lesions with increased incidence in DM.

DERMOPATHIES USUALLY ASSOCIATED WITH DIABETES MELLITUS (BOX 16.2)

Box 16.2: Dermopathies usually associated with diabetes mellitus (DM).

- Necrobiosis lipoidica
- Brown spots
- Lipoatrophies
- Glucagonoma syndrome
- Palmar sclerosis, Dupuytren's contractures, and limited joint mobility
- Scleredema
- Diabetic bulla.

Necrobiosis Lipoidica

Necrobiosis lipoidica (NL) is a chronic granulomatous inflammation of the skin with very characteristic lesions that appear most commonly on the anterior aspect of the legs, and are bilateral tending to be symmetrical. In 10% of the cases it may appear outside of the pretibial area, in the thighs, abdomen, breast or arms. NL is more common among Caucasians, women, and patients with DM-1. It used to be called necrobiosis lipoidica 'diabeticorum' but since it may also be found in nondiabetic individuals—although less common—it is now named only NL. It is not common (about 1% of all patients with DM), and its incidence seems to be decreasing for unknown reasons. The lesions are asymptomatic except for the cosmetic consequences, but they may develop ulcerations that can get infected. Initially they appear as erythematous and slightly raised especially around the periphery (inflammatory phase) (Fig. 16.1). With time they spread slowly leaving a pale or yellow center (lipoidica) with marked thinning of the skin and visible telangiectatic vessels (atrophic phase). In general they appear after the diagnosis of DM but occasionally they may precede it for a year or so. The onset is usually around the third decade, and it is unusual for NL to start after the age of 40 years.

It is very important to indicate that even its pathogenesis is unknown, NL is not associated with neuropathy, vasculopathy nor metabolic control. The histological picture varies with time (Figs. 16.2 and 16.3). Initially, it is a granulomatous inflammation surrounded by plasma cells and lymphocytes affecting both skin and subcutaneous tissue with a characteristic swelling and 'necrobiosis' of the collagen in the dermis giving the impression that it is a chronic inflammation against the local collagen. As the lesions extend in the periphery the skin in the center becomes atrophic, losing the subcutaneous tissue, and shows dilated vessels. By then the histology shows accumulation of lipids and scarring.

The diagnosis is mostly clinical, but if there are doubts a skin biopsy may be indicated—especially when NL appears outside of the classical pretibial location. The main differential diagnosis is with granuloma annulare that is not common in the legs but has a histological picture of granulomatous inflammation similar to NL. The histological differences are the absence of collagen necrobiosis and increased mucin deposition in the cases of granuloma annulare. The same area of the legs may show cutaneous sarcoidosis, necrobiotic xanthogranuloma or pretibial myxedema. In about 15% of the cases NL involutes and disappears, and in the rest it progresses for several years before it gets stable (Fig. 16.4).

There is no effective cure for NL, and unfortunately there are no well-controlled studies to validate the different treatments proposed over the years. As long as there are no ulcerations the

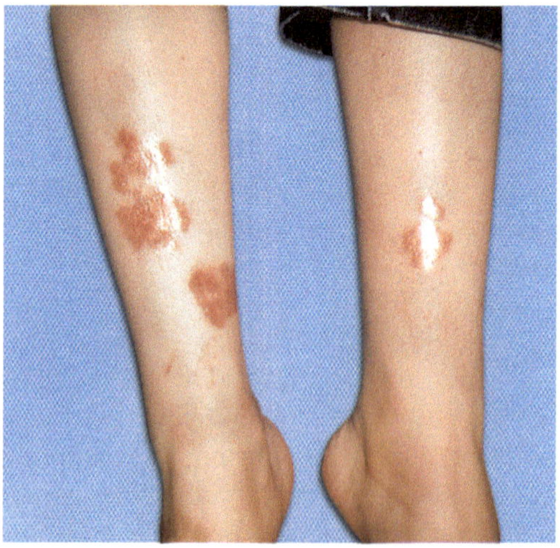

Fig. 16.1: Necrobiosis lipoidica in initial stages.

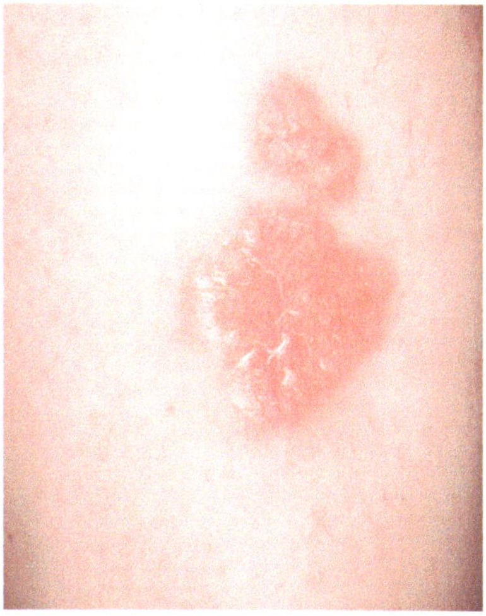

Fig. 16.2: Necrobiosis lipoidica, more advances stages.

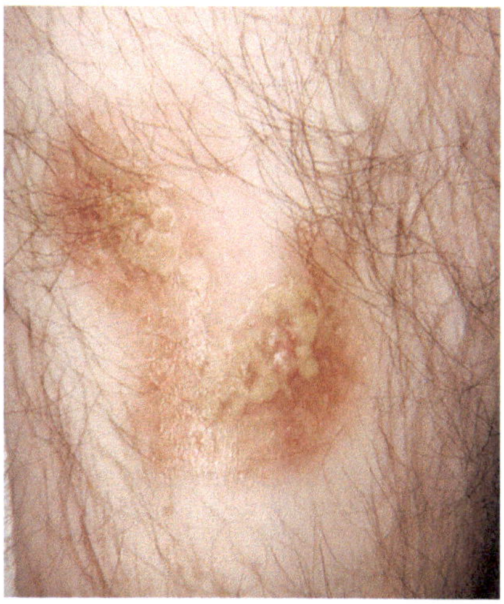

Fig. 16.3: Necrobiosis lipoidica with lipid accumulation.

only problem for the patients is a cosmetic one. If this is not a major concern the best approach for NL is benign neglect, protection against trauma (at times with 'shin pads' like they are used for football or field hockey), and follow-up. Glycemic control does not make any difference. The first line of treatment is the local application of a high potency steroid like clobetasol applied in the areas of local inflammation (reddish) and with nocturnal occlusion to improve results. Local steroids in any manner should be avoided in the areas already atrophic. Recently, a patient was treated successfully with infliximab, an anti-TNF (tumor necrosis factor) agent.

If these topical treatments do not show significant improvement intralesional injections with corticosteroids (usually triamcinolone acetonide) in the surrounding, reddish areas may be tried (Fig. 16.5). The clinical evidence of the benefit of these injections is lacking so far, and only successful sporadic cases have been reported. Multiple injections of these potent steroids

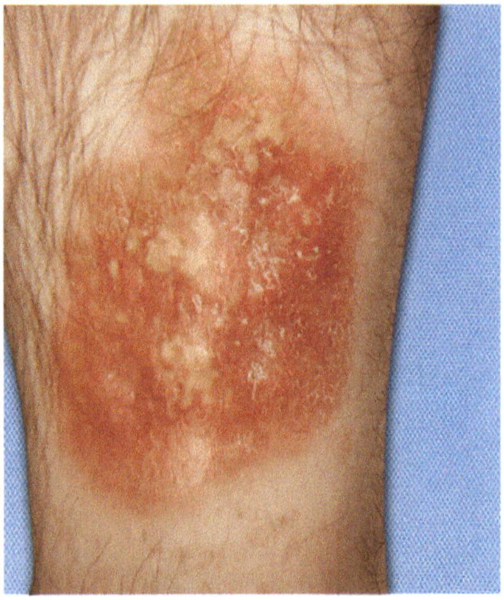

Fig. 16.4: Necrobiosis lipoidica in more advanced stages.

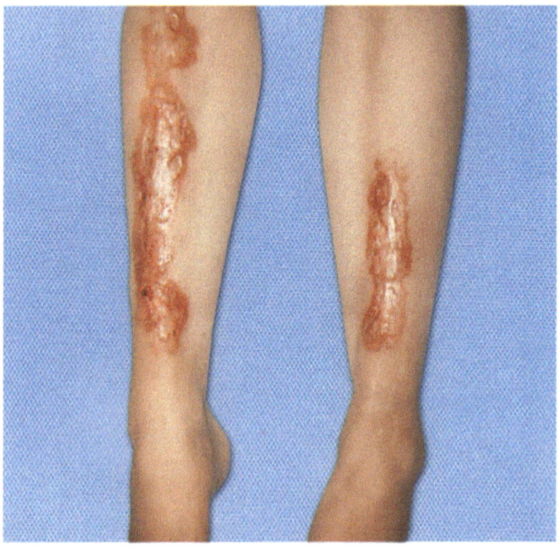

Fig. 16.5: Necrobiosis lipoidica with marked atrophy of the skin in the center.

may increase the blood glucose levels and they may cause local pain. Other therapies that have been used, although again with no clear evidence are topical tacrolimus, ultraviolet [Psoralen ultraviolet A (PUVA)] with or without local psoralen, and oral antimalarials (chloroquine or hydroxychloroquine).

The thinning and atrophy of the skin in this pretibial area makes it very susceptible to trauma increasing the chances of ulcerations that may become chronic, infected, and resistant to therapeutic interventions. Prevention is the first step with local protection and daily moisturizing of the affected skin. Once the ulceration appears, antibiotics, as local ointments or systemic, are indicated. Leg elevation and daily dressings also help (Figs. 16.6 to 16.8).

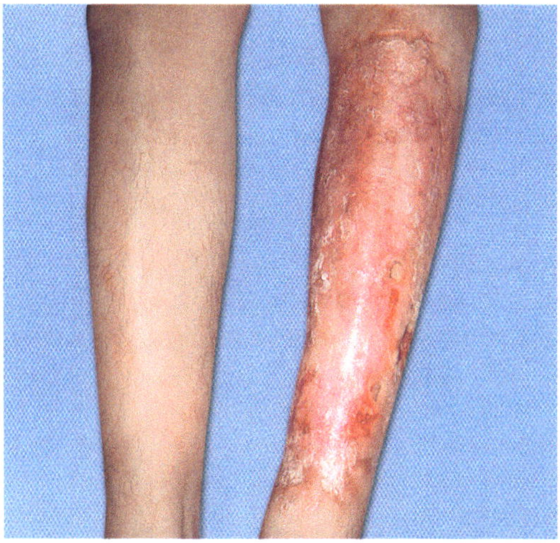

Fig. 16.6: Necrobiosis lipoidica complicated with ulcerations and infection.

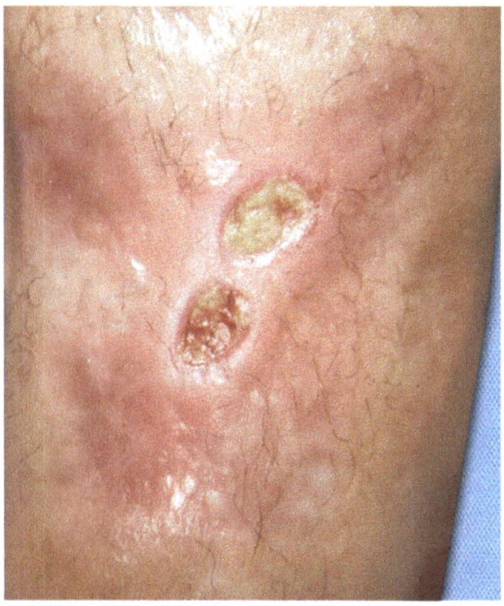

Fig. 16.7: Necrobiosis lipoidica with infected ulcerations.

Brown Spots

Brown spots, also known as 'diabetic dermopathy' (although they are more common in nondiabetic individuals) and 'shin spots', are the most common skin lesions in DM. They may be one or multiple, and are also more common in the legs. Like NL, they are asymptomatic but being smaller (<1 cm in diameter) very often they are overlooked by the patients. Brown spots are more frequent in men and in individuals with peripheral neuropathy or vascular disease. They are present in about 2% of the general population, increasing with age. The etiology is poor healing of trauma, infection or a surgical scar with hemosiderin and melanin pigmentation. The finding of brown spots along surgical scars (for example veins harvesting for coronary by-pass) is a clear indication that they are the result of poor healing. Very rarely they may disappear, and then only require reassurance. No treatment is indicated, and biopsies are not recommended. Differential diagnosis with the pigmentation of venous insufficiency is straight forward since the latter causes pigmented areas that are larger with decreased subcutaneous tissue tending to be circumferential, and in the lower parts of the legs only (Figs. 16.9 to 16.11).

Lipodystrophy

Lipodystrophy are areas of atrophy of the adipose tissue, at times combined with hypertrophy in other areas. They are usually discovered clinically because of changes in the subcutaneous tissue and skin (acanthosis nigricans) and associated metabolic abnormalities. Considering

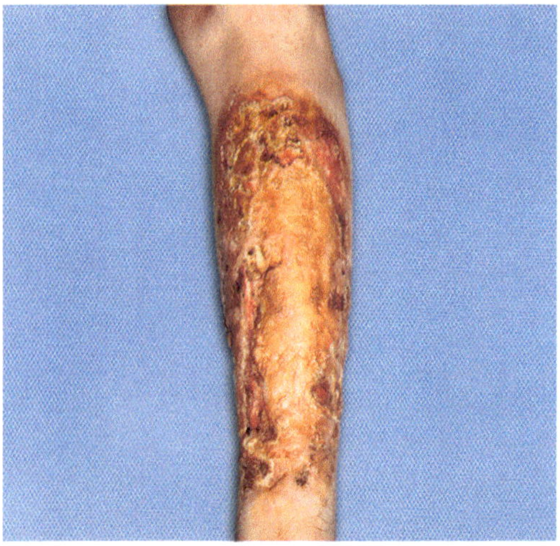

Fig. 16.8: Necrobiosis lipoidica in advanced stage with chronic ulcerations.

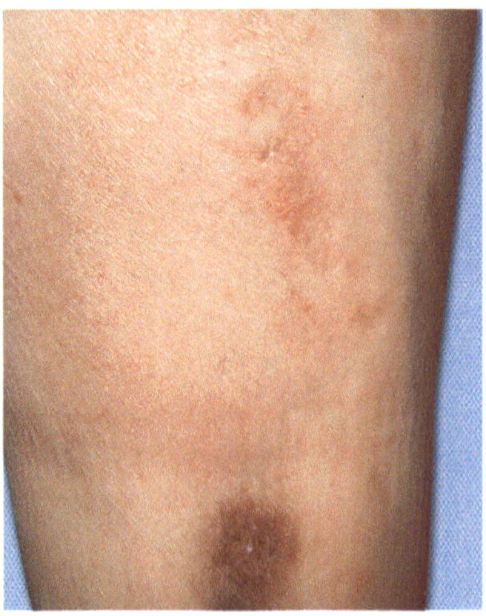

Fig. 16.9: Brown spot in the leg.

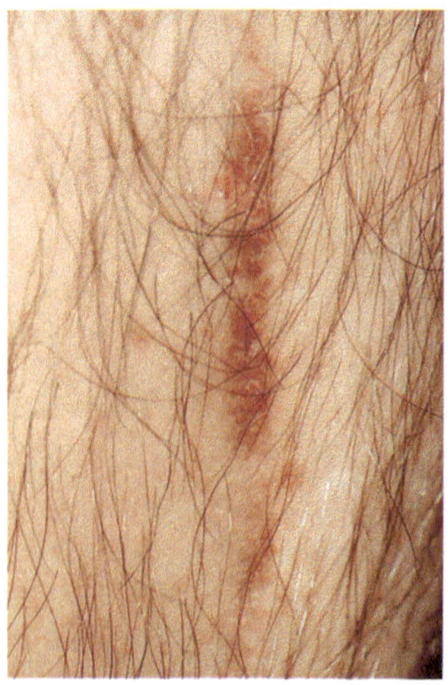

Fig. 16.10: 'Linear' brown spot after vein harvesting for a coronary by-pass.

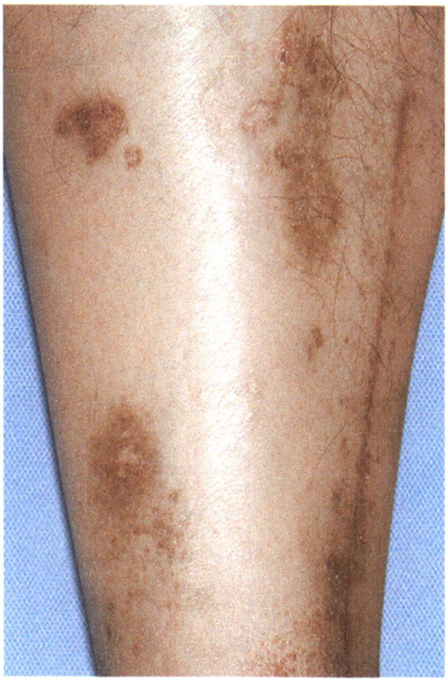

Fig. 16.11: Multiple brown spots in the leg with a 'linear' one on the medial aspect.

the subcutaneous tissue as a part of the skin and the most visible part of the adipose tissue, its complete assessment is very important in every patient. The well-known subcutaneous tissue distribution variations, gynecoid and android, should always be considered individuals with obesity, metabolic syndrome and diabetes. Generalized lipoatrophy cases are self-evident but partial lipodystrophies may go unnoticed (Figs. 16.12A to C).

These adipose atrophies cause serious metabolic abnormalities, usually with severe insulin resistance and hyperinsulinemia indicating the importance of the adipocytes in the intermediary metabolism. They are uncommon and present considerable clinical overlap making their precise diagnosis quite confusing, but with the new molecular techniques much has been learned, and we can now classify them better by their type of mutation, although in some cases the exact cause is still unknown. Like other dermatological lesions they can teach us about pathophysiology, in this case about the adipose tissue development, maintenance and its relation with the function of other organs.

The preservation of fat in some parts of the body in the generalized forms of lipodystrophy and the existence of partial lipodystrophies are indicating that the adipose tissue is not as homogeneous as we thought, and that there are areas with different development and maintenance guided by a complex system of molecular factors. The normal function of the adipose tissue (accumulation of stored fatty acids in the form of triglycerides to prevent excessive accumulation in nonadipose tissues) becomes very evident in these cases of lipodystrophy. When the adipose tissue has limited capacity as in the lipodystrophies, the fatty acids start accumulating in other organs especially in the liver and skeletal muscle leading to insulin resistance (lipotoxicity). This is a known phenomenon in obesity where the translocation of fatty acid is due to 'overflow' and adipositis. In the lipodystrophy, the translocation of fatty acids is even more exaggerated and the resulting insulin resistance may be extreme (Figs. 16.13 and 16.14).

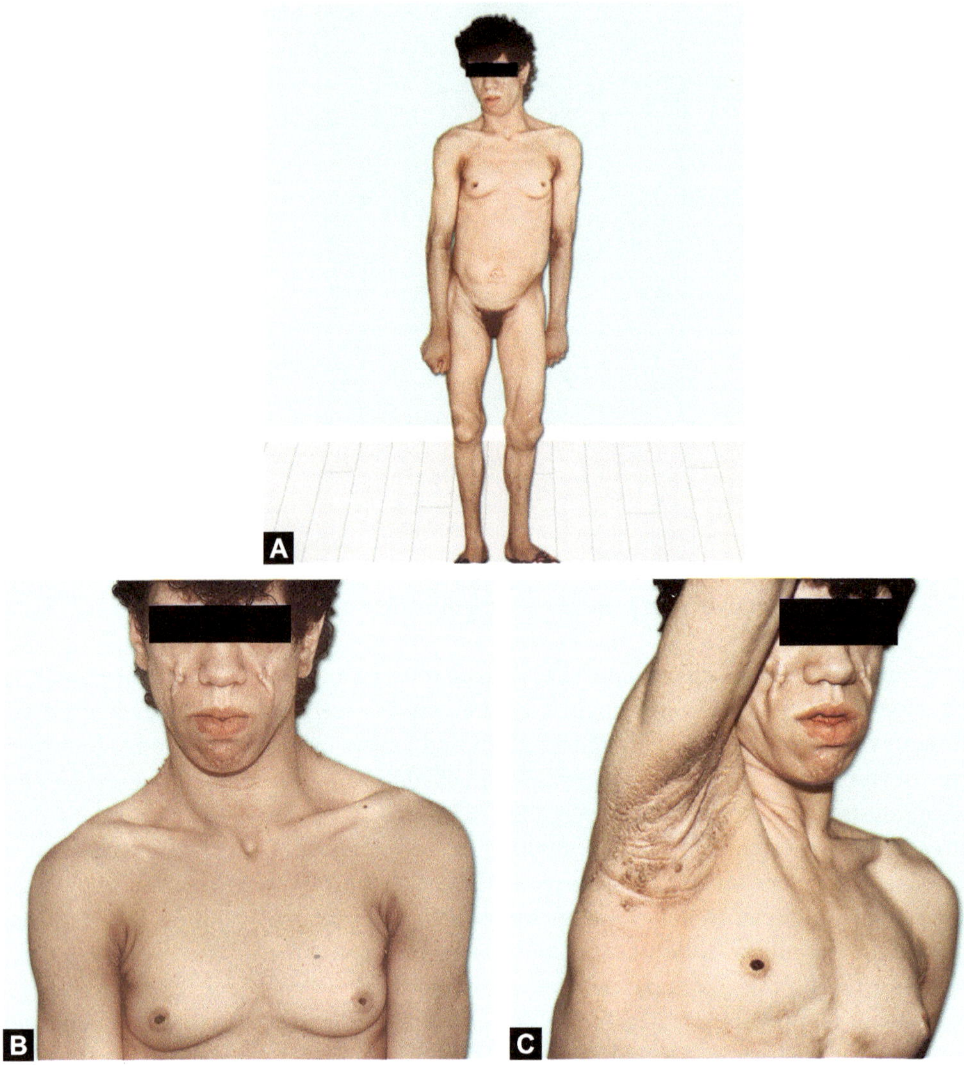

Figs. 16.12A to C: Congenital generalized lipoatrophic diabetes.
Source: From Dr Pedro de Pablo, Spain.

The chronic and severe insulin resistance caused by the lipodystrophy is accompanied by hyperinsulinemia and later on by hyperglycemia, hypertriglyceridemia, and low levels of HDL cholesterol. There is also fatty infiltration of the liver which is so severe that frequently leads to cirrhosis with portal hypertension. Overall, their clinical picture is one of the severe metabolic syndrome, and there is a direct relationship between the decrease in adipose mass and the metabolic abnormalities. The lipoatrophic forms of diabetes have both exaggerated translocation of fatty acids to non-adipose tissues, and the most severe forms of insulin resistance, without any chronic inflammation of the adipose tissue (adipositis). This suggests that in the pathogenesis of insulin resistance the translocation of fatty acids outside of the adipocytes may be more important that the adipositis caused by the obesity.

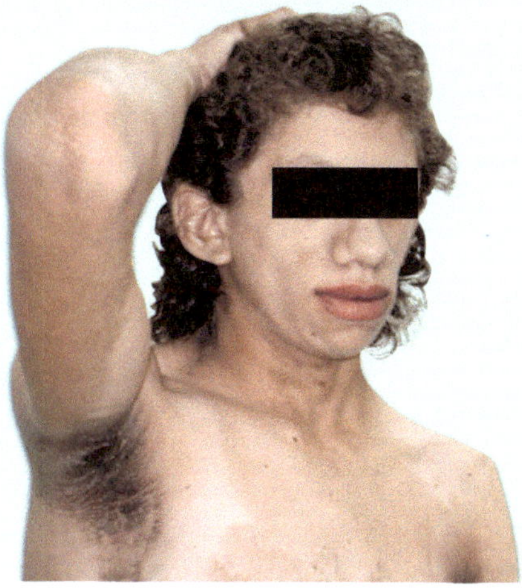

Fig. 16.13: Congenital generalized lipoatrophic diabetes with severe axillary acanthosis nigricans. *Source:* Dr Leila Araujo, Brazil.

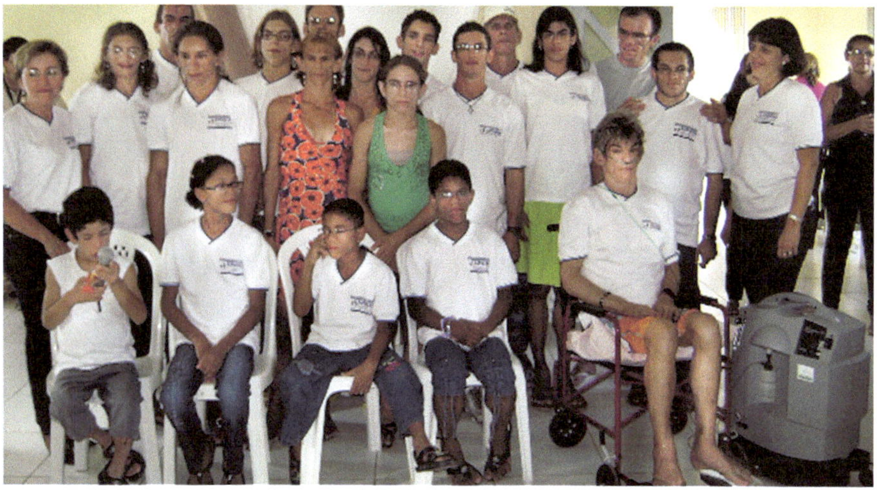

Fig. 16.14: Multiple cases of congenital lipoatrophic diabetes in an isolated village of Northern Brazil. *Source:* Dr Leila Araujo, Brazil.

The lipodystrophies can be classified as generalized or partial, and congenital or acquired (Boxes 16.3 and 16.4).

Congenital Generalized Lipodystrophies (Berardinelli–Seip Syndrome)

These are rare but very obvious conditions inherited usually as a recessive trait, and associated with consanguinity. Absence of subcutaneous tissue is apparent in the first years of life (Box 16.5). Even though there is almost complete absence of the subcutaneous and abdominal fat, the

Box 16.3: Complications of the lipodistrophies.

- Insulin resistance, usually severe
- Diabetes mellitus requiring large doses of insulin
- Rare ketosis and ketoacidosis
- Hypertriglyceridemia with low high-density lipoprotein (HDL) cholesterol
- Fatty liver, hepatomegaly
- Acute pancreatitis
- Low serum leptin levels
- Voracious appetite
- Increased metabolic rate
- Acanthosis nigricans
- Polycystic ovaries syndrome, hirsutism
- Prominent muscles and veins.

Box 16.4: Lipodystrophies.

- Generalized lipoatrophies
  - Congenital
  - Acquired
- Partial lipodystrophies
  - Congenital
  - Acquired.

Box 16.5: Congenital generalized lipodystrophies.

- Type 1: *AGPAT2* mutation, an acyltransferase
- Type 2: *BSCL2* mutation, 'Seipin'
- Type 3: Caveolin-1 mutation
- Type 4: *PTRF* mutation, caveolin-1 and 2
- Others without a known mutation.

amount of adipose tissue in perineum, mouth, tongue, orbits, palms, soles, and periarticular areas ('mechanical fat') are normal. Muscles and veins are quite prominent in part due to the absence of subcutaneous tissue ('anatomical preparations') but also because of a true hypertrophy.

There are four known mutations of the congenital generalized forms of lipodystrophy, but there are still rare cases of unknown etiology.

Acquired Generalized Lipodystrophy (Lawrence Syndrome)

It is less common than the congenital varieties and has the clinical characteristic of a subacute onset over a period of weeks or months, at times preceded by an acute febrile illness. Biopsies of the adipose tissue show a panniculitis, antibodies against different antigens in the adipose tissue have been found, and they have an increased association with autoimmune conditions (Hashimoto's thyroiditis, rheumatoid arthritis, hemolytic anemia, and chronic active hepatitis). All of these features are indicating the possibility of an autoimmune etiology. The physical examination is very similar to the congenital forms of lipodystrophies, so that the initiation after childhood and the subacute onset are important in the differential diagnosis (Box 16.6 and Figs. 16.15 to 16.17).

Congenital Partial Lipodystrophies

The atrophy of the fat tissue is characteristically limited to certain areas, and often there are other areas with lipohypertrophy. Several forms have been described and their phenotype at times may be overlooked (Box 16.7).

Box 16.6: Acquired generalized lipodystrophies.

- Similar to the congenital forms
- Appear in adolescents or young adults
  - In weeks or months
  - Autoimmune panniculitis
  - Other autoimmune conditions.

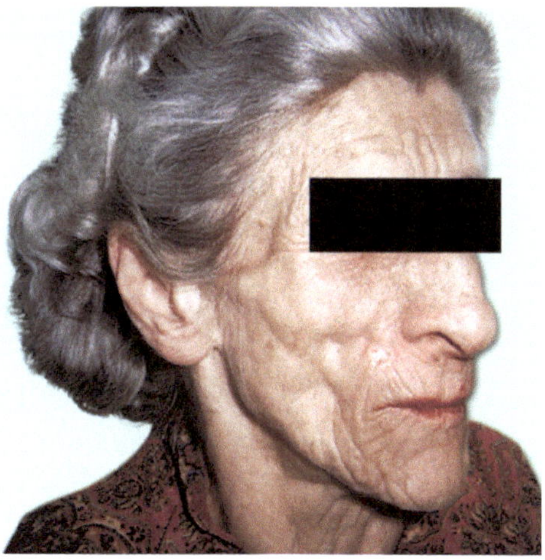

Fig. 16.15: Acquired generalized lipoatrophic diabetes with atrophy of the face fat and enophthalmos.

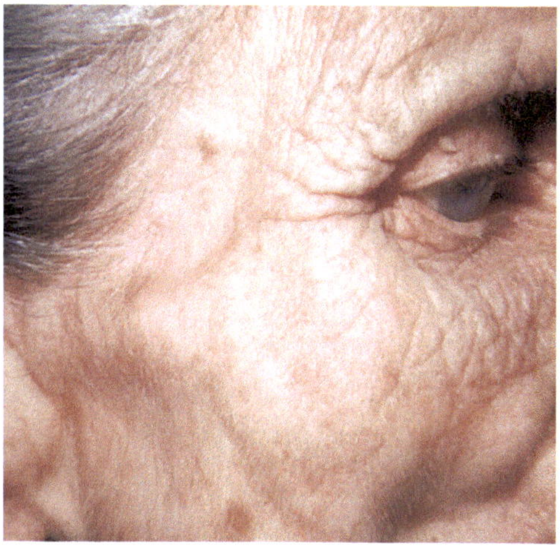

Fig. 16.16: Acquired lipodystrophy with enophthalmos and skin tags in the eyelids.

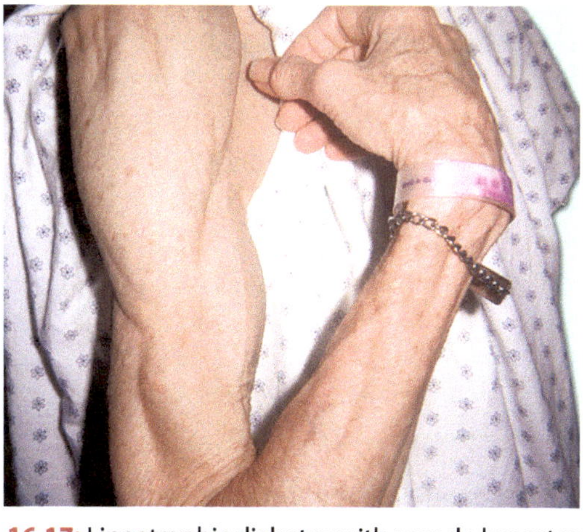

Fig. 16.17: Lipoatrophic diabetes with muscle hypertrophy.

Box 16.7: Congenital partial lipodystrophy.

- Type 1: Köbberling syndrome
- Type 2: Dunnigan syndrome, *LMNA* mutation
- Type 3: PPARG mutation
- Type 4: AKT2 mutation
- Type 5: *PLIN1* mutation
- Others.

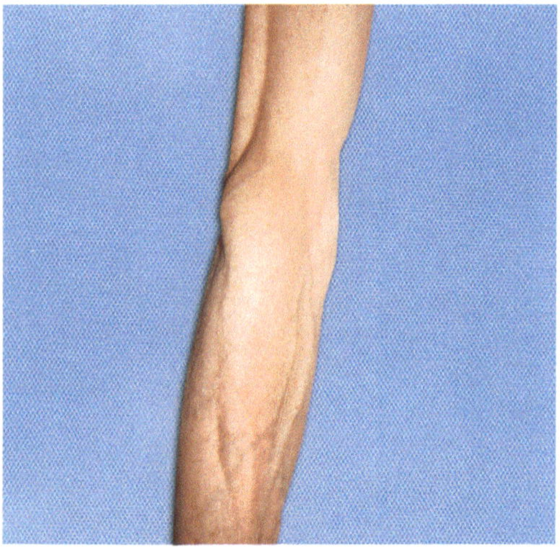

Fig. 16.18: Lipoatrophic diabetes with phlebomegaly.

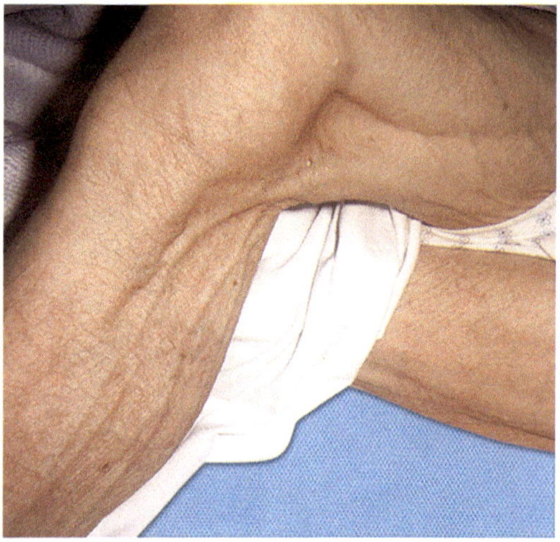

Fig. 16.19: Lipoatrophic diabetes with loss of the perimuscular fat and phlebomegaly.

Type 1 or Köbberling syndrome has been seen only in a few women, and is characterized by absent adipose tissue in the extremities and increased truncal fat. The molecular mechanisms of this form of partial lipodystrophy are still unknown. Type 2 or Dunnigan syndrome is associated with loss of fat in the extremities, abdomen and thorax, and increased fat deposition in the neck and supraclavicular areas. In some patients there is a clear demarcation of the areas of lipoatrophy in the extremities (Dunnigan's lines). Type 3, due to a mutation of the PPAR gamma receptor, is similar to the Dunnigan's variety but with less fat accumulation in the neck. Type 4 is due to a mutation in the *AKT2* gene that has multiple abnormalities and so far does not have a clear phenotype described. Type 5 also has similar areas of atrophy that the other congenital partial lipodystrophy and is due to a mutation in the perilipin 1 gene, an essential component of the lipid droplets in adipocytes. There are other types (accompanied by mandibulo-acral dysplasia, progeroid syndromes, etc.) that have not been well characterized nor in their clinical in molecular aspects (Figs. 16.18 to 16.22).

Acquired Partial Lipodystrophies

Acquired partial lipodystrophies are a mixed bag of syndromes with different causes and mechanisms that so far are not well understood (Box 16.8).

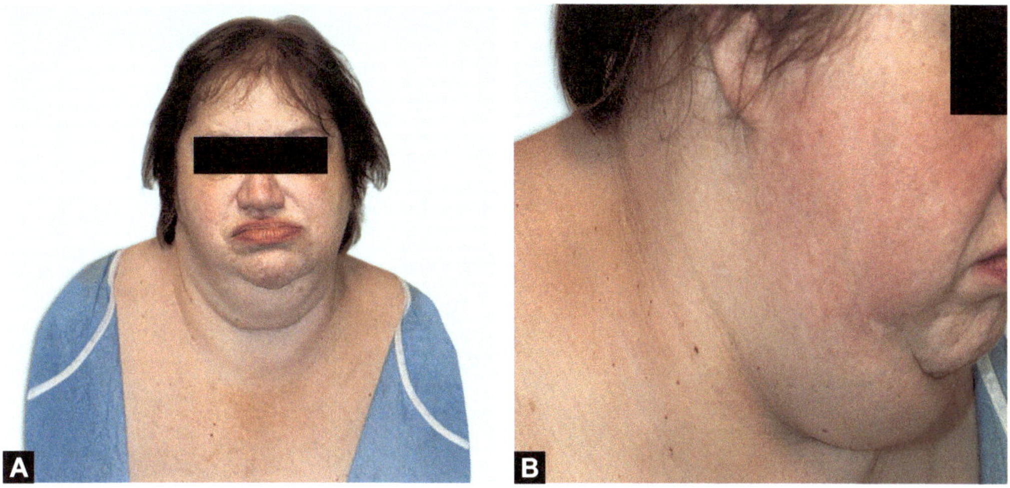

Figs. 16.20A and B: Dunnigan's congenital partial lipoatrophy with increased fat deposition in the neck and supraclavicular areas.

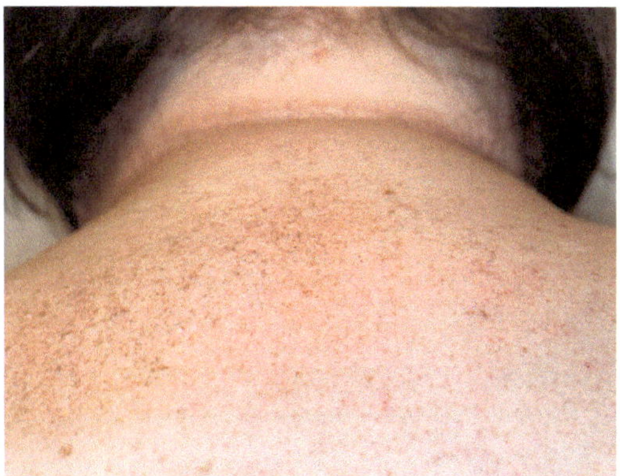

Fig. 16.21: Dunnigan's congenital partial lipoatrophy with increased fat deposition in the upper back (Buffalo hump).

The most common is the lipodystrophy associated to human immunodeficiency virus (HIV) therapy. The exact molecular mechanisms are not completely understood. Clinically it can be quite variable but in general it causes atrophy of the facial fat and hypertrophy in other areas especially in the posterior thorax or neck with abdominal obesity and metabolic syndrome. The Barraquer–Simons syndrome is much less frequent and it is characterized by fat atrophy in the upper body with increased adiposity in the lower body. These patients have an immunoglobulin called 'C3 nephritic factor' that is associated with a glomerulonephritis and other autoimmune disorders.

Localized atrophies and hypertrophies may also be seen from chronic insulin injections (much less since the purification of insulins) or simple injections of antibiotics, depot steroids and vaccines but they do not cause any metabolic abnormalities. Individuals who underwent

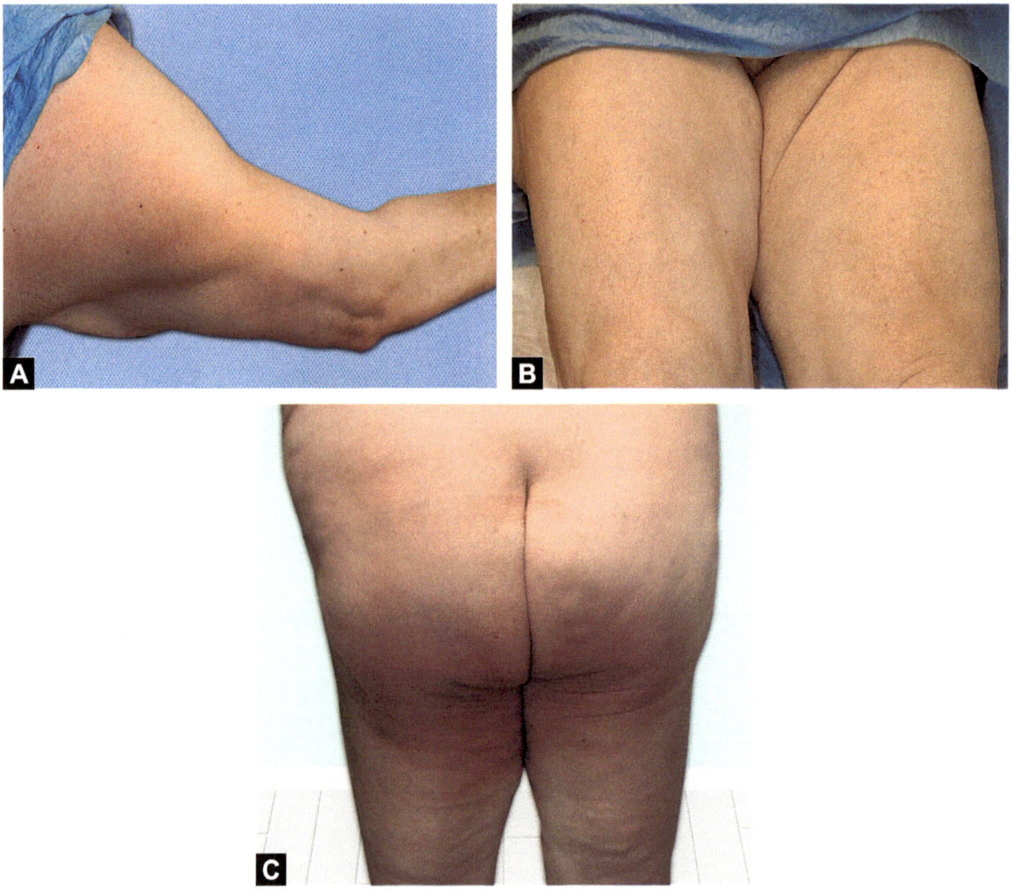

Figs. 16.22A to C: Dunnigan's partial lipodystrophy with a clear demarcation between the areas of atrophy and hypertrophy (Dunnigan's lines).

Box 16.8: Acquired partial lipodystrophy.

- Human immunodeficiency virus (HIV) therapy associated
- Barraquer–Simons syndrome
- Local atrophy and hypertrophy from insulin, antibiotics, or vaccine injections.

liposuctions may also develop areas of lipohypertrophy in other areas of the body (Figs. 16.23 and 16.24).

Glucagonoma Syndrome

Glucagonoma syndrome is an uncommon but very characteristic syndrome characterized by mild diabetes and a chronic skin inflammation, known as necrolytic migratory erythema (NME), caused by a neuroendocrine tumor of the pancreas that secretes glucagon. The rash begins as erythematous plaques in the extremities, face, and perineum followed by chronic crusting. Characteristically the rash does not respond to any of the usual dermatologic treatments. About

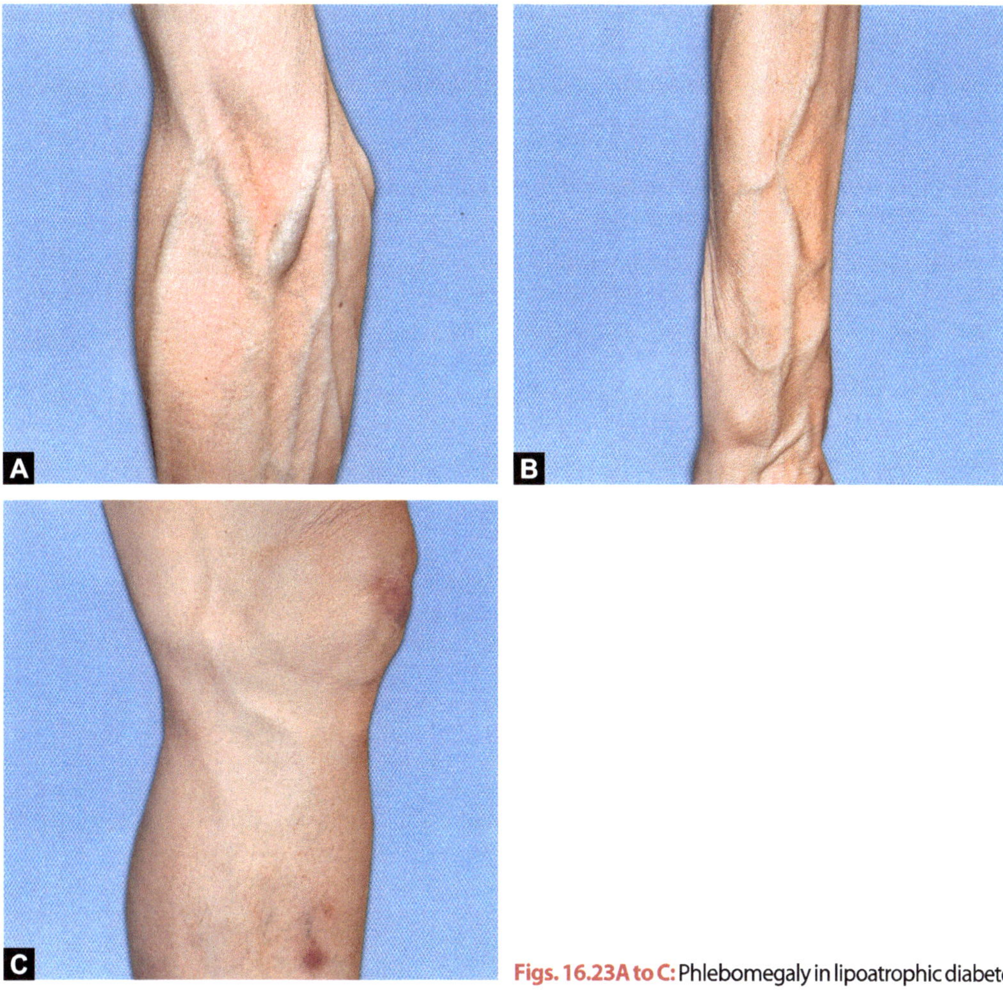

Figs. 16.23A to C: Phlebomegaly in lipoatrophic diabetes.

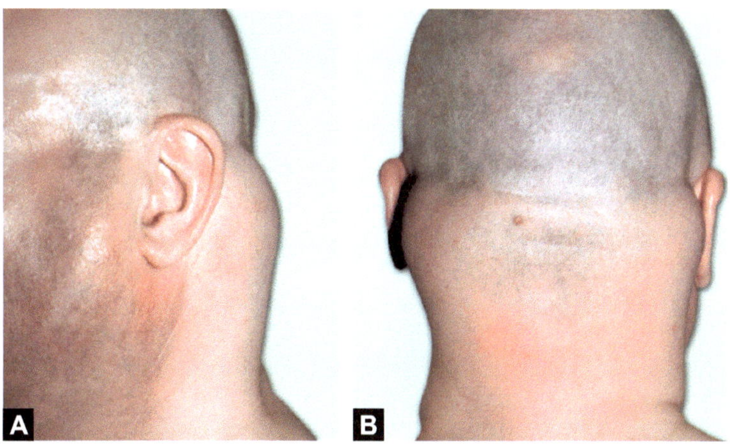

Figs. 16.24A and B: Areas of lipohypertrophy in a patient with human immunodeficiency virus (HIV)-lipodystrophy.

only-half of the patients have over diabetes mellitus. There is also anorexia and weight loss, glossitis and dystrophic changes of the nails. Some patients may also have diarrhea, venous thrombosis and psychiatric manifestations. Laboratory tests show anemia, a high erythrocyte sedimentation rate and levels of glucagon usually higher than 500 pg/mL. The diagnosis should then be confirmed with a CT, MRI, endoscopic ultrasound and/or angiograms. The tumors are usually more than 3 cm and toward the tail of the pancreas. They are usually sporadic but may also be part of an MEN-1 syndrome. Unfortunately, the diagnosis is often made when the tumor has already metastasized to the liver. Complete surgical removal of the tumor cures the NME, or it may also improve significantly with intravenous hyperalimentation (Figs. 16.25 to 16.28).

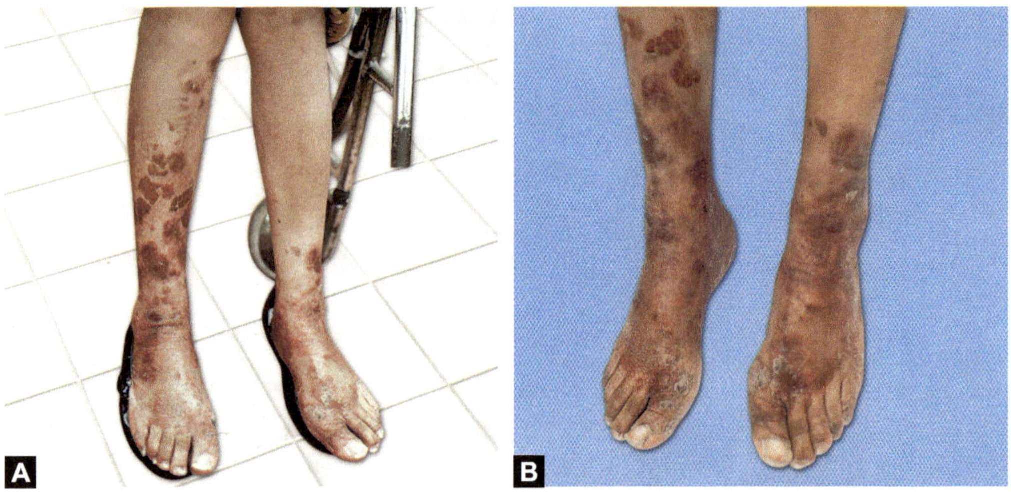

Figs. 16.25A and B: Necrolytic migratory erythema in the glucagonoma syndrome.

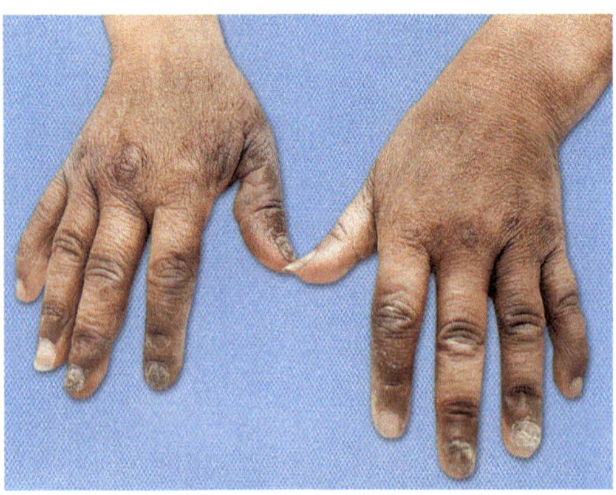

Fig. 16.26: Dystrophic nails in the glucagonoma syndrome.

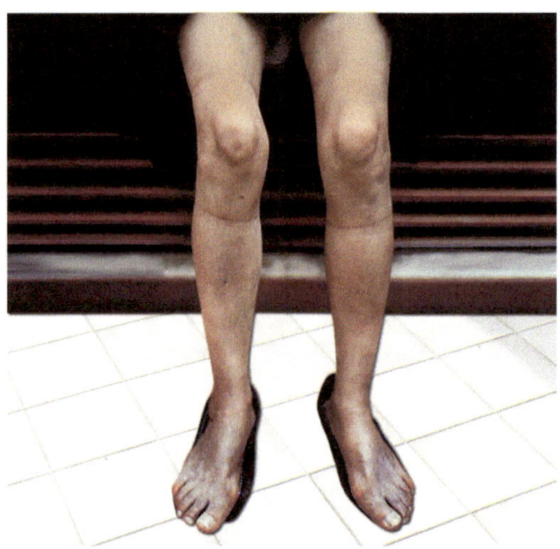

Fig. 16.27: Disappearance of the necrolytic migratory erythema after successful removal of the glucagonoma.

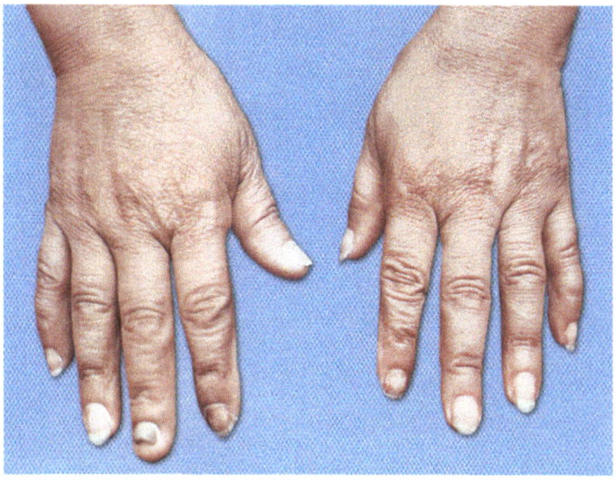

Fig. 16.28: Improvement in the nail dystrophy after the successful removal of the glucagonoma.

Box 16.9: Diabetic hand.

- Palmar sclerosis
- Dupuytren's contracture
- Limited joint mobility syndrome
- Flexion tenosynovitis.

Palmar Sclerosis, Dupuytren's Contracture and Limited Joint Mobility

They are past of a condition that increases the fibrosis in the palms also known as cheiroarthropathy, digital sclerosis, palmar fascia fibromatosis, and diabetic hand syndrome (Box 16.9). Chronic hyperglycemia increases the cross linkings between the collagen fibers of the palmar aspect of hands and fingers by a process of non-enzymatic glycation. Collagen is glycated more than other proteins because it has prolonged half-life of many years and is rich in serine and hydroxy-serine, amino acids with an extra amino group where glucose gets attached. The glycation thickens and shortens the collagen, and prolongs even more its half-life. This leads to a fibrosis of the palmar fascia that start to get attached to both the skin and tendon sheets, limiting the extension of the hand and fingers. In many patients this is easily palpable over the flexor tendons in the palms (Dupuytren's contracture). The flexion-contraction of the tendon sheets may get the tendon stuck and unable to extend the finger (tenosynovitis) (Box 16.10 and Figs. 16.29 to 16.37).

These changes in the hands are very common but almost completely asymptomatic. They increase with age, prolonged hyperglycemia, and duration of diabetes. By and large, once installed they have little or no improvement with improved glycemic control. The association with chronic diabetic complications is controversial, and it may just be due to the fact that palmar sclerosis and chronic complications are more common in patients with prolonged lack of glycemic control.

The hands of every patient with DM should be examined looking for these changes. The best way to find them is asking the patient to put both palms together in a praying position pressing

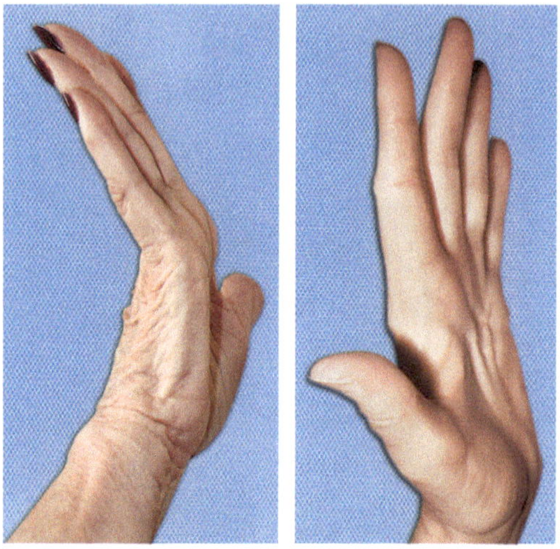

Fig. 16.29: A normal hand should have an extension at the metacarpophalangeal joints of more than 180°. The extension is limited with palmar fibrosis.

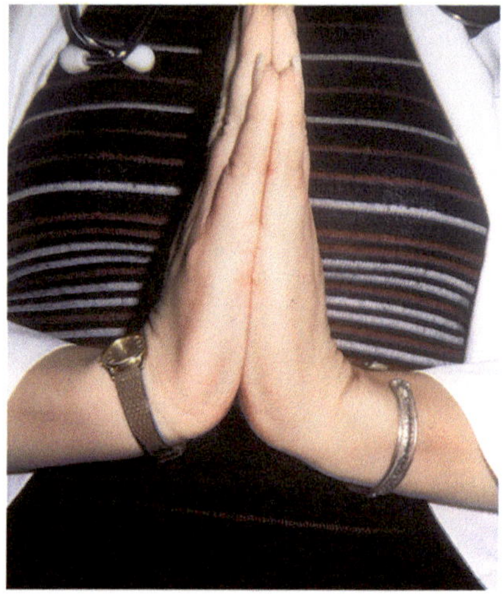

Fig. 16.30: With the hand in the 'praying position' there should be no light passing in between the palms.

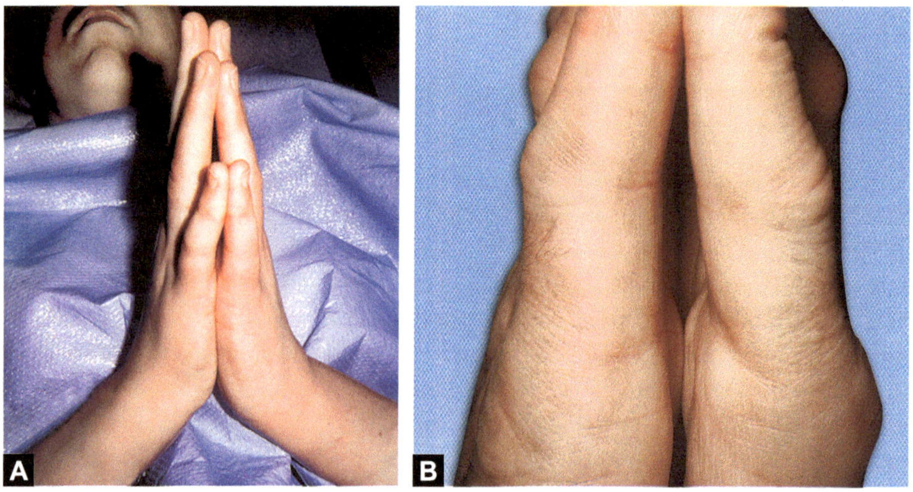

Figs. 16.31A and B: Palmar sclerosis, Grade 1, separation only at the levels of the fingers.

hard for a maximal cooptation ('praying sign'). In a normal individual there should be no light in between palms and fingers. With palmar fibrosis a progressive separation of the surfaces appears slowly, over the years, and in most cases the patients are not aware of it. The separation of the palms could be graded. Another maneuver to show the limited extension is to ask the patient to flatten the hand with pressure over a horizontal, firm surface. Most patients with this palmar separation also have Dupuytren's contracture (Figs. 16.37 to 16.39).

Dupuytren's contracture is more common among Northern Europeans, and much less among Asians and individuals of African descent. It affects preferentially the palmar area of

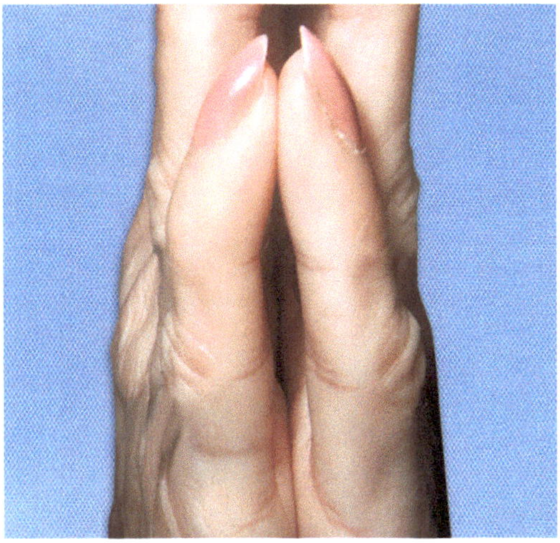

Fig. 16.32: Palmar sclerosis, Grade 2, greater separation at the fingers.

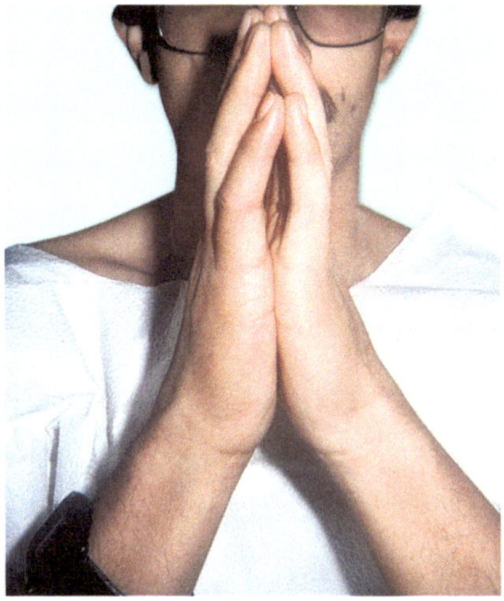

Fig. 16.33: Palmar sclerosis, Grade 2, with even greater separation at the fingers.

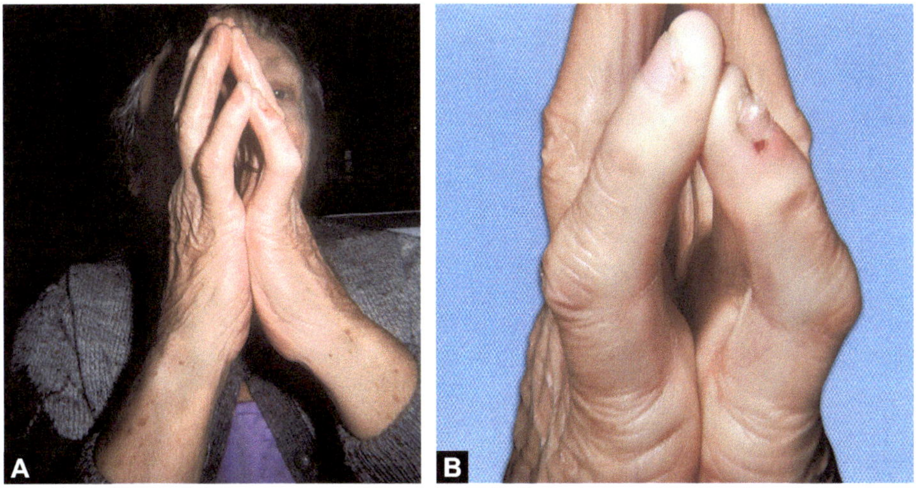

Figs. 16.34A and B: Palmar sclerosis, Grade 3, with exaggerated separation at the fingers.

the flexor tendons of the second and third fingers never the index or first finger. They may also be seen in nondiabetic individuals with hepatic cirrhosis (especially alcoholic), epilepsy (with chronic treatment with phenytoin and barbiturates), syndromes of fibrosclerosis, manual laborers, and in families with a hereditary component. It tends to be most marked in the hand that is used more commonly (left in left handed individuals). Rarely, they also may be found in the middle of the soles, medially, also completely asymptomatic (Plantar Dupuytren's). The diagnosis is mostly clinical, and there is no need for biopsies. Palmar fibrosis with a positive 'praying sign' may also be seen in nondiabetic individuals with aging, severe osteoarthritis of the hands and collagen vascular diseases (scleroderma, dermatomyositis, etc.).

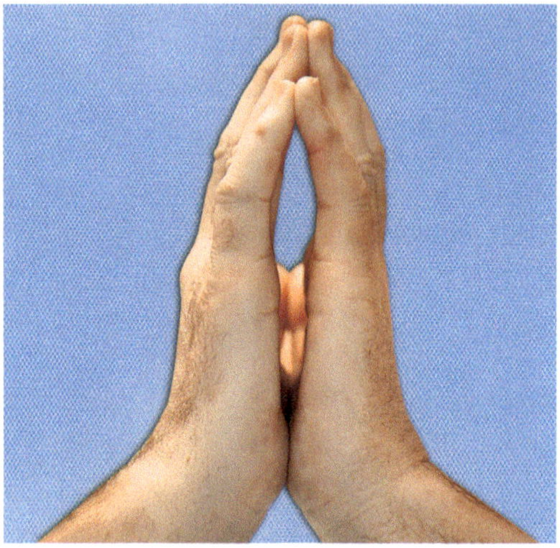

Fig. 16.35: Palmar sclerosis, Grade 4, with clear separation at the level of the palms.

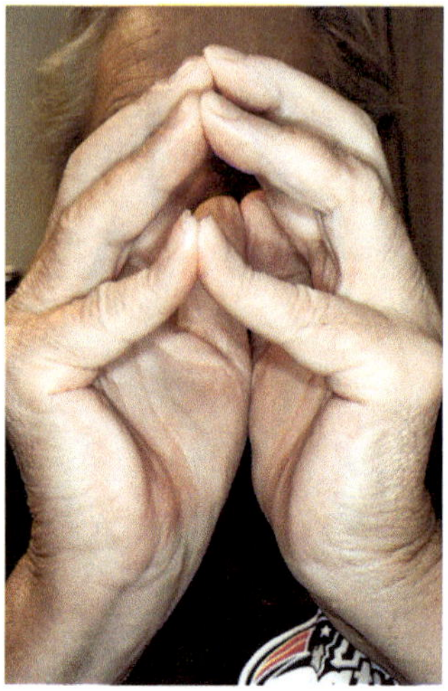

Fig. 16.36: Palmar sclerosis, Grade 4 with extreme separation of fingers and palms.

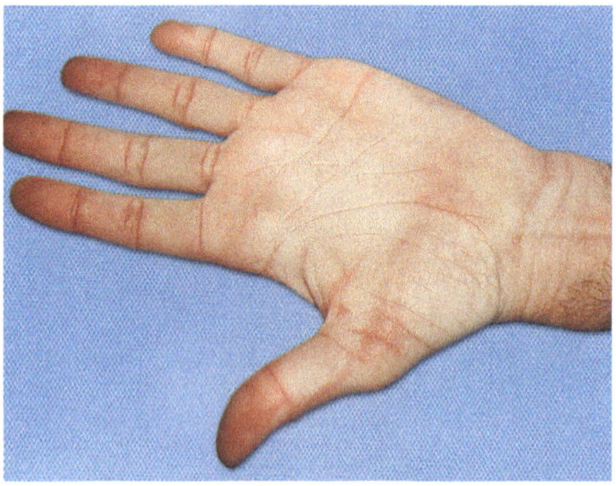

Fig. 16.37: Palmar sclerosis showing that in full extension there is blanching of the skin and the skin lines appear red.

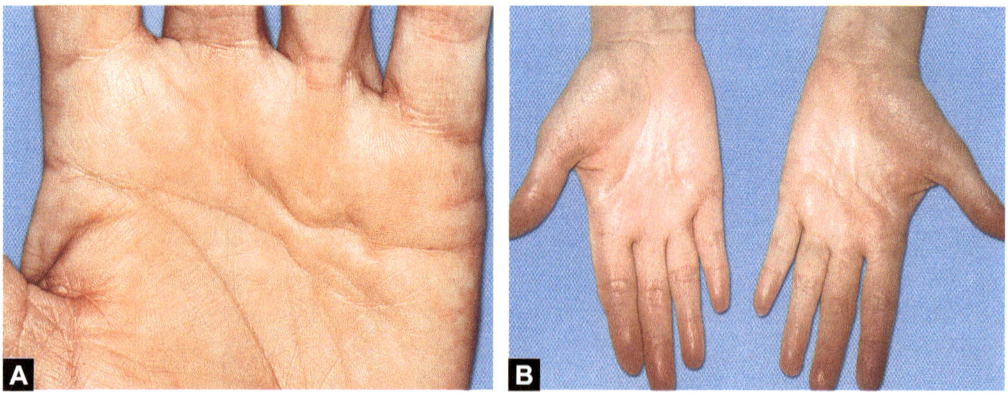

Figs. 16.38A and B: Dupuytren's contracture.

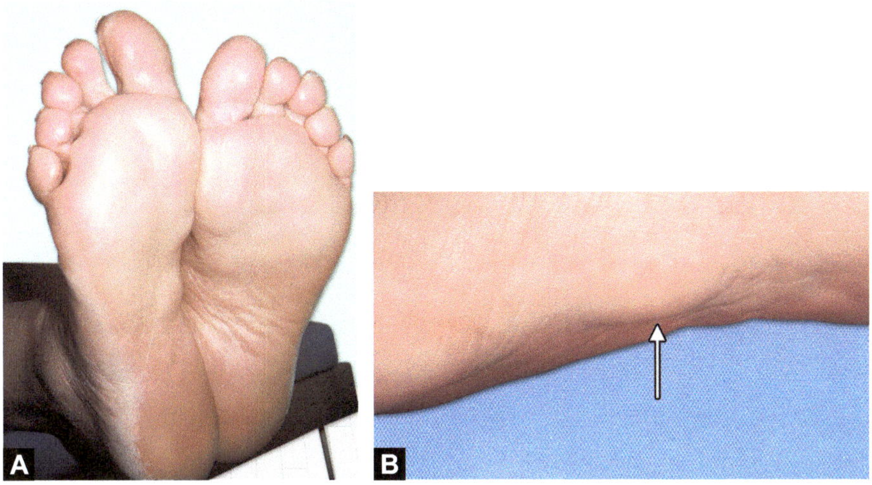

Figs. 16.39A and B: Plantar Dupuytren's contracture.

Palmar fibrosis and Dupuytren's contracture rarely require treatment. Physical therapy and local corticoid injections usually do not offer long-term improvement. More recently, in situ injections with collagenases from *Clostridium hystoliticum* are being used mostly for cosmetic or professional (musicians) reasons. In severe cases that interfere with the hand functions plastic surgery is indicated usually with good results in centers of experience. Flexor tenosynovitis, on the other hand, with fingers getting continuously 'stuck' in flexion and unable to extend, requires surgery more often and usually with good results. In the feet, a similar shortening of tendons occurs frequently, but on the extensor tendons and causes 'hammer toes' (see Chapter on 'The Diabetic Foot') (Figs. 16.40 and 16.41).

Scleredema

Scleredema is a skin lesion of diabetes that 'is not seen but felt'. It requires to palpate and pinch the skin in the back of the thorax. This is very easy to do and the skin in that area should be as soft as other areas of the body in normal individuals. In persons with uncontrolled diabetes of long duration the skin in that area becomes indurated and it cannot be pinched. It is more common in men and it tends to improve very slowly with glycemic control.

Diabetic Bulla

Uncommon lesions that tend to appear in hands and feet after prolonged periods of uncontrolled hyperglycemia. They are painless and their size is variable with some of them up to several centimeters. They contain serous material. It takes months to heal and the effect of glycemic control on their healing is not known. It is better not to open them and keep them covered to prevent spontaneous ruptures and subsequent infection.

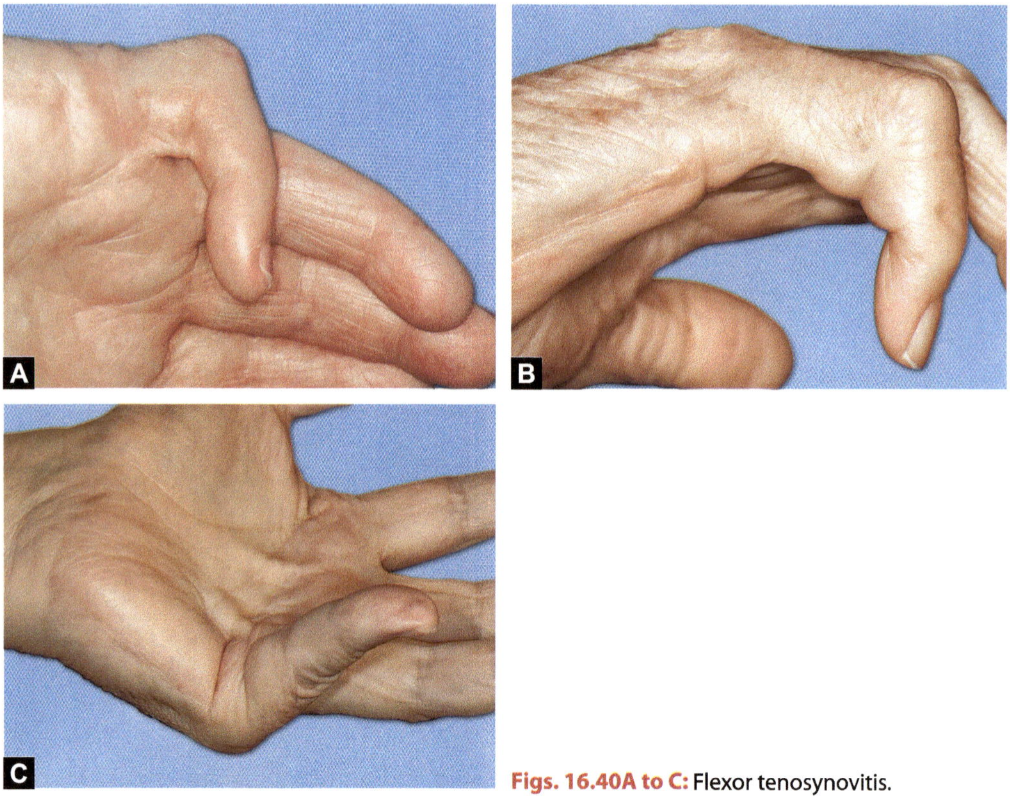

Figs. 16.40A to C: Flexor tenosynovitis.

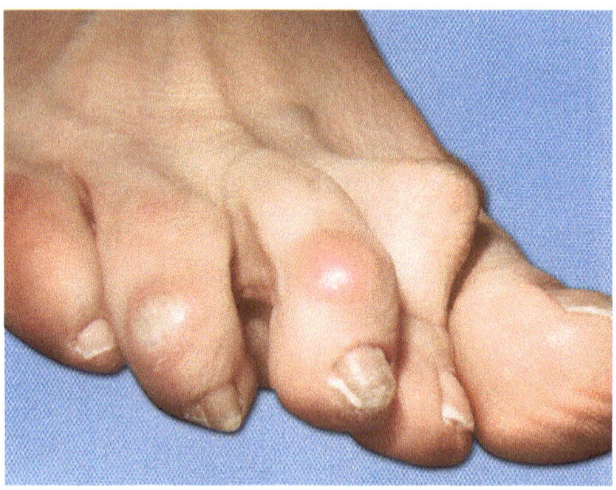

Fig. 16.41: Retraction of the extensor tendons of the feet with "hammer toes" causing calluses over the interphalangeal joints.

LESIONS DUE TO METABOLIC ALTERATIONS (BOX 16.10)

Xanthoma

Xanthomas are yellowish accumulations of lipid laden macrophages under the skin in individuals with severe hyperlipidemia. They are quite infrequent nowadays with available treatments but they may still be seen in some of the congenital severe hyperlipidemias, cerebrotendinous xanthomatosis, and familial sitosterolemia. According to their site and appearance they have been classified as planar (flat), tuberous, or tendinous. Xanthelasma palpebrarum is the most common form of planar xanthomas but they are neither necessarily associated with dyslipidemias nor cardiovascular risk. The most common places of the tendinous variety are along the Achilles' tendon, dorsum of the forearms and elbows, and in the hands. In general they tend to respond well to lipid lowering treatments (Figs. 16.42A and B).

Box 16.10: Lesions due to metabolic alterations.

- Xanthoma
- Eruptive xanthoma
- Carotenodermia.

Eruptive Xanthoma

Eruptive xanthomas are acute eruptions associated with the 'chylomicronemia syndrome' that appear when plasma triglycerides levels exceed 1000 mg/dL. Eruptive xanthomas are yellowish, small papules that appear suddenly in many parts of the body, particularly on the elbows and buttocks. They are surrounded by an inflammatory reaction that, at times, leads to the erroneous diagnosis of a skin infection. The pathology shows the deposition of large amounts of chylomicrons in histiocytes of the skin. It is frequently accompanied by lipemia retinalis (creamy color retina with whitish vessels) (tomato soup appearance), and acute pancreatitis. The very high level of triglycerides may interfere with the laboratory determination of the amylasemia, giving lower results.

The cause of the familial chylomicronemia syndrome is impaired triglyceride metabolism that may be primary (familial hypertriglyceridemia), but more frequently is secondary to uncontrolled DM, at times as part of the syndrome of ketoacidosis. The treatment consists of insulin, fibrates, metformin, and if tolerated, nicotinic acid (Figs. 16.43A and B).

Carotenodermia

Carotenodermia is the yellowish discoloration of the skin especially in the palms and soles. The differential diagnosis with jaundice is very simple because carotenodermia does not appear in

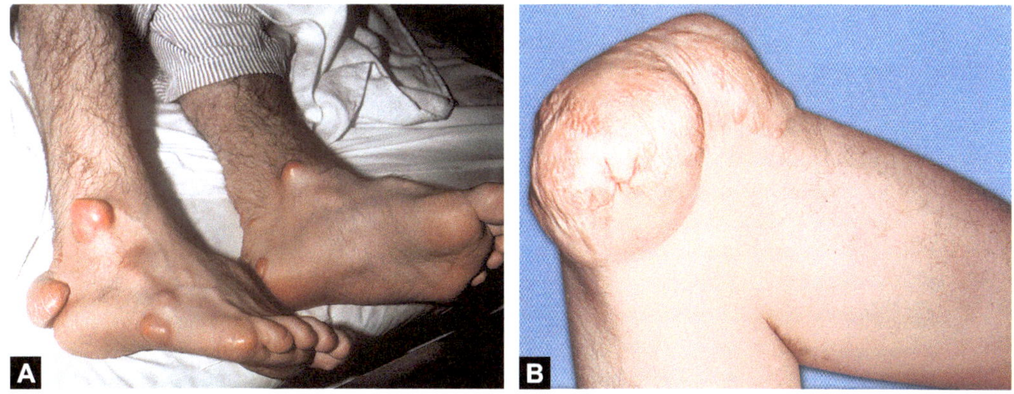

Figs. 16.42A and B: Xanthomas.

the sclera. Prolonged hyperglycemia may cause carotenodermia, but it may also be seen with hypothyroidism, anorexia nervosa, and high intake of vegetables (vegetarians), not necessarily only pigmented ones like carrots and tomatoes. Inside of the chlorophyll of the green vegetables there are plenty of carotenoids (Fig. 16.44).

SKIN INFECTIONS MORE COMMON IN DIABETES (BOX 16.11)

Candidiasis

Infections with Candida are quite common in patients with DM especially if it is out of control. Humidity, heat and high levels of glucose facilitate the growth of this fungus especially in folders of the skin (submammary, groin, and axilla) where they are called *intertrigo*. Less commonly they may appear in the intergluteal or perineal area extending to the scrotum. Initially, they are

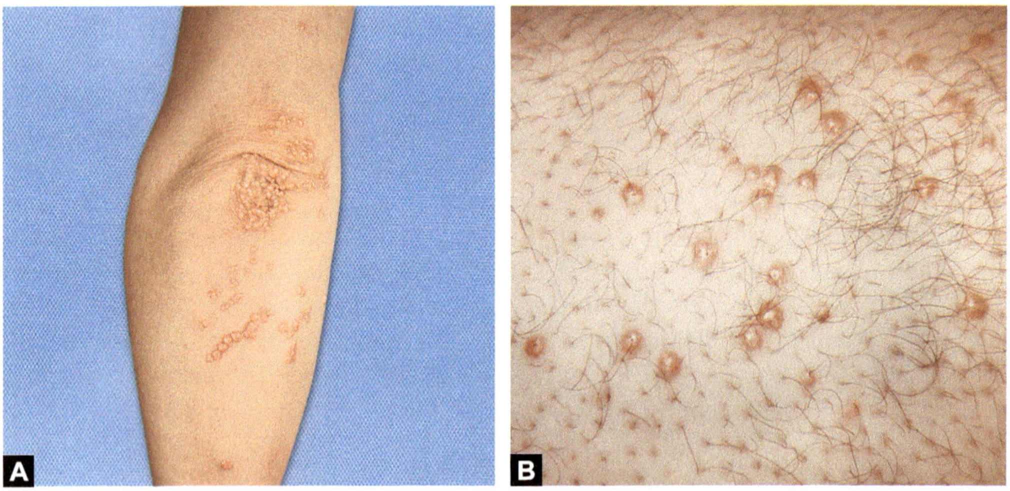

Figs. 16.43A and B: Eruptive xanthomas.

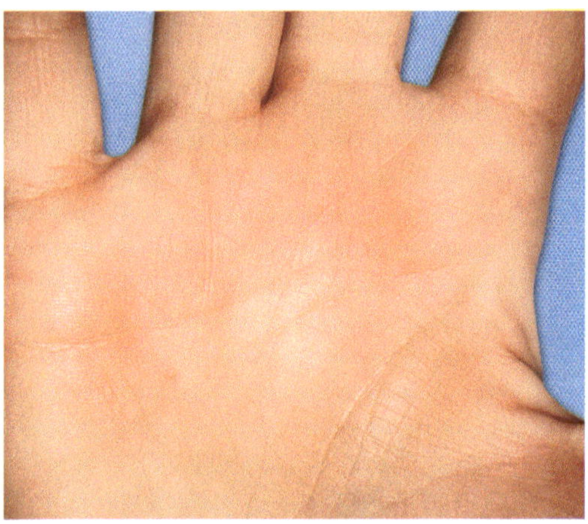

Fig. 16.44: Carotenodermia.

Box 16.11: Skin infections more common in diabetes.

- *Candidiasis*:
  - Intertrigo
  - Vulvovaginitis and balanitis
  - Erosio interdigitalis
- *Fungal*: Tinea pedis and onychomycosis
- *Bacterial*:
  - Abscess, cellulitis, and impetigo
  - Hidradenitis suppurativa
  - Foot infections.

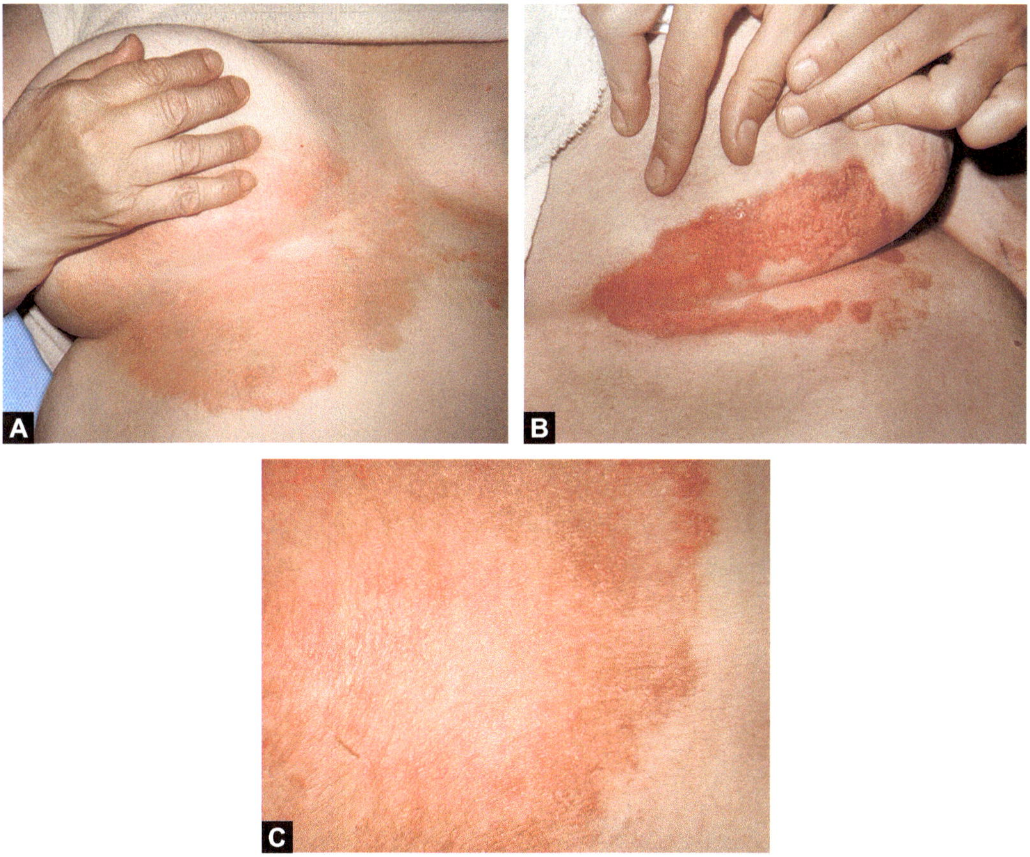

Figs. 16.45A to C: Intertrigo.

erythematous plaques with small pustular lesions in the periphery. They may or may not be pruritic. The lesions extend slowly with time without clearing areas at the center like in other mycosis. As they become chronic they may take a psoriasiform aspect with white plaques, and they become less symptomatic (Figs. 16.45 to 16.49).

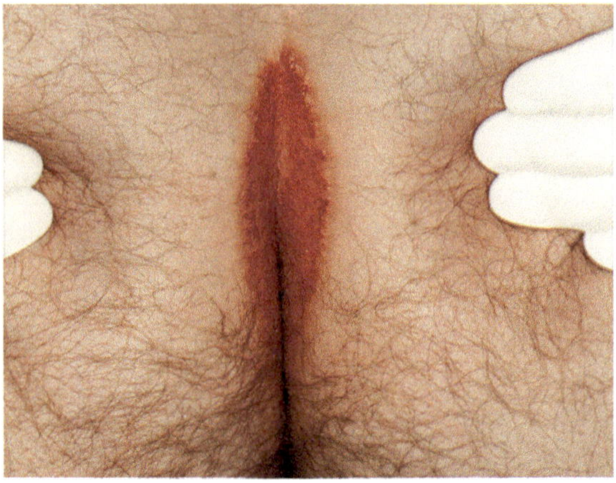

Fig. 16.46: Intergluteal intertrigo.

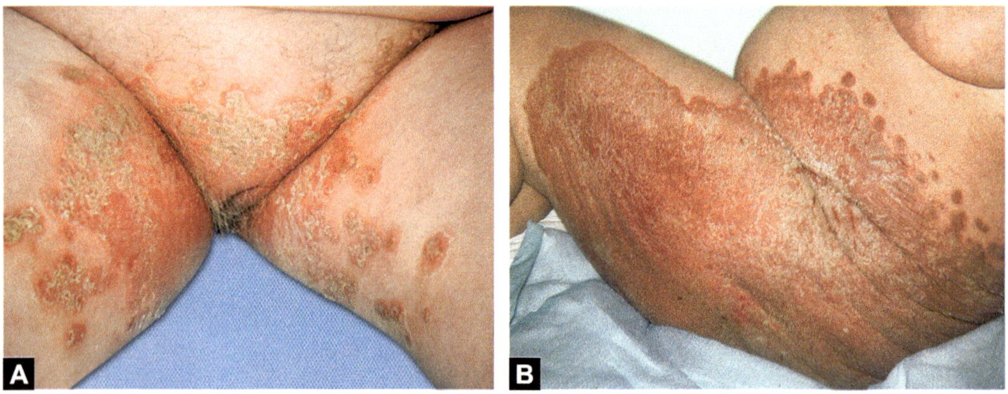

Figs. 16.47A and B: Chronic intertrigo in a patient with urinary incontinence.

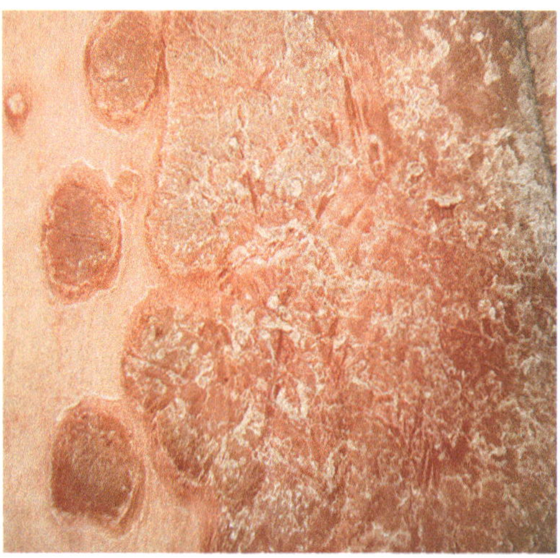

Fig. 16.48: Chronic intertrigo with psoriasiform scales.

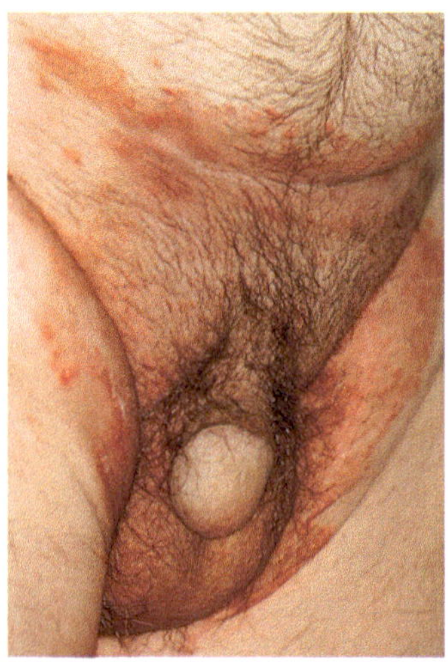

Fig. 16.49: Inguinal intertrigo.

Vulvovaginitis

Vulvovaginitis is also quite common among women with diabetes, and at times is the presenting symptom. The glycosuria creates an environment very favorable for the fungal growth, and for that reason this type of infections may also be seen in women taking SGLT-2 inhibitors. On physical examination, the vulva and variable parts of the vagina appear red with a white, cheese material that is quite characteristic. Control of blood glucose is very important for the treatment. Most cases of recurrent vulvovaginal candidiasis are due to persistent hyperglycemia and glycosuria.

Less common are cases of *balanitis* among men. It tends to happen more often in non-circumcised individuals and it may be very pruritic. Again, at times it is the symptom that leads to the diagnosis of diabetes. Usually the glans and the internal parts of the prepuce are very red and may have white, cheese material, occasionally with superficial ulcerations (Figs. 16.50 and 16.51). *Erosio interdigitalis* is more common in the hands of diabetic individuals who have

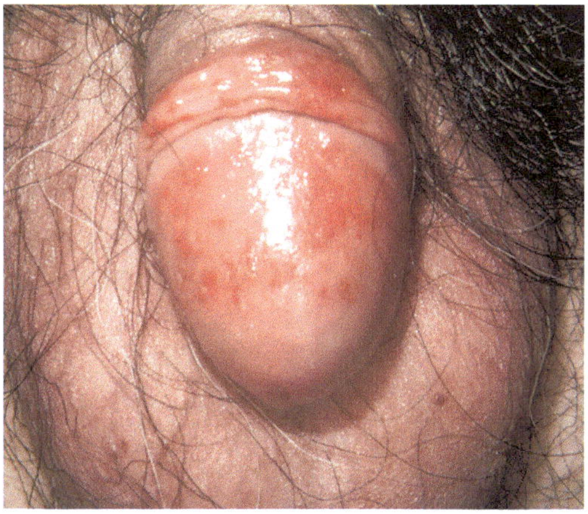

Fig. 16.50: Balanitis.

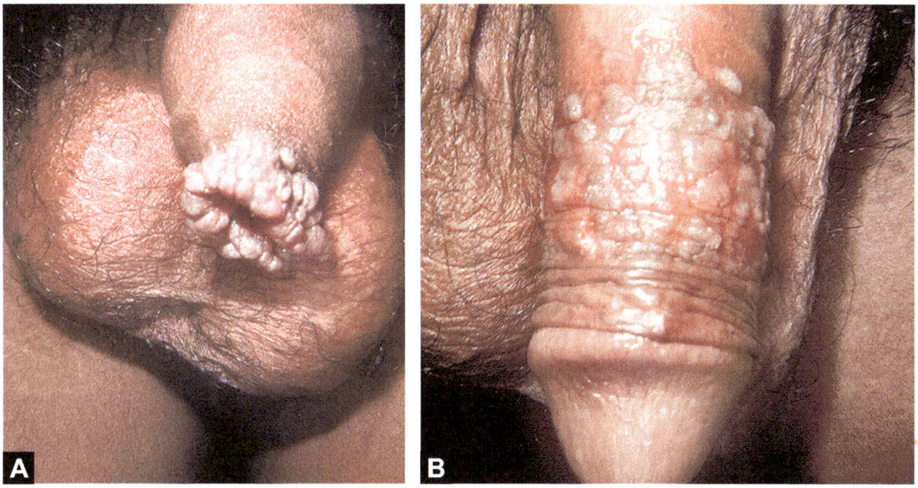

Figs. 16.51A and B: Chronic balanitis.

continuous exposure to water and detergents. One or more interdigital spaces may be involved at the metacarpal fold. The lesions again are erythematous with superficial erosions, and usually quite symptomatic with pruritus. In general, patients with DM do not have an increased frequency of invasive candidiasis.

The treatment of these skin candidiasis in persons with DM is usually quite simple. Local antifungal (ketoconazole, clotrimazole, or miconazole creams), keeping the area dry to the point of using a hair dryer directed to the area after baths, and glycemic control are usually sufficient. If the lesions are very pruritic a mild steroid ointment may be applied with the antifungal creams. In recurrent or recalcitrant cases, especially of vulvovaginitis, oral antifungal agents such as itraconazole or fluconazole, may be administered for two or more days.

Tinea pedis or athlete's foot is not necessarily more frequent in DM but they may be the cause of the beginning of an infection in the toes and foot. For that reason it should be looked for and treated as part of the prevention of a 'diabetic foot.' Most of them are interdigital and less commonly plantar when it extends to the soles. Again, hygiene and dryness are very important for the treatment and prevention.

Onychomycosis

Onychomycosis is a frequent problem in the general population and not necessarily more frequent among individuals with DM. It is a chronic infection mostly of the toenails caused by several dermatophytes that increases with age. It causes nail thickening, discoloration and separation of the nail bed usually in several toes. Very often it is close to impossible to make a differential diagnosis with onychogryphosis (nail thickening and curvature without a fungal infection), even with KOH preparations and cultures. Again the problem, outside of cosmetic is that it may cause problems with the skin of the toes, and in a foot with decreased circulation and/or innervation it may lead to serious problems. Once the nail infection is established it is very difficult to eradicate. Treatments with oral antifungals are widely publicized in the media but in reality they are not very effective, have the problem of interactions with other medications (statins), and liver toxicity. Podiatry care (trimming of toenails) and local antifungals applied daily are occasionally effective. Daily application of Vick's VapoRub 'balsamic ointment' is an inexpensive treatment that has been effective in some patients although it does not have any proven clinical evidence.

BACTERIAL INFECTIONS OF THE SKIN

Abscess, Cellulitis, and Impetigo

Although the pathogenic mechanisms are not clear so far, patients with chronic hyperglycemia tend to have more bacterial infections and particularly in the skin. The host defense problems most frequently encountered with hyperglycemia seem to be decreased adherence and intracellular killing in neutrophils that seem to improve with blood glucose control. Decreased circulation and innervation, skin thinness and dryness, and stasis dermatitis in obese patients are also conditions that may lead to 'secondary impetiginization.' Careless, repeated use of needles used in insulin administration may also cause local abscesses at the site of injections.

Diabetic patients also are more frequently carriers of *Staphylococcus* including methicillin-resistant strains, in the skin and nasal orifices, but often the skin infections are polymicrobial. Simple skin infections may get complicated with necrotizing fasciitis, Fournier's gangrene, surgical wounds, and foot infections. Prolonged, severe hyperglycemia may be a factor of severe skin infections, and severe skin infections can be the source of glycemic decompensations and ketoacidosis.

Hidradenitis Suppurativa

Hidradenitis suppurativa is a chronic inflammation of the hair follicles (the name is a misnomer) in areas of skin friction, mostly axilla and groin, more common in obese young women with metabolic syndrome. It starts as an obstruction of the hair follicles' pores with a secondary infection and abscess formation. In chronic cases there are sinus tract formation, and hypertrophic scars. The treatments are frequently quite frustrating, and consist of surgical drainage and antibiotics.

Foot infections frequently start as innocuous skin infections (see Chapter on 'Diabetic Foot').

SKIN COMPLICATIONS OF TREATMENTS (BOX 16.12)

Sulfonylureas

Very rarely nowadays treatment with sulfonylureas may cause an allergic reaction with a generalized erythematous rash and pruritus that tend to appear within the first days.

Insulin Injections

Insulin injections may cause localized or generalized allergic reactions. If the injection technique is not very good some patients may get hematomas or even abscesses, particularly if they were using nondisposable equipment. Very high doses of insulin may cause a localized area of acanthosis nigricans. Areas of localized lipoatrophy or lipohypertrophy used to be much common when insulins were not highly purified but they may still be seen nowadays even with insulin analogs particularly in children and adolescents. The patients should be instructed not to inject in the same sites and particularly avoid sites that already have lipohypertrophy (they look like an easy site) because the absorption of insulin from these areas may be erratic and it may increase the hypertrophy (Figs. 16.52 to 16.59).

Glucagon-like Peptide 1 Analogs Injections

Rarely cause local problems but occasionally they may produce an allergic reaction (Fig. 16.60).

Box 16.12: Skin complications of treatments.

- Sulfonylureas
- Insulin injections
- Glucagon-like peptide 1 (GLP-1) agonists.

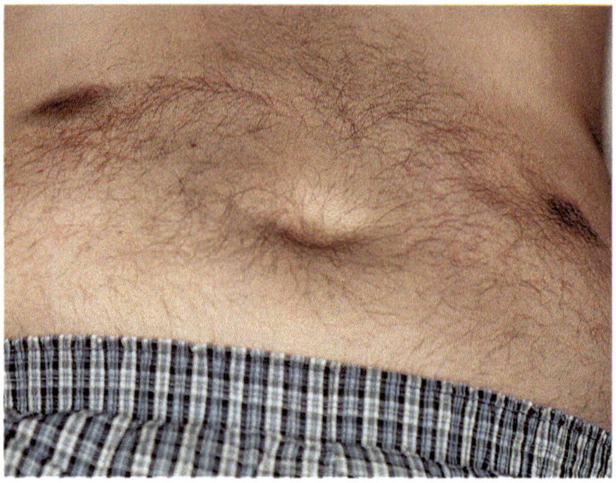

Fig. 16.52: Insulin hematomas.

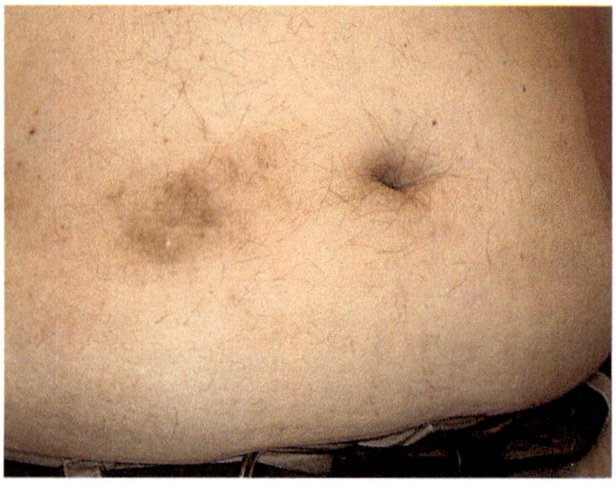

Fig. 16.53: Insulin injection site acanthosis from very large doses.

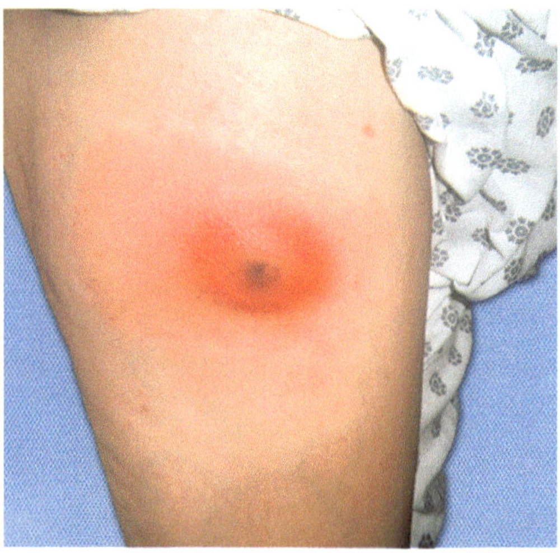

Fig. 16.54: Abscess at the site of insulin injection with poorly sterilized equipment.

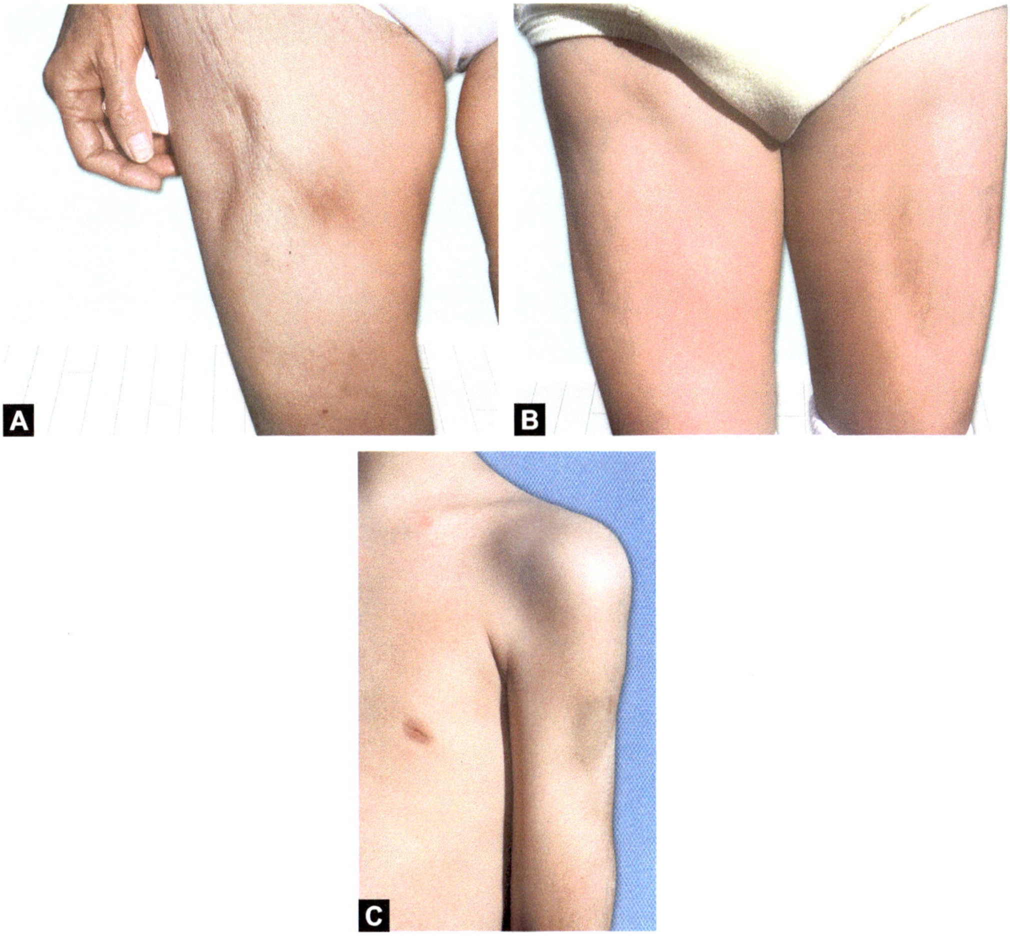

Figs. 16.55A to C: Insulin lipoatrophy.

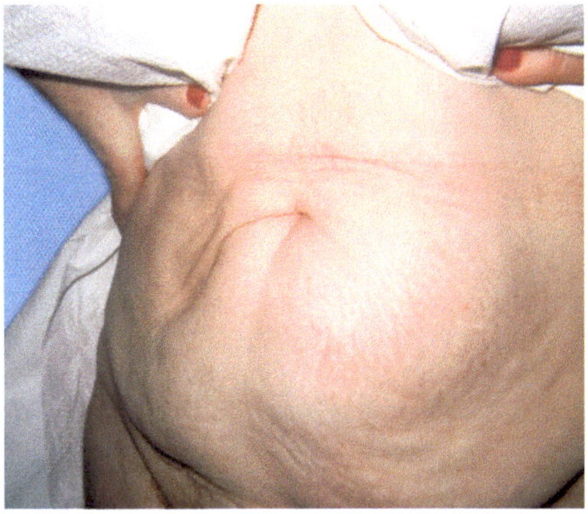

Fig. 16.56: Areas of insulin lipoatrophy and lipohypertrophy in the abdomen.

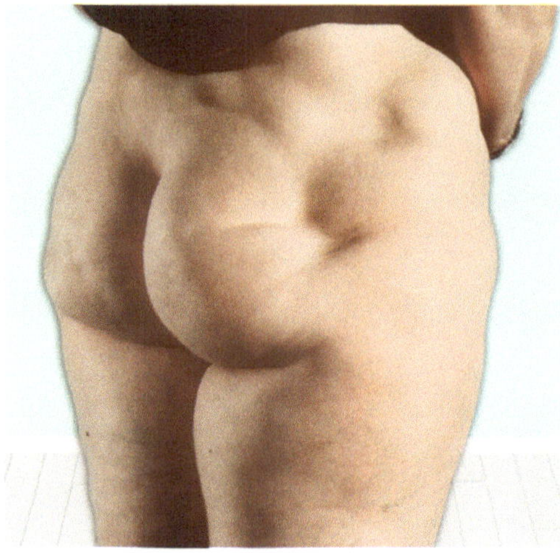

Fig. 16.57: Insulin lipoatrophy in a patient who was injecting in the buttocks.

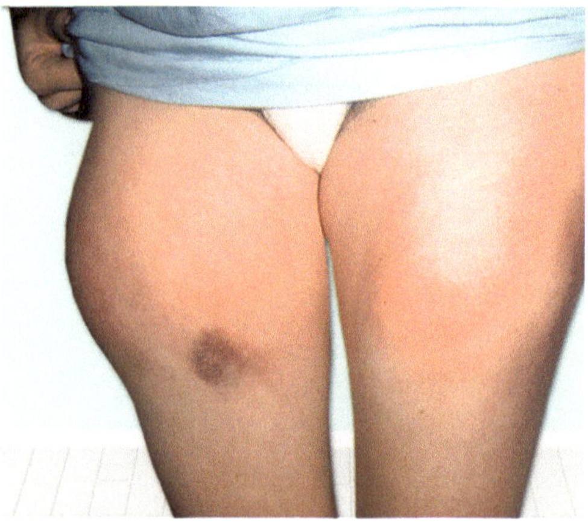

Fig. 16.58: Insulin lipohypertrophy in the thighs.

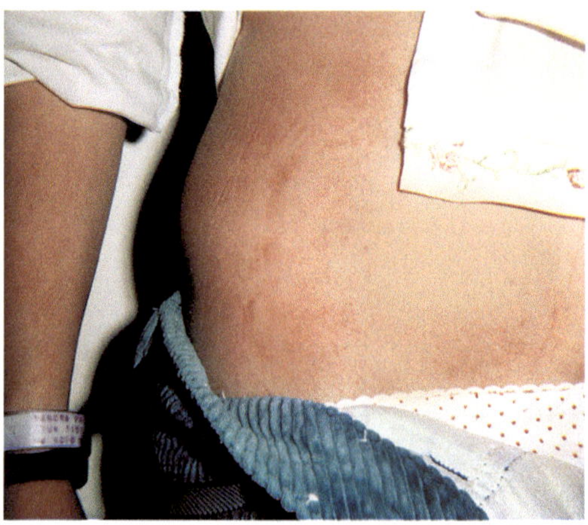

Fig. 16.59: Insulin lipohypertrophy at the side of the abdomen.

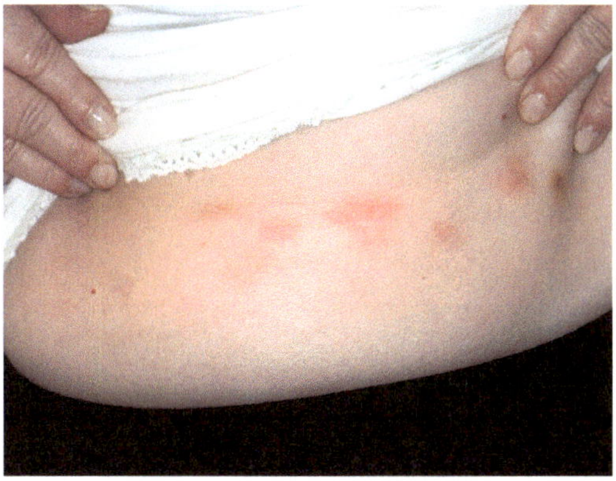

Fig. 16.60: Local reaction at the site of liraglutide injection.

Box 16.13: Skin lesions with increased incidence in diabetes mellitus (DM).

- Vitiligo
- Acanthosis nigricans and skin tags
- Psoriasis
- Punctures from glycemic monitoring
- Darkening of the skin
- Kaposi's sarcoma
- Blue toe syndrome
- Calciphylaxis.

SKIN LESIONS WITH INCREASED INCIDENCE IN DIABETES MELLITUS (BOX 16.13)

Vitiligo

Vitiligo is present in 1% of the total population, but it is more common in persons with autoimmune disorders such as DM-1, Hashimoto's thyroiditis, Addison's disease, pernicious anemia, premature ovarian failure, and hypoparathyroidism. It is an acquired, patchy loss of the skin pigmentation, bilateral 'trying to be symmetrical,' that starts in acral areas (hands and feet) progressing slowly to flexor, genital, and periorificial areas. It may also appear around surgical scars and has very clear borders. It is usually asymptomatic, but occasionally it gets irritated with sun exposure, and it can be cosmetically devastating to the individual. One of the many mysteries of vitiligo is the fact that being a 'systemic' autoimmune condition it attacks only well-circumscribed areas of the skin respecting the rest, but that is exactly what happens with the islets in DM-1 and in Hashimoto's thyroiditis, areas destroyed intermixed with areas completely spared (Figs. 16.61 to 16.68).

Biopsies are usually not necessary but when done they show absence of melanocytes and occasional chronic inflammation at the borders. In light-skinned individuals the patches are more obvious during the summer because of increased contrast with sun-tanned skin. In dark-skinned persons, the depigmented areas are more noticeable during the entire year. The

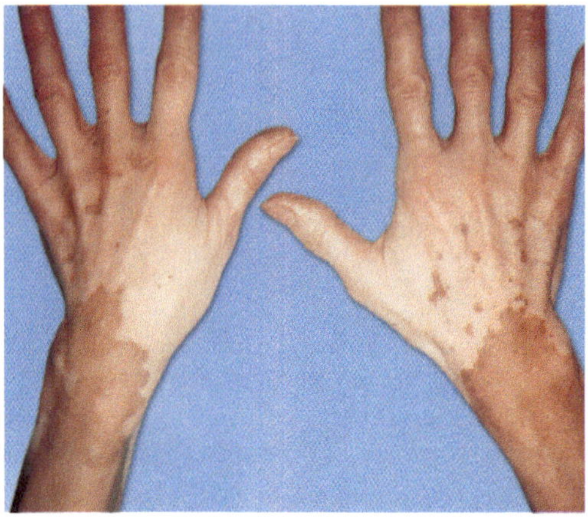

Fig. 16.61: Typical lesions of vitiligo with well-delineated borders.

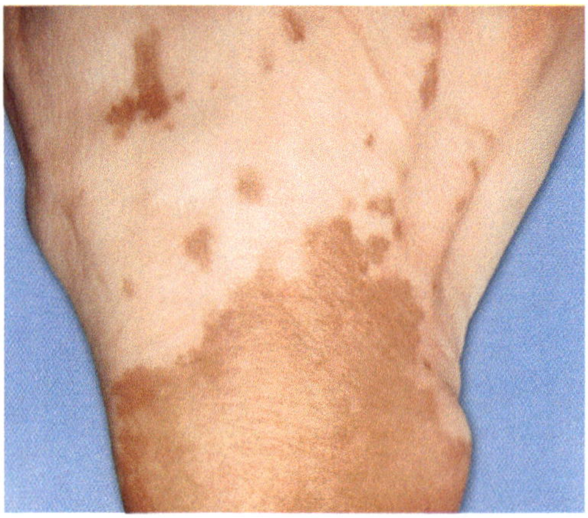

Fig. 16.62: Vitiligo with well-delineated borders.

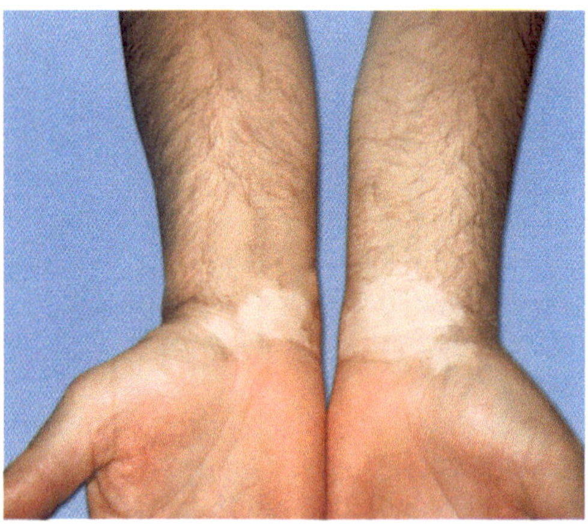

Fig. 16.63: Vitiligo is bilateral and "tries to be symmetrical".

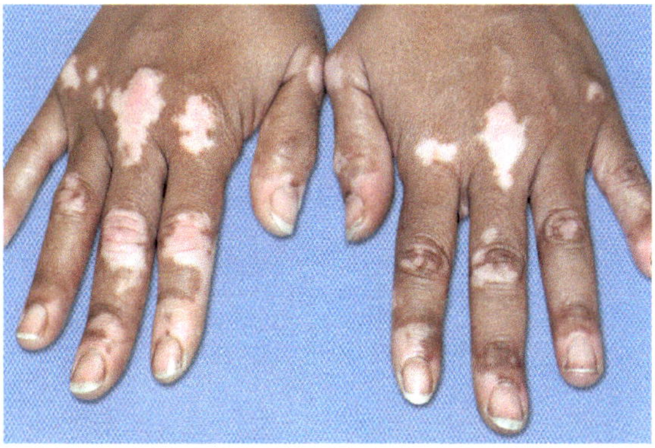

Fig. 16.64: Vitiligo in the dorsum of the hands and fingers.

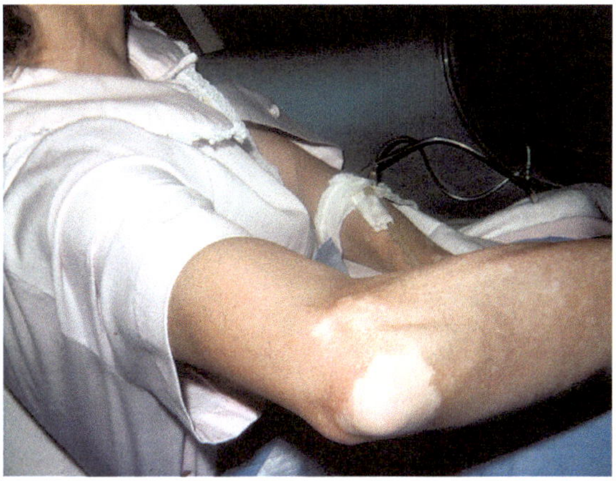

Fig. 16.65: Elbow is another site for vitiligo to appear.

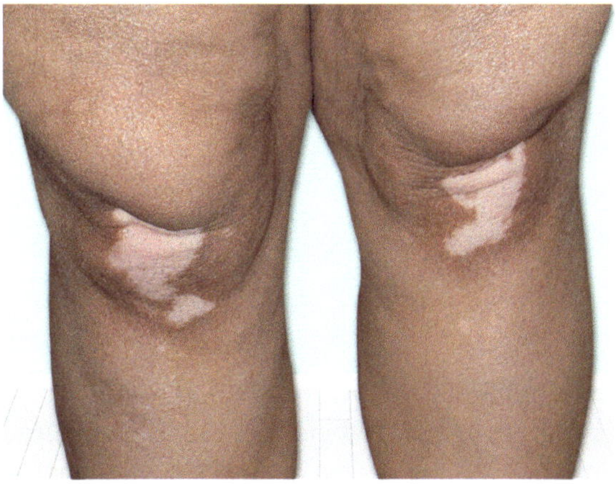

Fig. 16.66: Vitiligo over the anterior aspect of the knees.

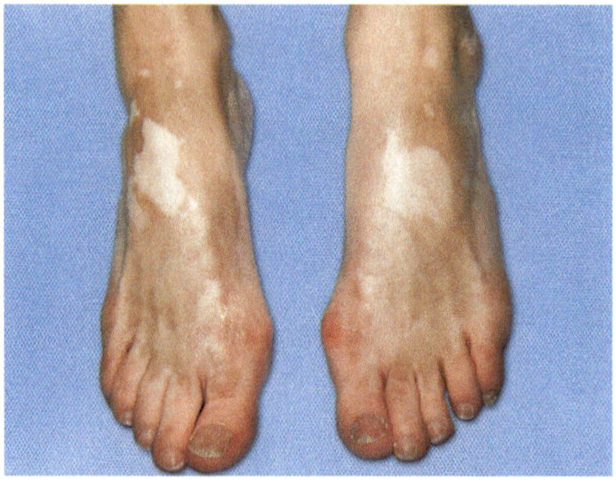

Fig. 16.67: Vitiligo on the dorsum of the feet.

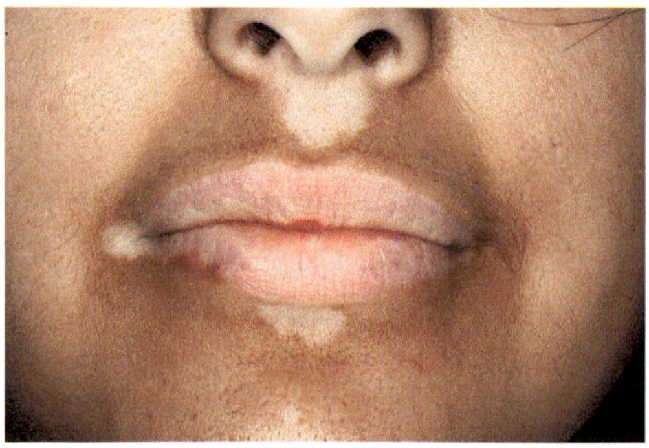

Fig. 16.68: Periorificial vitiligo.

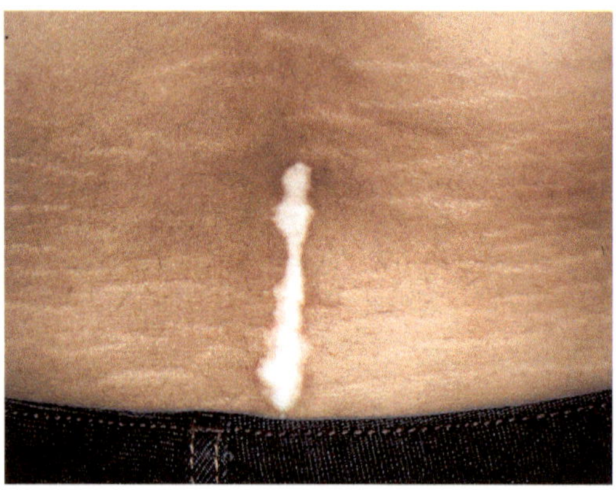

Fig. 16.69: Vitiligo at the site of a surgical scar (cesarean section).

lesions progress slowly in the peripheries with periods of rapid expansion and others when they remain stable. The treatment consists in repigmentation programs that are usually only partially effective, and has to be done by experienced dermatologists (Figs. 16.69 to 16.76).

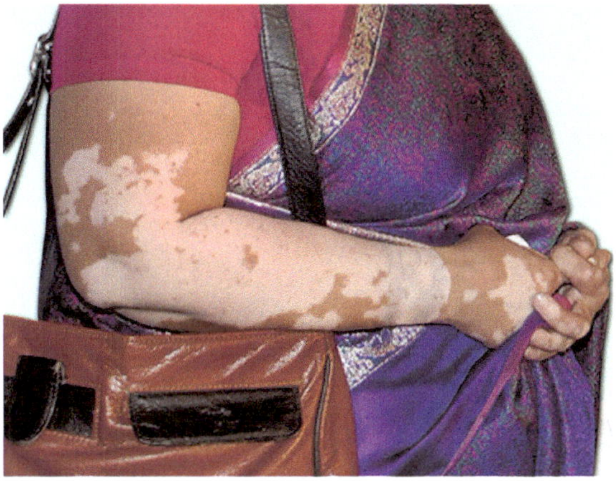

Fig. 16.70: Vitiligo over the arm and forearm.

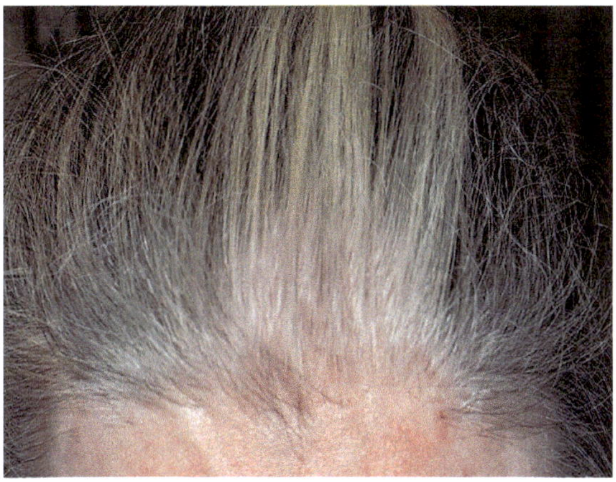

Fig. 16.71: Leukotrichia, a band of depigmented hair in the scalp.

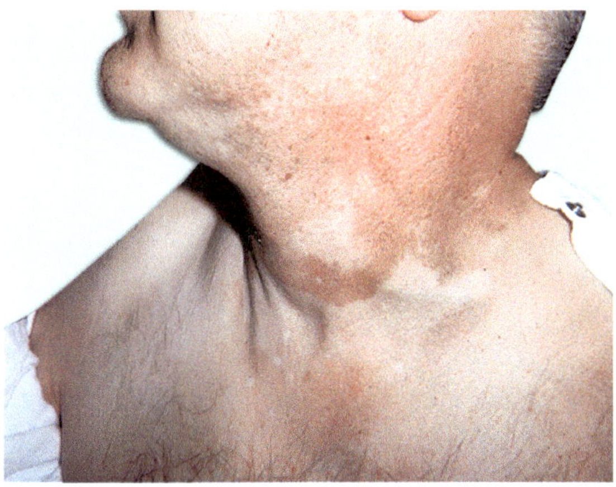

Fig. 16.72: Vitiligo over the anterior neck in a patient with Hashimoto's thyroiditis.

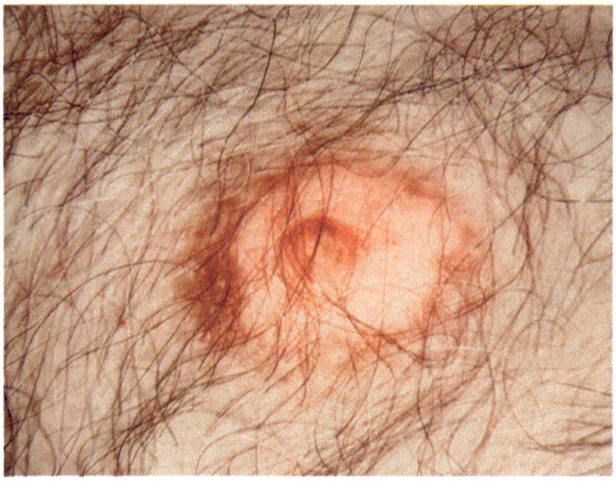

Fig. 16.73: Vitiligo of the nipple.

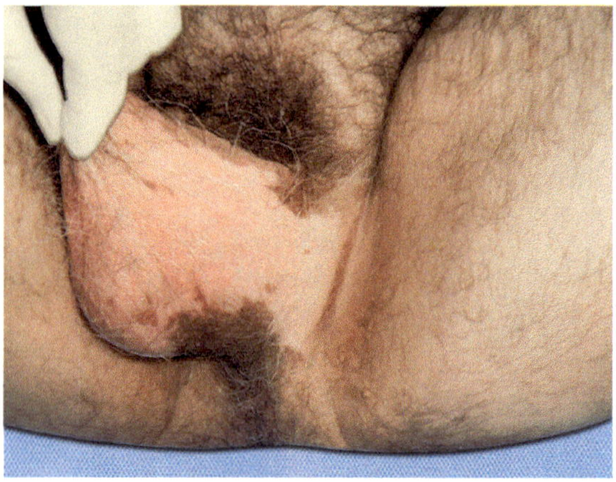

Fig. 16.74: Vitiligo of the scrotum.

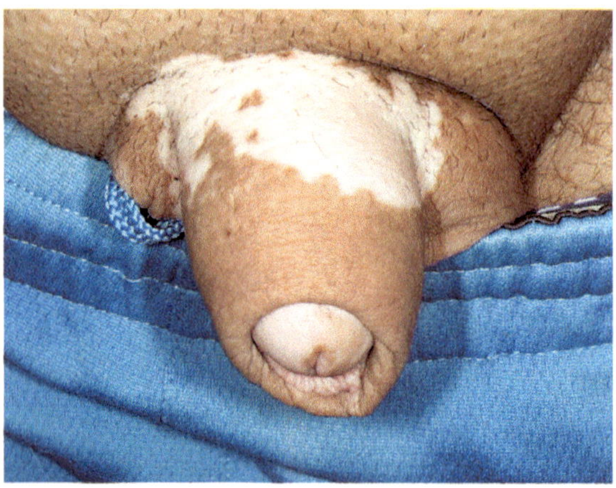

Fig. 16.75: Vitiligo of the penis.

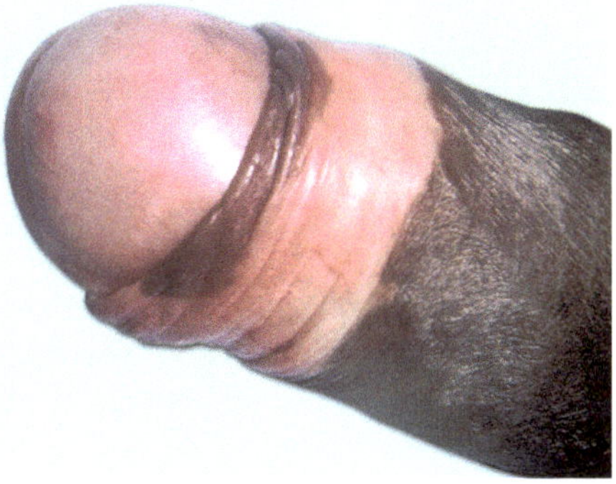

Fig. 16.76: Vitiligo of the glands and prepuce.

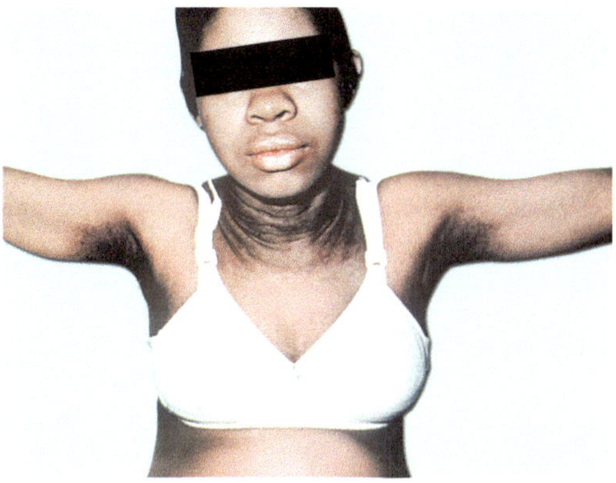

Fig. 16.77: Acanthosis nigricans of neck and axillae.

Acanthosis Nigricans

Acanthosis nigricans is a thickening and darkening of the skin that appears slowly, symmetrically and without any symptoms mostly in flexural folds. Clinically it is a marker of chronic insulin resistance with increased serum levels of insulin, although rarely it may be due to other circulating trophic factors like in the cases of 'malignant' acanthosis nigricans. It may also appear in predisposed patients after receiving glucocorticoids, nicotinic acid or growth hormone therapy. The two pathogenic factors are: (1) the severity of the insulin resistance and (2) the intrinsic tendency of the skin pigmentation, so it is less common in Nordic individuals and more common in persons with darker skin. There is a correlation with time and severity of the insulin resistance with the most severe cases of acanthosis nigricans found in patients with extreme insulin resistance such as in the lipoatrophic DM (Figs. 16.77 and 16.78).

The lesions appear more frequently in the back and side of the neck, axilla, inframmary, and inguinal folds. It may also be seen in elbows, knuckles, knees, dorsum of fingers and toes and in the perineal area. It may also appear at insulin injection sites. It is also very common in individuals without DM but with obesity or polycystic ovaries. Weight loss particularly after bariatric surgery leads to a slow improvement of these lesions. From a clinical point of view, the presence of acanthosis nigricans in a person with DM particularly in adolescents is a clear indication of DM-2 in the differential diagnosis with DM-1. Otherwise, it is mostly a cosmetic concern and the only possible treatment is weight loss (Figs. 16.79 to 16.90).

Skin Tags or Acrochordons

Skin tags or acrochordons are pedunculated, small benign skin lipofibromas that appear in the same areas as acanthosis nigricans, and they also tend to be pigmented according to the basic color of the skin. They have the same relationship with obesity and insulin resistance. Skin tags are asymptomatic although at times they may get irritated or bleed with friction. No treatment

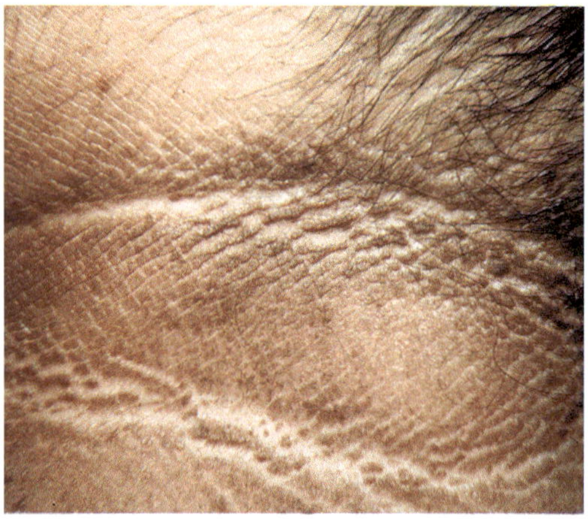

Fig. 16.78: Close view of acanthosis nigricans showing the thickening and darkening of the skin.

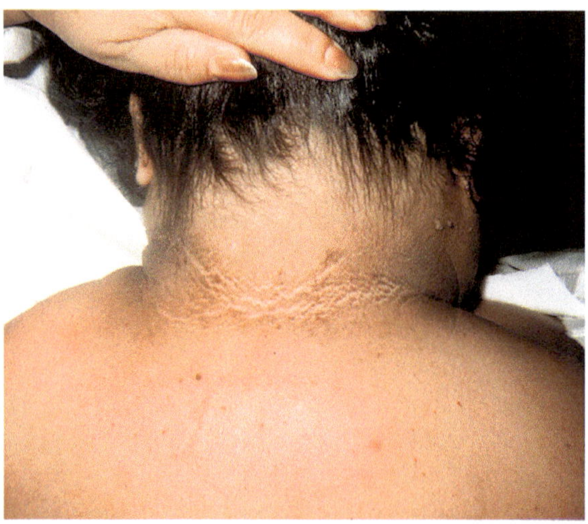

Fig. 16.79: The back of the neck is the most common site of acanthosis nigricans.

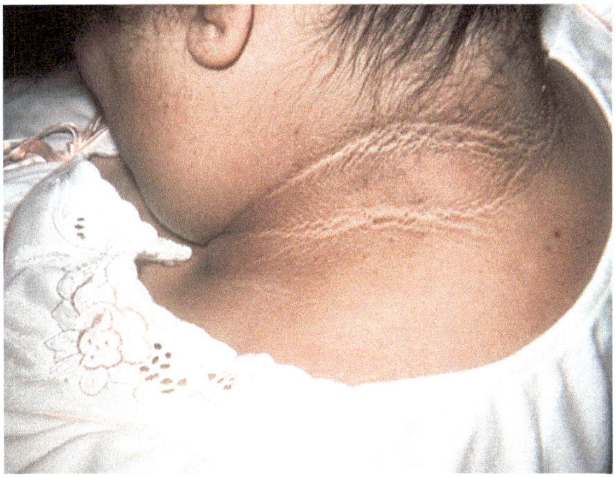

Fig. 16.80: The sides of the neck is another common site of acanthosis nigricans.

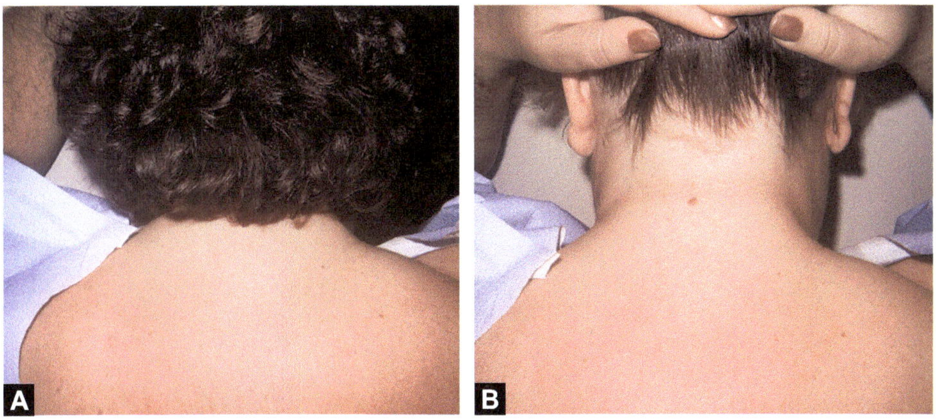

Figs. 16.81A and B: At times it is necessary to lift the hair in the back of the head to find acanthosis nigricans.

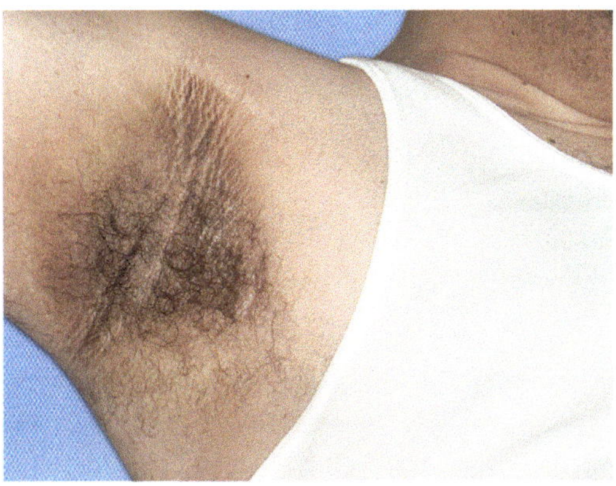

Fig. 16.82: Axillary acanthosis nigricans.

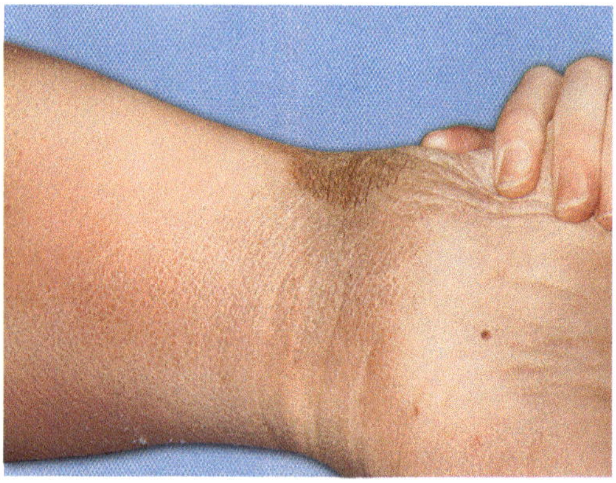

Fig. 16.83: Acanthosis nigricans of the wrist is not very common.

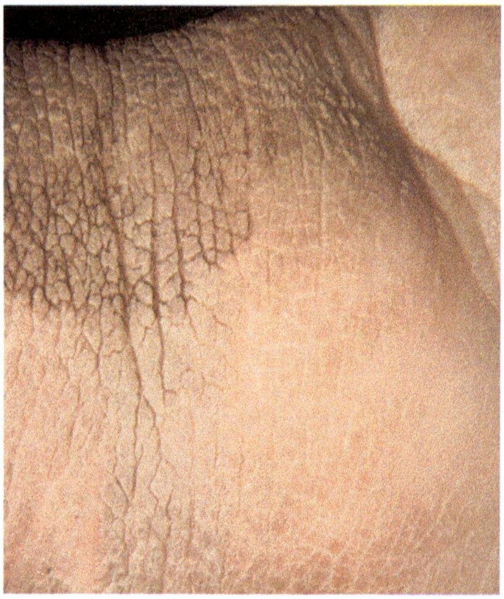

Fig. 16.84: Acanthosis nigricans of the wrist with marked hypertrophy and a 'verrucous' aspect.

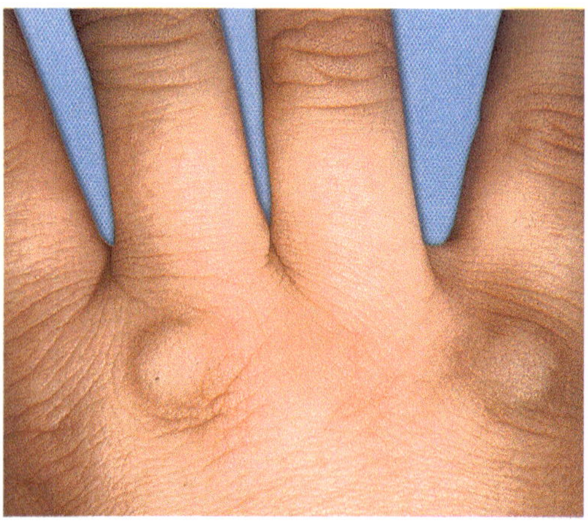

Fig. 16.85: Acanthosis nigricans of the knuckles.

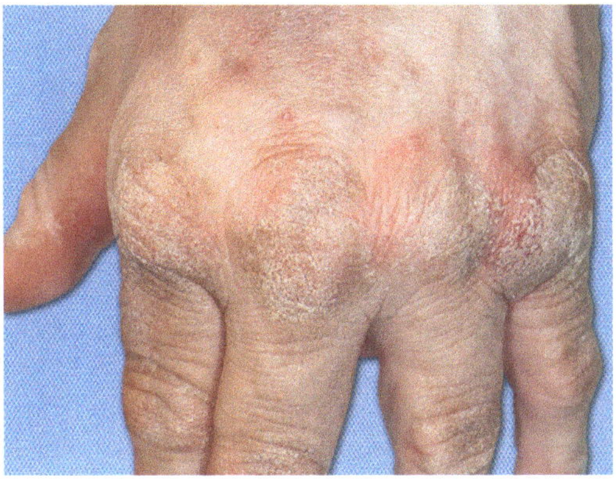

Fig. 16.86: Acanthosis nigricans of the knuckles with a 'verrucous' appearance.

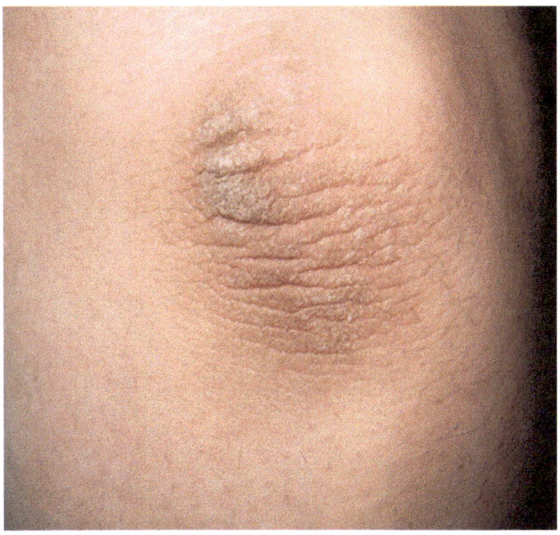

Fig. 16.87: Acanthosis nigricans of the knee.

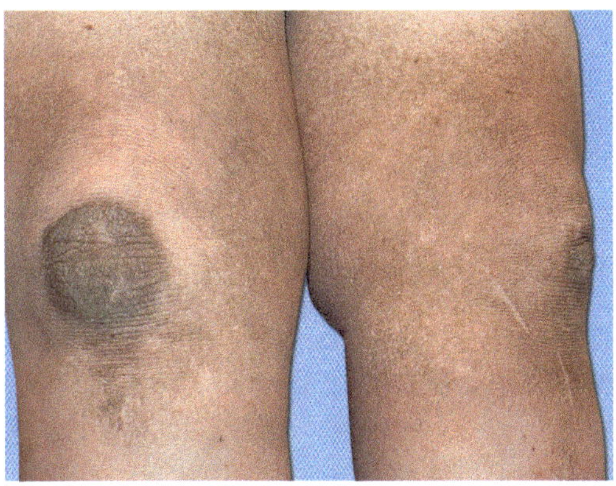

Fig. 16.88: Acanthosis nigricans of the knee, more severe.

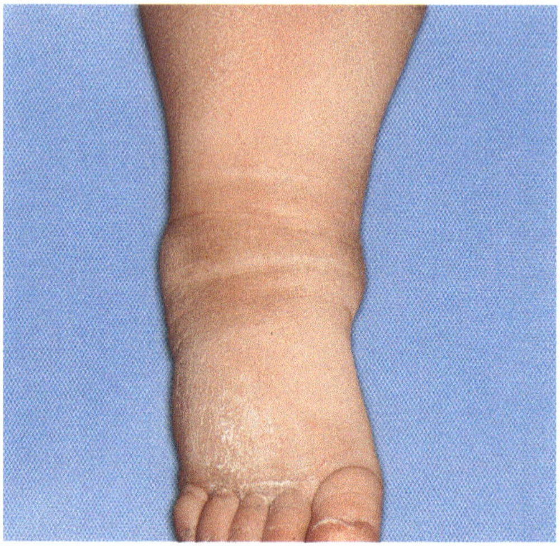

Fig. 16.89: Acanthosis nigricans of the dorsum of the feet.

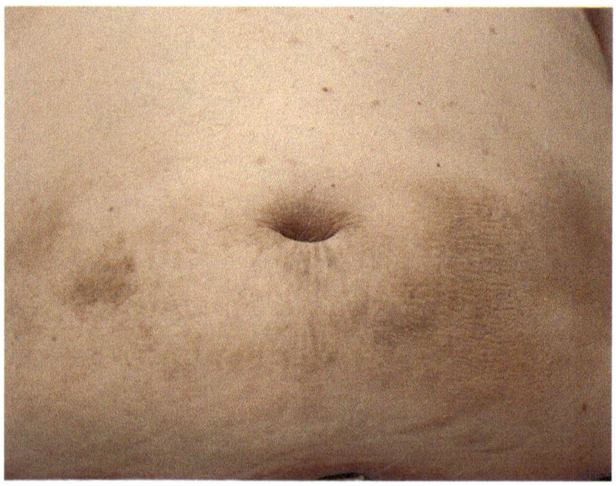

Fig. 16.90: Acanthosis nigricans of the abdomen at sites of insulin injection in large doses.

is usually necessary but in some cases, usually for cosmetic reasons, they may be removed with cryotherapy or simple surgery (Figs. 16.91 to 16.96).

Psoriasis

Psoriasis is a chronic inflammation of the skin with red and scaly lesions that appear more commonly in elbows and knees, and is more frequent in persons with a family history and with obesity. It is more common among Caucasians and less among Africans and Asians. Its course can be quite variable and capricious but with a tremendous cosmetic and emotional toll for the individual. The lesions are due to an inflammation and hyperproliferation of the skin that causes the characteristic redness with whitish plaques. It may also appear in knuckles, scalp, trunks, periumbilical, and intergluteal areas. They are usually asymptomatic although in periods of increased activity they may become pruritic. Psoriatic plaques may also appear

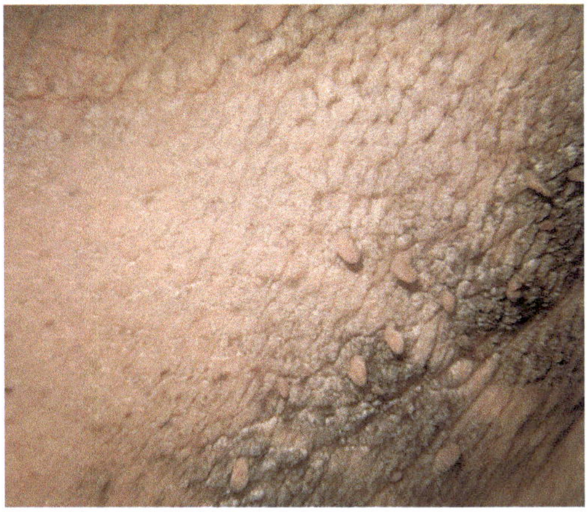

Fig. 16.91: Areas of acanthosis with skin tags.

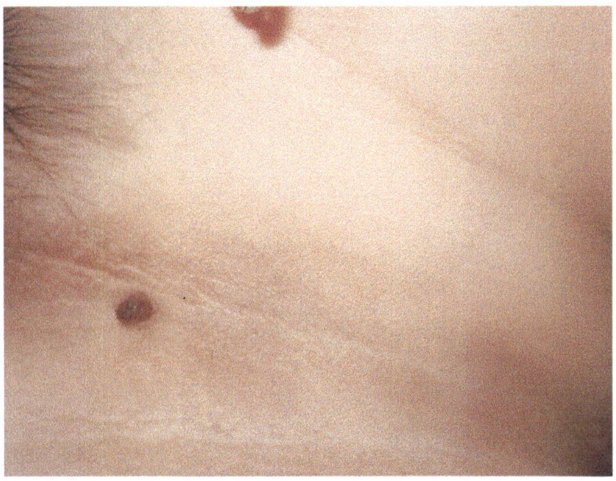

Fig. 16.92: Acanthosis nigricans with a skin tag on the side of the neck.

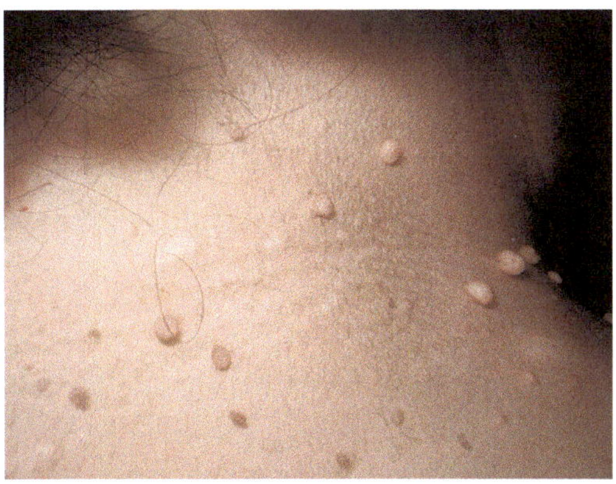

Fig. 16.93: Multiple skin tags.

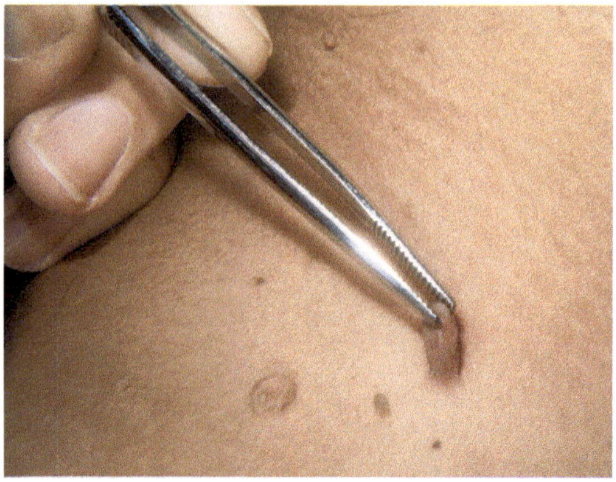

Fig. 16.94: Skin tags may be pedunculated.

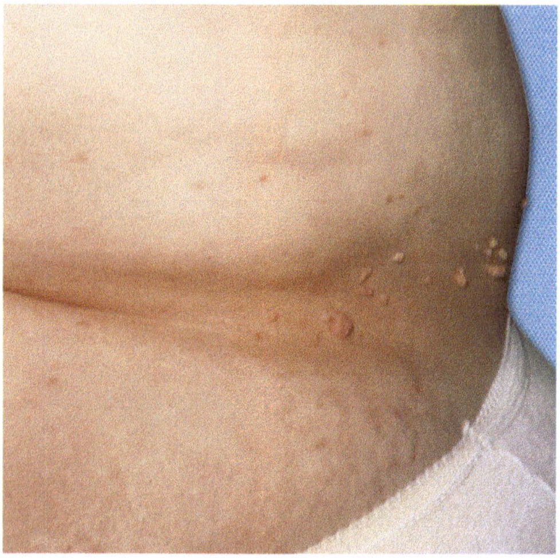

Fig. 16.95: Multiple skin tags at the side of the abdomen.

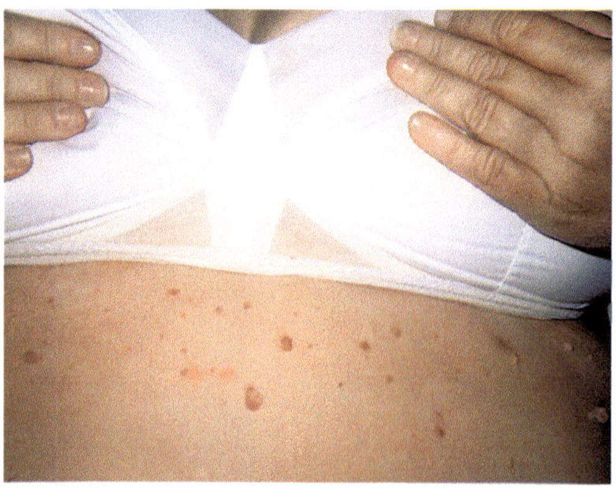

Fig. 16.96: Multiple submammary skin tags.

in the areas of trauma or injury (Kobner reaction) including insulin injection sites. It may also cause characteristic pitting of the nails, and 10% of patients may develop psoriatic arthritis (Figs. 16.97 to 16.102).

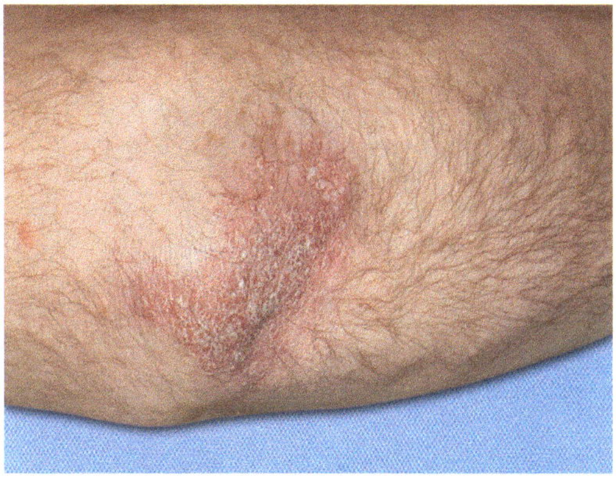

Fig. 16.97: Typical psoriatic lesions of the elbow.

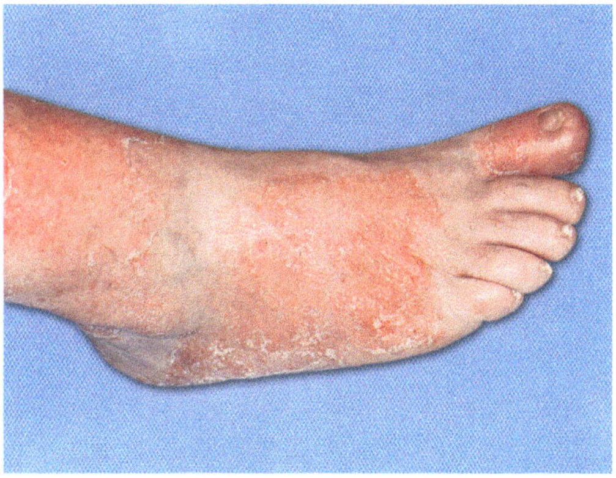

Fig. 16.98: Psoriasis affecting the dorsum of the foot and big toe (with acute psoriatic arthritis).

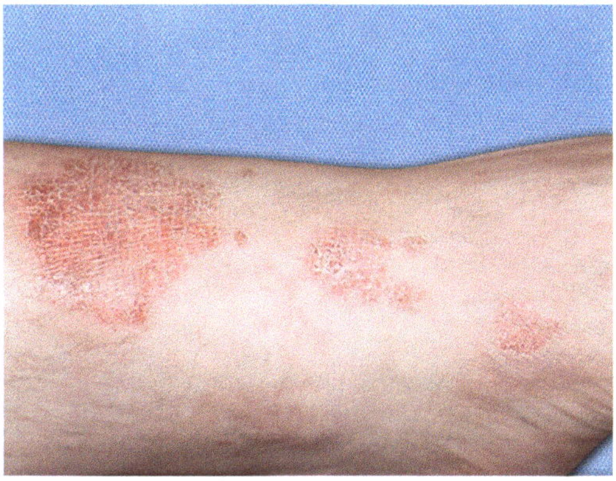

Fig. 16.99: Psoriatic plaques in the front of the leg.

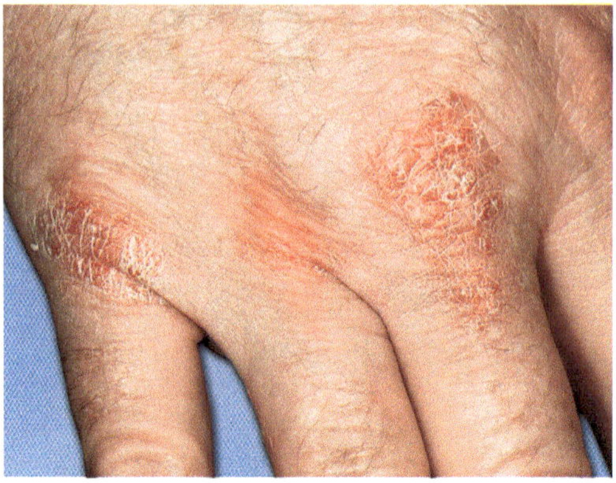

Fig. 16.100: Typical pearly white areas in psoriatic plaques on the dorsum of the hand.

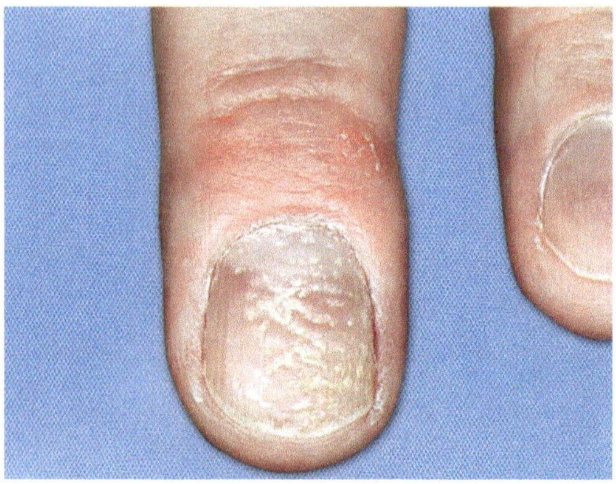

Fig. 16.101: "Pitting" of the nails in psoriasis.

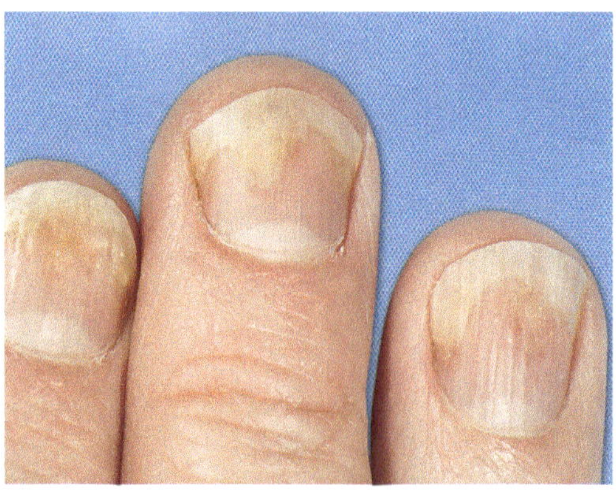

Fig. 16.102: Onycholysis in psoriasis. It may also be seen in prolonged thyrotoxicosis but without the "pitting" of the nails.

Because of its association with obesity, psoriasis is more common in patients with DM-2, metabolic syndrome and hypertension. Simple cases of psoriasis may be treated with topical steroids, keratolytics, retinoids, vitamin D derivatives, or immunomodulators. Phototherapy, methotrexate and the new 'biologicals' may be used in recalcitrant cases. Treatments with GLP-1 analogs have been shown to improve the psoriatic lesions, and treatment of psoriasis with TNF-alpha inhibitors tends to decrease insulin resistance and the risk of DM-2, and may predispose to hypoglycemias in patients treated with antidiabetic medications.

Punctures from Glycemic Monitoring

Patients who need to do frequent blood glucose monitoring and puncture their fingertips several times a day may develop pigmented lesions in the nondominant hand. These lesions may also appear in the thenar or hypothenar areas of the palm if the blood samples are obtained there (Figs. 16.103 and 16.104).

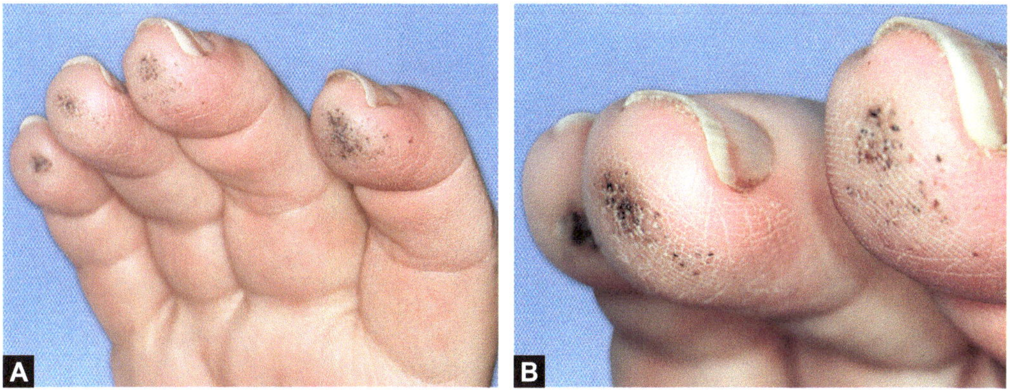

Figs. 16.103A and B: Punctures in the fingers from blood glucose monitoring.

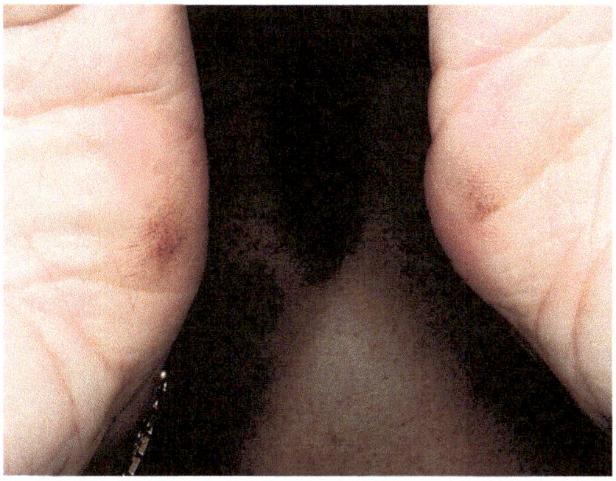

Fig. 16.104: Puncture marks in the hypothenar areas of the palms, a good place to obtain blood with less pain.

Darkening of the Skin

In a person with DM may just be due to simple sun or ultraviolet light exposure but it may also be due to hemochromatosis or the onset of Addison's disease in a patient with DM-1 (Figs. 16.105 and 16.106).

Kaposi's Sarcoma

"In its "classical" form, not the ones associated with HIV infections, is more common" among patients with DM who are older and of Mediterranean origin. It is characterized by 'beefy' nodules usually in the feet or hands that are painless and grow very slowly over years. Indolent lesions do not require treatment but larger ones may require surgery or radiotherapy (Figs. 16.107 to 16.109).

Blue Toes or Cholesterol Embolization Syndrome

Blue toes or cholesterol embolization syndrome is a painful discoloration of the toes with livedo reticularis due to embolization of cholesterol pieces from an ulcerated plaque usually in the

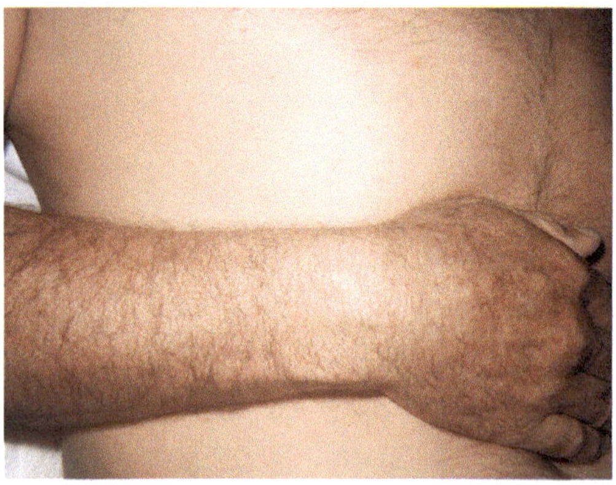

Fig. 16.105: Diffuse darkening of the skin in a person with hereditary hemochromatosis.

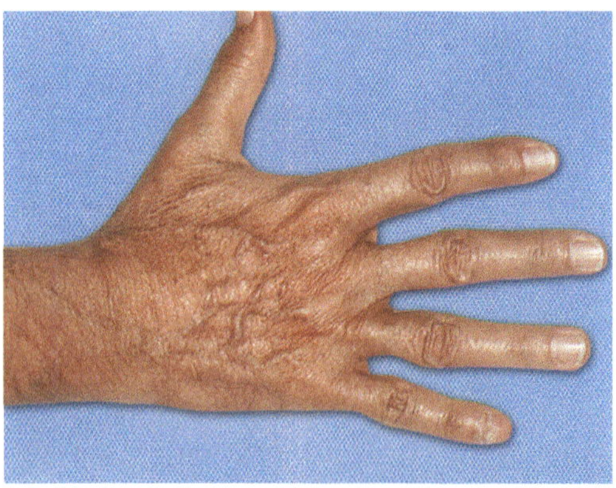

Fig. 16.106: Darkening of the skin in a patient with hereditary hemochromatosis.

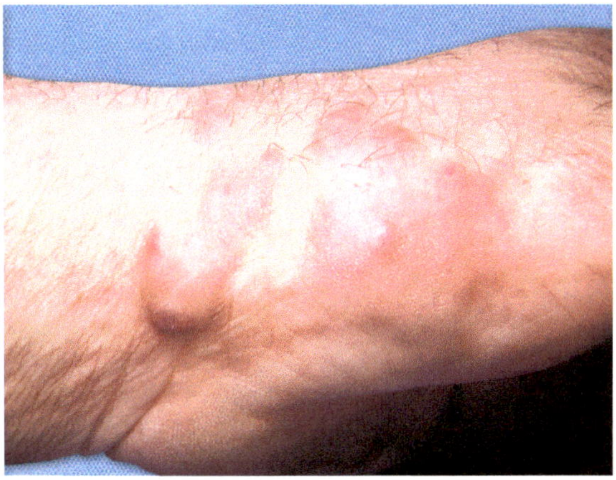

Fig. 16.107: Classical Kaposi's sarcoma with "beefy" lesions in the wrist.

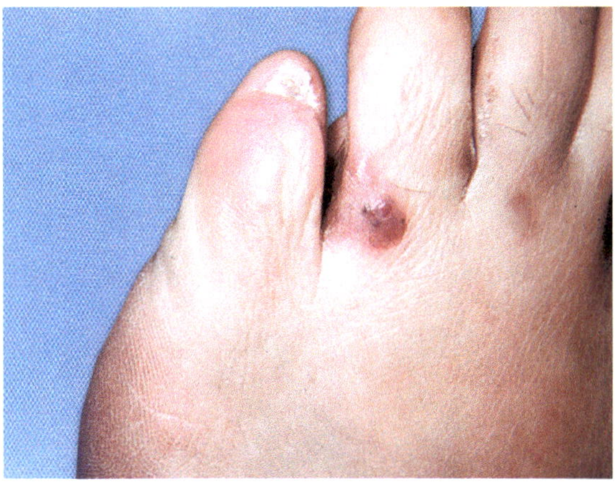

Fig. 16.108: "Classical" Kaposi's sarcoma with lesions in the toes.

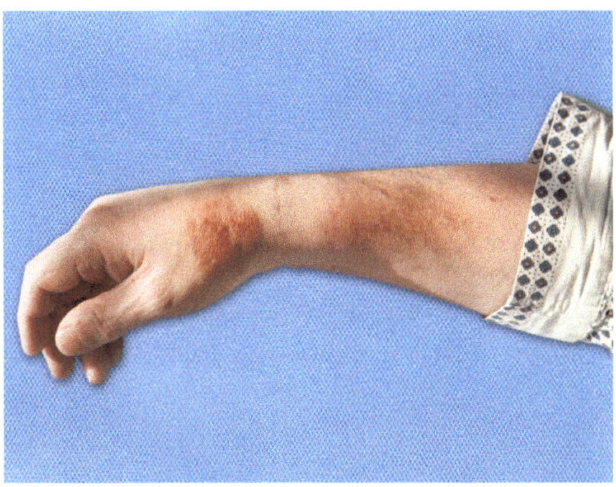

Fig. 16.109: "Classical" Kaposi's sarcoma lesions in the wrist.

aorta or femoral arteries (see Chapter on 'Diabetic Foot'). It may appear spontaneously or after endovascular procedures and thrombolysis (Figs. 16.110 and 16.111).

Calciphylaxis

Calciphylaxis also called calcific uremic arteriolopathy is a thrombosis of subcutaneous arterioles due to precipitation of calcium salts causing severe ischemia and necrosis of the skin in patients

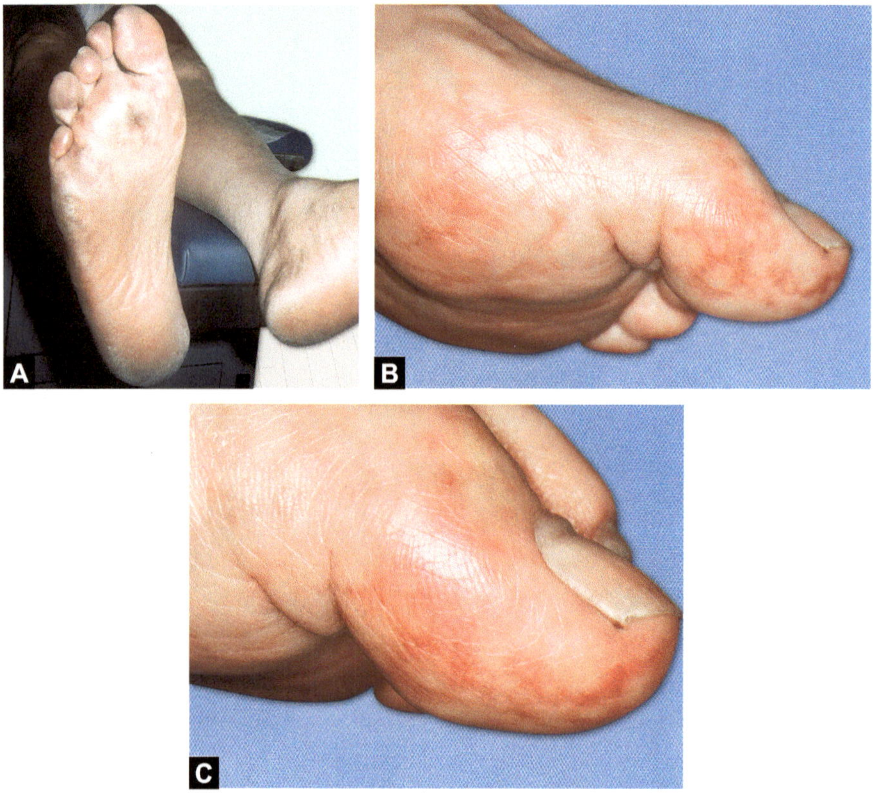

Figs. 16.110A to C: Cholesterol embolization syndrome.

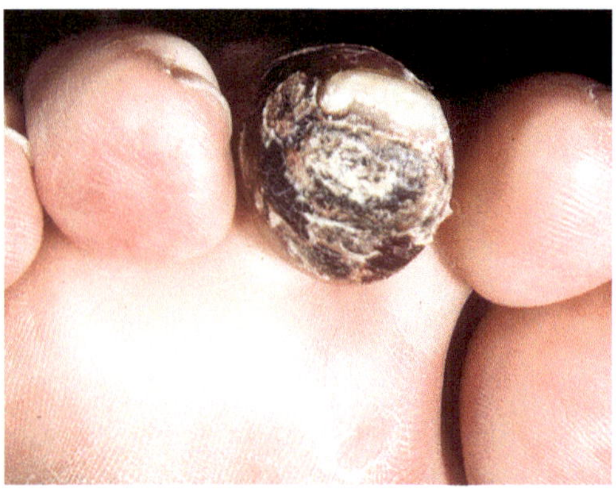

Fig. 16.111: Necrotic toe in a patient with calciphylaxis.

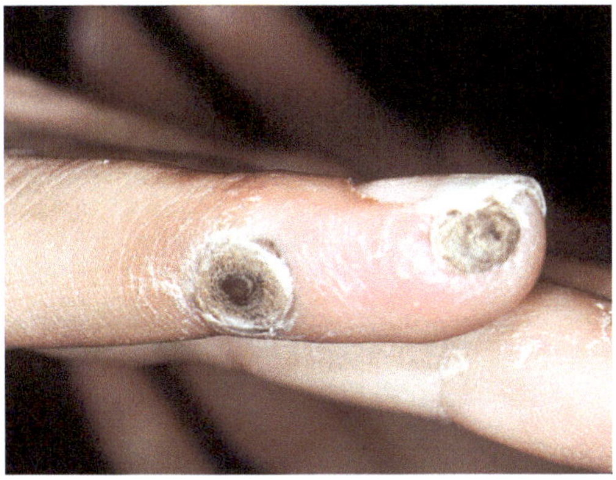

Fig 16.112: Calciphylaxis with finger lesions.

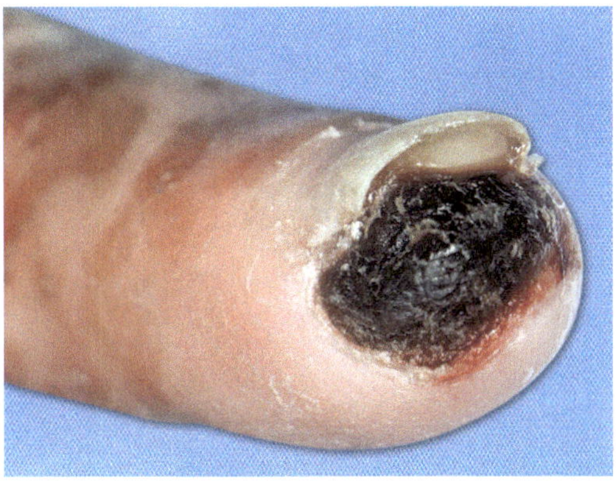

Fig 16.113: Calciphylaxis with necrotic areas in the fingers.

with renal failure, most commonly also with DM, hypercalcemia and hyperphosphatemia (Ca × P Product > 55) (Figs. 16.112 and 16.113). The lesions may appear anywhere in the body but are more frequent in the extremities. They look like dark areas of necrosis, of different sizes, well circumscribed, tender to touch and with a black eschar. Plain X-rays or CT may show calcifications in the superficial arteries to help the diagnosis. Its pathogenesis and treatment are still controversial, and it is a condition with extreme pain and a high mortality rate.

BIBLIOGRAPHY

1. Basoulis D, et al. Anti-TNFα treatment for recalcitrant ulcerative necrobiosis lipoidica diabeticorum: A case report and review of the literature. Metabolism. 2016;65:569-73.
2. Chatterjee S. Neck pain, stiffness, and periorbital edema in a man with diabetes. JAMA. 2016;315(11):1159-60.
3. Cruz-Bautista I, Lerman I, Perez-Enriquez B, et al. Diagnostic challenge of glucagonoma: case report and literature review. Endocr Pract. 2006;12(4):422-6.
4. Erfurt-Berge C, Seitz AT, Rehse C, et al. Update on clinical and laboratory features in necrobiosis lipoidica: a retrospective multicenter study of 52 patients. Eur J Dermatol. 2012;22(6):770-5.

5. Gerrits E, Landman GW, Nijenhuis-Rosien L, et al. Limited joint mobility syndrome in diabetes mellitus: A minireview. World J Diabetes. 2015;6:1108-12.
6. Gupta-Ganguli M, Cox K, Means B, et al. Does therapy with anti-TNF-alpha improve glucose tolerance and control in patients with type 2 diabetes? Diabetes Care. 2011;34(7):e121.
7. Jeonq HS, Dominguez AR. Calciphylaxis: Controversies in Pathogenesis, Diagnosis and Treatment. Am J Med Sci. 2016;351(2):217-27.
8. Kohorst JJ, Kimball AB, Davis MD. Systemic associations of hidradenitis suppurativa. J Am Acad Dermatol. 2015;73(5 Suppl 1):S27-35.
9. Leaf DA. Chylomicronemia and the chylomicronemia syndrome: a practical approach to management. Am J Med. 2008;121(1):10-2.
10. Nigwekar SU et al. Calciphylaxis: Risk factors, Diagnosis and Treatment. Am J Kidney Dis. 2015;66(1):133-46.
11. Patni N, Garg A. Congenital generalized lipodystrophies—new insights into metabolic dysfunction. Nat Rev Endocrinol. 2015;11(9):522-34.
12. Pennington M, Yeager J, Skelton H, et al. Cholesterol embolization syndrome: cutaneous histopathological features and the variable onset of symptoms in patients with different risk factors. Br J Dermatol. 2002;146(3):511-7.
13. Talan DA, Mower WR, Krishnadasan A, et al. Trimethoprim-Sulfamethoxazole versus placebo for uncomplicated skin abscess. N Eng J Med. 2016;374:823-32.
14. Troillet N, Carmeli Y, Samore MH, et al. Carriage of methicillin-resistant Staphylococcus aureus at hospital admission. Infect Control Hosp Epidemiol. 1998;19(3):181-5.
15. Wilbur MB, Daum RS, Gold HS. Skin abscess. N Engl J Med. 2016;374:882-4.

CHAPTER 17

Cardiovascular Outcomes in Type 2 Diabetes Mellitus

Nandhakumar Vasu, S Mullasari Ajit, Sunil Sathe

INTRODUCTION

Cardiovascular (CV) disease (CVD) is a major cause for morbidity and mortality in patients with type 2 diabetes mellitus (t-2DM). Diabetic patients without a history of prior myocardial infarction (MI) have the same risk of developing an MI as nondiabetic patients who have already had an MI.[1] Though hyperglycemia was considered as the pathogenic mechanism for CVD in t-2DM, subsequent evidence showed that, tight glycemic control or optimal glycemic control actually resulted in poor CV outcomes.[2-8] Even in prediabetics or the so called impaired glucose tolerant patients, CV safe antidiabetic drugs significantly reduced fatal MI, nonfatal MI and stroke, despite not requiring tight glycemic control.[9,10] Several mechanisms namely glucotoxicity, lipotoxicity, oxidative stress, endoplasmic reticulum stress and amyloid deposition are linked with pathogenesis of t-2DM and collectively they make the final pathway for tissue inflammation. Multiple cell stressors, particularly glucose lead to the generation of reactive oxygen species which inturn causes tissue inflammation.[11] Tissue inflammation plays a major role in pathogenesis of atherosclerosis and contributes to poor CV outcomes. The spectrum of CVD in t-2DM patients can vary from macrovascular to microvascular disease; coronary artery disease (CAD), carotid artery disease, cerebrovascular disease, renal artery stenosis, aortic aneurysm and stenosis, peripheral vascular disease (PVD), microvascular angina (MVA), dilated cardiomyopathy (DCM), heart failure (HF) with preserved ejection fraction (HFpEF).

CARDIOVASCULAR OUTCOME OF ANTIDIABETIC DRUGS BEFORE 2008

There is a 2–4 folds increase in the risk of CAD and 6–7 years decrease in life expectancy in t-2DM patients as compared to the nondiabetic group.[12] Prior to 2008, when US Food and Drug Administration (FDA) and the European Medicines Agency (EMA) issued guidance to set out CV outcomes based expectations for the development of newer antidiabetic drugs, major clinical trials were focussed on tight versus less stringent glycemic control to predict CV outcome. Though few individual trials failed to show the benefit of tight glycemic control, meta-analyses did indicate a modest reduction in nonfatal MI.[13-21] Action to control cardiovascular risk in diabetes (ACCORD) trial showed increased CV mortality with the tight glycemic control strategy and similarly no reduction in CV mortality was shown in the VADT trial. This leads to less stringent glucose lowering, especially in older patients with high CV risk.[22-25] The antidiabetic drugs which were approved before 2008 guidance were focused on HbA1C reduction along with safety data from mid term phase 2 and 3 randomized contolled trials (RCT). As these trials were conducted on recent onset diabetic patients with low CV risk, CV safety of these drugs were unreliable.[26,27]

Cardiovascular safety of antidiabetic drugs became a major concern after two landmark meta-analyses of muraglitazar and rosiglitazone, belonging to a family of peroxisome proliferator-activated receptor agonists, published in year 2000. Muraglitazar was found to increase more than twice the CV complications including HF and death.[28] Rosiglitazone, a thiazolidinedione (TZD) showed a 43% increased risk of MI and 64% increased risk of death.[29] Pioglitazone, another TZD, has been shown to reduce the secondary composite endpoint of all-cause mortality, nonfatal MI and stroke in t-2DM who were at high risk of macrovascular events in the PRO-active (prospective pioglitazone clinical trial in macrovascular events) study.[30] The older generation drugs tolbutamide and phenformin were shown to increase CV risk in comparison to insulin or placebo, though these trials were underpowered for events.[31-33] The UKPDS trial randomized patients to receive either intensive therapy or standard care with diet. The former group received insulin, sulfonylurea or metformin. At 10 years follow-up, CV associated risk reduction was greater in the intensive therapy group. On subanalysis, metformin subgroup outperformed the insulin or sulfonylurea subgroups (MI = 39% vs. 15%; all-cause mortality = 36% vs. 13%).[34] Meta-analyses of metformin was initially not promising, as the studies included in meta-analysis were done with the sulfonylurea combination. CV risk actually did not increased significantly 10 years after the end of the study.[35,36] Metformin has been shown to reduce cyclophilin A expression in human monocyte-derived macrophages and thus function as a suppressor of proinflammatory effects of cyclophilin A in high glucose conditions by attenuating its expression and repressing cyclophilin A induced decrease in AMPK-1 activity in macrophages.[37] Three trials studied the CV outcome of insulin treatment. BARI 2D trial, which compared insulin providing and insulin sensitizing strategies found no difference in CV outcome.[38] Though HEART 2D trial did not show difference in CV outcome between basal and postprandial insulin treatment strategies, post-hoc analysis showed a positive effect of postprandial control of hyperglycemia in older patients.[39-41] The ORIGIN trial randomized patients with prediabetes and t-2DM with CVD risk factors to standard glucose control or insulin glargine. There were no differences in primary CV outcome.[42]

CARDIOVASCULAR OUTCOME OF DIABETES MELLITUS AND SYSTEMIC HYPERTENSION

Prevalence of systemic hypertension (SHT) is twice as frequent in patients with diabetes as in those without, more so in industrialized nations, as populations are older and both t-2DM and SHT incidences increase with age. Death certificates show that hypertensive disease had been implicated in 4.4% of deaths coded to diabetes, and diabetes was involved in 10% of deaths coded to hypertensive disease.[43,44] Association of SHT with t-2DM increases the mortality to 7.2 fold. More than 75% of adults with DM have blood pressure more than or equal to 130/80 mm Hg or were using medications for SHT in a study.[45] In patients with t-2DM and SHT, the high CV risk requires an integrated therapeutic intervention in the order of effective antihypertensive therapy, statin, optimal glycemic control and antiplatelets.[46]

CARDIOVASCULAR OUTCOME OF NEWER ANTIDIABETIC DRUGS

As the number of CV events emanating during a typical phase 2 or 3 trial is usually insufficient for statistical confidence, FDA suggested in 2008, that separate CV outcomes trials (CVOT) are necessary, as metaanalyses could not rule out CV risk.[47] Specific CVOT outcome trial must set a goal for a hazard ratio (HR) of less than 1.8 with two sided 95% confidence interval (CI) in order to get the approval for a new drug. The post-approval trials require a risk ratio of 1.3 for major adverse cardiac events (MACE). It is mandated that trials should be conducted for at least 2 years for CV safety data and include high risk populations, like the elderly, those with renal impairment and those with advanced disease.[48] Insulin is excluded from the CV safety evaluation as it is a known life saving therapy for type 1 diabetes mellitus and during diabetic ketoacidosis. Some of the newer insulin formulations have been studied in CVOT trials.[49] The newer group of antidiabetic drugs have been extensively studied in CVOT trials, namely dipeptidyl peptidase-4 (DPP-4) inhibitors, sodium-glucose cotransporter-2 (SGLT2) inhibitors, glucagon-like peptide 1 (GLP-1) receptor agonists, TZD, α-glucosidase inhibitors. Figure 17.1 depicts the timeline of CVOT of various newer antidiabetic drugs.

MACE Composite Endpoint

Primary outcome of various newer antidiabetic drugs from the respective CVOT is shown in Table 17.1. Though CV death, MI and stroke are the major adverse cardio cerebrovascular

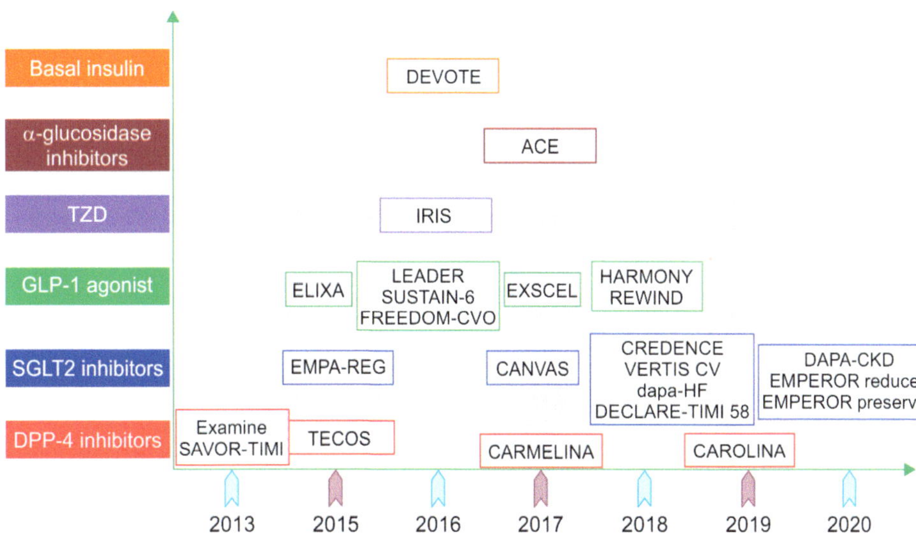

Fig. 17.1: Cardiovascular outcome trials of antidiabetic drugs.

Table 17.1: Cardiovascular outcome results of newer antidiabetic drugs in comparison to placebo.

Study	*Composite MACE HR (95% CI)*	*MACE Event rate (%)*	*CV death HR (95% CI)*	*MI HR (95% CI)*	*Stroke HR (95% CI)*	*UA HR (95% CI)*	*HF HR (95% CI)*
DPP-4 Inhibitors							
SAVOR TIMI 53[51]	1.00 (0.89–1.12) p = 0.99	7.3	1.03 (0.87–1.22) p = 0.72	0.95 (0.80–1.12) p = 0.52	1.11 (0.88–1.39) p = 0.38	1.19 (0.89–1.60) p = 0.24	1.27 (1.07–1.51) p = 0.007
EXAMINE[53]	0.96 (≤1.16) p = 0.315	11.3	0.85 (0.66–1.10) p = 0.212	1.08 (0.88–1.33) p = 0.47	0.91 (0.55–1.50) p = 0.71	0.90 (0.60–1.37) p = 0.632	1.19 (0.90–1.58) p = 0.220
TECOS[54]	0.98 (0.89–1.08) p = 0.65	9.6	1.03 (0.89–1.19) p = 0.71	0.95 (0.81–1.11) p = 0.49	0.97 (0.79–1.19) p = 0.76	0.90 (0.70–1.16) p = 0.42	1.00 (0.83–1.20) p = 0.98
GLP-1 receptor agonist							
ELIXA[55]	1.02 (0.89–1.17) p = 0.81	13.4	0.98 (0.78–1.22) p = 0.85	1.03 (0.87–1.22) p = 0.71	1.12 (0.79–1.58) 0.54	1.11 (0.47–2.62) 0.81	0.96 (0.75-1.23) 0.75
LEADER[57]	0.87 (0.78–0.97) p = 0.01	13.0	0.78 (0.66–0.93) p = 0.007	0.86 (0.73–1.00) p = 0.046	0.86 (0.71–1.06) p = 0.16	0.98 (0.76–1.26) p = 0.87	0.87 (0.73–1.05) p = 0.14
SUSTAIN-6[58]	0.74 (0.58–0.95) p<0.001/0.02	6.6	0.98 (0.65–1.48) p = 0.92	0.74 (0.51–1.08) p = 0.12	0.61 (0.38–0.99) p = 0.04	0.82 (0.47–1.44) p = 0.49	1.11 (0.77–1.61) p = 0.57
EXSCEL[61]	0.91 (0.83–1.00) p = 0.06	11.4	0.88 (0.76–1.02) p = N.A	0.97 (0.85–1.10) p = N.A	0.85 (0.70–1.03) p = N.A	N.A	0.94 (0.78–1.13) p = N.A
SGLT-2 inhibitors							
EMPA-REG OUTCOME[56]	0.86 (0.74–0.99) p = 0.04	10.5	0.62 (0.49–0.77) p<0.001	0.87 (0.70–1.09) p = 0.23	1.18 (0.89–1.56) p = 0.26	0.99 (0.74–1.34) p = 0.97	0.65 (0.50–0.85) p = 0.002
CANVAS[60]	0.86 (0.75–0.97) p = 0.02	26.9	0.87 (0.72–1.06) p = N.A	0.89 (0.73–1.09) p = N.A	0.87 (0.69–1.09) p = N.A	N.A	0.67 (0.52–0.87) p = N.A
α-glucosidase inhibitor							
ACE[62]	0.98 (0.86–1.11) p = 0.73	14.4	0.89 (0.71–1.11) p = 0.29	1.12 (0.87–1.46) p = 0.38	0.97 (0.70–1.33) p = 0.83	1.02 (0.82–1.26) p = 0.87	0.89 (0.63–1.24) p = 0.48
Basal Insulin							
DEVOTE[59]	0.91 (0.78–1.06) p<0.0001	8.5	0.96 (0.76–1.21) p = 0.71	0.85 (0.68–1.06) p = 0.15	0.90 (0.65–1.23) p = 0.50	0.95 (0.68–1.31) p = 0.74	N.A

(CI: confidence interval; CV: cardiovascular; DPP: dipeptidyl peptidase; GLP: glucagon like peptide; HF: heart failure; HR: hazard ratio; MACE: major adverse cardiac cerebrovascular event; MI: myocardial infarction; NA: not available; SGLT: sodium glucose cotransporter; UA: unstable angina) event (MACE) events in all the studies, unstable angina (UA) was additionally included in TECOS and ELIXA trials. In the Saxagliptin (SAVOR-TIMI 53),[50,51] Alogliptin (EXAMINE),[52,53] sitagliptin (TECOS)[54] and Lixisenatide (ELIXA)[55] treatment, the primary composite MACE endpoint did not differ from placebo, making these drugs noninferior in CV safety. In the EMPA-REG OUTCOME trial, the primary endpoint occurred in 10.5% of the empagliflozin, a SGLT-2 inhibitor treated patients as compared to 12.1% in the placebo group (HR 0.86; $p = 0.04$ for superiority).[56] A similar superiority outcome was also noted in established CV disease subgroup of LEADER trial patients, who were treated with liraglutide, a GLP-1 agonist (13% vs. 14.9%; HR 0.87; $p = 0.01$ for superiority).[57] Mortality benefit was seen in both EMPA-REG OUTCOME and LEADER trials. Semaglutide, another GLP-1 receptor agonist have been shown to be superior to placebo in primary composite outcome of SUSTAIN-6 trial (6.6% vs. 8.9%, HR: 0.74; $p<0.001$).

Non-fatal stroke was the reason for decrease in MACE in the SUSTAIN-6 trial.[58] In the DEVOTE study, degludec insulin was compared with glargine, where MACE occurred in 8.5% of degludec group versus 9.3% of glargine group (HR 0.91; $p<0.001$ for noninferiority).[59] Canagliflozin was shown to reduce the MACE when compared to placebo in CANVAS trial (26.9% vs. 31.5%, $p < 0.001$ for noninferiority; $p = 0.02$ for superiority).[60] EXSCEL investigators showed that once weekly exenatide was non inferior to placebo in CV safety but not superior in terms of efficacy ($p< 0.001$ for noninferiority; $p = 0.06$ for superiority).[61] Primary outcome was met by 14.4% of acarbose group vs. 14.7% of placebo group in ACE trial ($p = 0.73$).[62]

All-cause Mortality

All-cause mortality was observed in 5.3% of degludec group in comparison to 5.8% of glargine group in DEVOTE trial (HR 0.91; $p = 0.35$)[59] thus revealing no difference. Treatment with canagliflozin or acarbose as compared to placebo did not reduce all cause mortality in CANVAS trial or ACE trial respectively.[60,62] Eventhough EXSCEL trial showed a trend toward decrease in all cause mortality in once weekly exenatide group (6.9% vs. 7.9%), it was not statistically significant.[61]

Cardiovascular Death

EMPA-REG OUTCOME and LEADER trials showed decrease in CV death when compared to placebo.[56,57] Other trials with newer drugs did not decrease the CV death compared to placebo treatment though they were non inferior. Degludec insulin was non inferior to Glargine insulin in tem of CV death (3.6% vs. 3.7%; HR 0.96; $p = 0.71$).[59] 4.6% ($n = 340$) patients treated with exenatide died when compared to 5.2% ($n = 383$) in the placebo arm in EXSCEL trial (HR 0.88; 95% CI 0.76–1.02).[61] Though statistically not significant, participants those who were treated with canagliflozin had lower CV mortality when compared to placebo in the CANVAS trial.[60] In the ACE study 4.4% of patients died of CV causes in the acarbose group and 5.0% in the placebo group ($p = 0.29$).[62]

Fatal/Non-fatal Myocardial Infarction

Non-fatal MI, the second component of primary endpoint was seen in 3.8% of degludec group versus 4.4% of glargine group ($p = 0.15$) in DEVOTE study.[59] In CANVAS trial statistically non significant reduction in fatal or non-fatal MI was observed (11.2 vs. 12.6 participants per 1,000 patient years).[60] EXCSEL trial revealed that 6.6% of once weekly exenatide group developed fatal or non-fatal MI versus 6.7% of placebo group.[61] In ACE trial the secondary outcome was met by 122 (3.7%) patients of acarbose treated group versus 108 (3.3%) of placebo group ($p = 0.38$).[62] Though all the trials showed non inferiority for fatal or non-fatal MI, none revealed superiority.

Fatal and/or Non-fatal Stroke

In the DEVOTE trial non inferiority was confirmed for degludec insulin regarding the primary endpoint nonfatal stroke. 2.1% of glargine insulin group versus 1.9% of degludec insulin group met the primary endpoint (HR 0.90; 95% CI 0.65–1.23; $p = 0.50$).[59] 7.9% of patients treated with canagliflozin group and 9.6% of patients treated with placebo developed fatal and non-fatal stroke in the CANVAS trial. Though there was a trend towards decrease in fatal and non-fatal stroke in canagliflozin treated arm, it was statistically not significant.[60] Fatal and non-fatal stroke occurrences were same in both once weekly exenatide group in comparison with placebo (2.5% vs. 2.9%).[61] Similarly reduction of stroke events were not different between the groups in ACE trial.[62] EMPAREG-OUTCOME trial revealed a trend towards an increased stroke incidence.[56] But SUSTAIN-6 trial showed a significant reduction of stroke rates in semaglutide treated patients.[58]

Unstable Angina

The significance of unstable angina (UA) was not same in different trials. EMPAREG-OUTCOME, SAVOR-TIMI and EXAMINE studies included it as part of secondary composite end-point.[51,53,56] TECOS and ELIXA trials included UA in their primary endpoints, whereas LEADER and SUSTAIN-6 included it as part of an extended primary composite end-point.[54,55,57,58] In the DEVOTE study, UA was included as the extended primary outcome. In both groups 1.9% of participants were hospitalized for UA.[59] UA was included as a five point MACE and was independently evaluated as a secondary outcome in the ACE study. 174 patients developed UA after being treated with acarbose and 170 patients of the placebo group (5.3% vs. 5.2%; $p = 0.87$).[62] CANVAS and EXSCEL program did not analyze UA.[60,61]

Heart Failure Hospitalization

EMPAREG-OUTCOME study showed statistically significant decrease in HF hospitalization in empagliflozin treated patients when compared to placebo (2.8% vs. 4.5%; $p<0.001$).[56] LEADER trial showed a nonsignificant decrease in HF hospitalization in patients treated with liraglutide.[57] The rate of HF hospitalization was not different between the treatment arm and placebo in SUSTAIN-6, TECOS, EXAMINE and ELIXA trials.[53-55,58] But treatment with saxagliptin was found to increase hospitalization rates for HF in SAVOR-TIMI trial (3.5% vs. 2.8%; $p = 0.007$).[51] Canagliflozin was superior to placebo in CANVAS study (5.8 vs. 8.7 participants per 1,000 patient years) in preventing HF hospitalization.[60] There is no difference between the groups in EXSCEL trial, in which 219 patients (3.0%) in treatment arm and 231 patients (3.1%) in placebo group had HF hospitalization.[61] Like EXSCEL study, ACE trial also did not show significant difference between the groups (2.0% vs. 2.2%; $p = 0.48$).[62]

Kidney Disease

The kidney injury outcome was analyzed in different ways in various CVOTs. EMPA-REG OUTCOME trial showed slower progression of kidney disease in empagliflozin treated patients than placebo ($p<0.001$).[56] ELIXA and TECOS trial did not analyze the renal outcome.[54,55] EXAMINE trial mentioned only about initiation of dialysis.[53] Detailed renal end points were discussed in SAVOR-TIMI trial including doubling of creatinine level, initiation of dialysis, renal transplantation or creatinine more than 6 mg/dL. There was no difference between the treatment arm and placebo.[51] In the LEADER trial the incidence of composite renal and microvascular outcomes was lower in liraglutide arm, due to significantly lower rate of nephropathy events ($p = 0.003$). The renal outcome included in the LEADER trial are new onset micro-albuminuria or the doubling of the serum creatinine level and an eGFR less than or equal to 45 mL/min/1.73 m^2, need for continuous renal-replacement therapy or death from renal disease.[57] The renal outcome in SUSTAIN-6 trial consisted of persistent microalbuminuria, doubling of the serum creatinine level and eGFR less than or equal to 45 mL/min/1.73 m^2, need for continuous renal-replacement therapy. Semaglutide treated patients had a lower risk than placebo treated patients (3.8% vs. 6.1%; $p = 0.005$).[58] Acute kidney injury occurred in 1.8% of degludec insulin treated and 2.5% of glargine insulin treated patients. In CANVAS-R, renal outcomes were specifically analyzed. Albuminuria progression was less frequent in canagliflozin treated patients.

Peripheral Vascular Disease

Either amputations or non-traumatic amputations were analyzed in different CVOTs. CANVAS trial showed that the incidence of amputations were higher in canagliflozin group than placebo group (6.3 vs. 3.4 participants per 1,000 patient years).[60] But the subgroup analysis revealed that the relative risk was comparable between the groups. Once weekly exenatide treated patients underwent non-traumatic amputations similar to placebo group in EXSCEL trial (1.7% in both groups).[61]

Revascularization of Coronary Artery Disease

Table 17.2 summarizes the primary outcome of various CAD revascularization trials. COURAGE trial compared death and nonfatal MI as the primary outcome between optimal medical therapy (OMT) with or without PCI for stable coronary disease in 2,287 patients with a median follow-up of 4.6 years. Nearly one-third of patients in both groups were diabetics (32% in PCI group; $n = 367$ vs. 35% in optimal medical therapy; $n = 399$). On subgroup analysis of diabetic patients, event rates were same in both groups (0.25% in PCI vs. 0.24% in optimal medical therapy; $p = 0.33$).[63] 10 year follow-up of Bypass Angioplasty Revascularization Investigation trial (BARI) showed, the PTCA group had higher repeat revascularization than the coronary artery bypass graft (CABG) group (76.8% vs. 20.3%, $p<0.001$), but angina rates in both groups were similar. The results were primarily driven by the diabetic subgroup in which the CABG assigned group had higher survival than the PTCA group (PTCA 45.5% vs. 57.8%, $p = 0.025$).[64] BARI 2D study randomized 2,368 patients to medical management or revascularization with either PCI or CABG. The mean duration of follow-up was 5.3 years. Patients with diabetes

Table 17.2: Cardiovascular outcome in revascularization of coronary artery disease.

Study	*Number of diabetics*	*Duration of follow-up*	*Intervention*	*Primary outcome*	*Result*
COURAGE[63]	32% (n = 367) in PCI group; 35% (n = 399) in OMT group	4.6 years	PCI vs OMT	MACE	PCI 0.25% vs OMT 0.24% p = 0.33
BARI[64]	PTCA-173 CABG-180	10.4 years	PTCA vs CABG	MACE	PTCA 57.8% vs CABG 45.5% p = 0.025
BARI 2D[65]	2,368	5.3 years	Revascularization vs OMT	Survival	88% vs 88%, p = 0.97
				Freedom from CVD	77% vs 76%, p = 0.70
			Insulin providing vs Insulin sensitizing	Survival	88% vs 88%, p = 0.89;
				Freedom from CVD	78% vs 75%, p = 0.13
Onuma et al.[66] (ARTS-I, II)	367	5 years	BMS vs SES vs CABG	MACE	BMS 53.6% vs SES 40.5% vs CABG 23.4%; p<0.01 for SES vs BMS p<0.01 SES vs CABG
FREEDOM[67]	1,900	5 years	PCI with DES vs CABG	MACE (all cause death, nonfatal MI and nonfatal stroke)	PCI with DES –26.6% vs. CABG-18.7%; p = 0.005
CARDia[68]	510	1 year	PCI with stent vs CABG	MACE (death, MI and stroke)	PCI 13% vs CABG 10.5% (p = 0.39)
EXCEL[70]	548 diabetics with ULMCA disease, PCI with EES-286 and CABG-268	3 years	PCI with EES and CABG in diabetics vs nondiabetics	MACE (death, MI and stroke)	19.9% vs 13%; HR =1.6; 95% CI, 1.25–2.04

(BMS: bare metal stent; CABG: coronary artery bypass surgery; CVD: cardiovascular disease; DES: drug eluting stent; EES: everolimus eluting stent; MACE: major adverse cardio cerebrovascular event; MI: myocardial infarction: OMT: optimal medical treatment: PCI: percutaneous coronary intervention: PTCA: percutaneous transluminal coronary angioplasty; SES: sirolimus eluting stent: ULMCA: unprotected left main coronary artery) and angiographic CAD demonstrated similar mortality rates with prompt revascularization therapy and medical therapy (Survival: 88% vs. 88%, p = 0.97; freedom from CVD event: 77% vs. 76%, p = 0.70). There was no difference in clinical outcomes between groups receiving insulin sensitization treatment vs. insulin providing treatment (survival: 88% vs. 88%, p = 0.89; freedom from CVD event: 78% vs. 75%, p = 0.13). The study revealed that in low risk patients selected for PCI there was no benefit with revascularization, but among high risk patients who underwent CABG, major CV events were less when compared to medical therapy (22% vs. 31%, p = 0.01). Non-fatal MI occurred less frequently in CABG treated patients (7%) than in the medical therapy group (15%).[65] Onuma Y et al. studied the 5 years follow-up of coronary revascularization in diabetic patients with multivessel coronary artery disease from Arterial Revascularization Therapy Study (ARTS) I and II trials and concluded that there was no mortality difference among PCI with bare metal stent (BMS), PCI with siroloimus eluting stent (SES) and CABG groups, but the rate of MACE was higher in PCI with BMS group (BMS 53.6% vs. SES 40.5% vs. CABG 23.4%; p<0.01 for SES vs. BMS and SES vs. CABG). The rate of MI was higher in BMS arm, where as it was much lower in both CABG and PCI with SES arms (BMS 11%, SES 4.8%, CABG 5.2%, p = 0.04 for SES vs. BMS and p = 0.76 for SES vs. CABG). The rate of repeat revascularization was lower in CABG arm than the SES arm (SES 33.2% vs. CABG 10.7%, p < 0.001). Though revascularization rate of SES was lower than the BMS initially, at 5 years it approached that of BMS group.[66] FREEDOM trial evaluated strategies for multivessel revascularization in patients with diabetes. 1,900 patients were randomized to undergo either PCI with drug eluting stent (DES) or CABG. The composite primary outcome of all cause death, non-fatal MI and non-fatal stroke occurred more in the PCI with DES group at 5 years follow-up (PCI with DES-26.6% vs. CABG-18.7%; p = 0.005). The better outcome in CABG group was primarily driven by reduction in MI (p<0.001) and all cause death (p = 0.049). But stroke was more in CABG group (PCI 2.4% vs. CABG 5.2%; p = 0.03).[67] Coronary Artery Revascularization in Diabetes (CARDia) trial compared the safety and efficacy of PCI with stenting against CABG in patients with t-2DM and symptomatic CAD. At 1 year follow-up, the primary composite of death, MI and stroke was 13% in PCI group and 10.5% in CABG group (p = 0.39). Whereas the secondary outcome, which included repeat revascularization with the primary outcome was 19.3% in PCI group versus 11.3% in the CABG group (p = 0.02).[68] TUXEDO-India investigators randomized 1,830 patients with t-2DM and CAD who were undergoing PCI to receive either Paclitaxel-eluting stent or an everolimus eluting stent. At 1 year there were more target vessel failure in Paclitaxel group (5.6% vs. 2.9%; p = 0.38 for noninferiority).[69] EXCEL trial compared 3 year outcome of PCI with Everolimus eluting stent (EES) versus CABG in left main coronary artery (LMCA) disease. Diabetic subgroup analysis showed that out of 548 patients with diabetes and unprotected LMCA disease, 286 were underwent PCI with EES and 268 underwent CABG. At 3 years, risk of death, stroke or MI was higher in diabetic subgroup than without diabetes (19.9% vs. 13%; HR = 1.6; 95% CI, 1.25–2.04). Death, stroke, MI and unplanned revascularization were worse in patients with diabetes who were treated with insulin, as compared with those not treated with insulin or patients without diabetes (26.6% vs. 25.9% vs. 19%; P < 0.01).[70] Borges N et al. concluded after analyzing the diabetic subgroup data of EXCEL and NOBEL trials, that CABG is preferable in the presence of diabetes in unprotected LMCA or complex lesions (SYNTAX score > 33) included distal left main lesions.[71] In a systematic review and meta-analyses of long-term mortality in t-2DM patients who were treated by CABG, eleven studies with 12,955 patients were included. The mortality was significantly higher in patients with t-2DM with OR: 1.54, 95% CI: 1.37–1.72, P < 0.00001; OR: 1.53, 95% CI: 1.36–1.72, P<.00001; and OR: 1.53, 95% CI: 1.26–1.87, P < .0001 at 1–15, 5–15, and 7–15 years, respectively. They concluded that t-2DM is an independent risk factor for mortality in post-CABG patients, yet it is the best revascularization strategy in these patients.[72] The subgroup analysis of FREEDOM and ARTS II studies showed that long-term outcome of left internal mammary artery (LIMA) graft is better than SVG graft to left anterior descending coronary artery (LAD) among the CABG group.[66,67]

Coronary Physiology

Liu Z et al., studied the CV outcome of deferred lesions by FFR in diabetic patients (n = 180) and compared it with nondiabetic groups (n = 450). Patients with diabetic and FFR more than 0.85 had a twofold higher risk of death and MI than nondiabetics (HR 2.20; 95% CI: 1.19–4.01, p = 0.015).[73] Kennedy MW et al. included 294 patients with DM into FFR negative (>0.80) medical treatment group (n = 205) and FFR positive (≤ 0.80) complete revascularization group (n = 89) and they were followed for a mean period of 32.6±18.1 months. The former group had higher MACE rate (44% vs. 26.6%; p = 0.02). They concluded that patients with DM and with previous MI (p = 0.03), deferred revascularization is associated with poor medium-term outcomes. Combining FFR with intravascular imaging techniques may be required to guide the treatment strategy in these patients with rapidly progressing atherosclerosis.[74] Cook et al. studied the FFR/iFR discordance in angiographically intermediate stenosis using Doppler derived coronary flow measurements. FFR disagreed with iFR in 14% (n = 50 of 366) of stenosed vessels, in which 22 were FFR+/iFR– and 28 were FFR–/iFR+. In comparison to patients with FFR+/iFR– discordant stenosis, patients with FFR–/iFR+ discordant stenosis had a significantly higher prevalence of diabetes. The discordance of FFR in diabetes is due to coronary microvascular dysfunction.[75]

CONCLUSION

The risk of developing MI in t-2DM patients without prior history of MI is numerically the same as that of nondiabetic patients with previous history of MI. The risk of developing CVD in t-2DM patients is 2–4 folds higher than the general population. Since 2008 the newer molecules for t-2DM need to prove CV safety and existing antidiabetic drugs except insulin need to prove its safety for FDA approval.

Following the FDA/EMA regulations for CV safety in 2008, newer antidiabetic drugs have shown in a number of CVOTs their CV safety. Some drugs, such as empagliflozin, semaglutide and liraglutide have shown additional CV protection in addition to glucose lowering effect primarily by decrease in CV death and HF hospitalization. In a t-2DM with high CV risk it is advisable to start a SGLT-2 inhibitor along with metformin, as GLP-1 agonist needs to be given as an injectable.

The ideal revascularization strategy for multivessel CAD, more so with left ventricular dysfunction in t-2DM patient is CABG as the better CV outcome was primarily driven by reduction in all cause death, MI and repeat revascularization though there was a rise in stroke rate. Though the subgroup analysis of COURAGE trial showed the noninferiority of OMT over PCI in both diabetic and nondiabetic groups, recent coronary physiology studies reveal the rapid progressive nature of coronary atherosclerosis in t-2DM. The addition of intravascular image guidance to coronary physiology can predict and improve outcomes in CAD revascularization strategies, though large multicentre RCT with long-term follow-up will be needed to prove this.

REFERENCES

1. National Cholesterol Education Program (NCEP) Expert Panel on Detection, Evaluation, and Treatment of High Blood Cholesterol in Adults (Adult Treatment Panel III). Third Report of the National Cholesterol Education Program (NCEP) Expert Panel on Detection, Evaluation, and Treatment of High Blood Cholesterol in Adults (Adult Treatment Panel III) final report. Circulation. 2002;106:3143.
2. Levine SA. Coronary thrombosis: its various clinical features. Medicine. 1929;8:245-418.
3. Cruickshank N. Coronary thrombosis and myocardial infarction with glucosuria. Br Med J. 193;1: 618-9.
4. Kuusisto J, MykkänenL, PyöräläK, et al. NIDDM and its metabolic control predict coronary heart disease in elderly subjects. Diabetes. 1994;43:960-7.
5. Andersson D, Svärdsudd K. Long-term glycemic control relates to mortality in type II diabetes. Diabetes Care. 1995;18:1534-43.
6. Gall M-A, Borch-Johnsen K, Hougaard P, et al. Albuminuria and poor glycemic control predict mortality in NIDDM. Diabetes. 1995;44:1303-9.
7. Gerstein HC, Miller ME, Genuth S, et al, Long-term effects of intensive glucose lowering on cardiovascular outcomes. N Engl J Med. 2011;364:818-28.
8. Nissen SE, Wolski K. Effect of rosiglitazone on the risk of myocardial infarction and death from cardiovascular causes. N Engl J Med. 2007;356:2457-71.
9. Kernan WN, Viscoli CM, Furie KL, et al. Pioglitazone after ischemic stroke or transient ischemic attack. N Engl J Med. 2016;374:1321-31.
10. Young LH, Viscoli CM, Curtis JP, et al. Cardiac outcomes after ischemic stroke or TIA: effects of pioglitazone in patients with insulin resistance without diabetes. Circulation 2017;135:1882-93.
11. Donath MY, Shoelson SE. Type 2 diabetes as an inflammatory disease. Nat Rev Immunol. 2011;11: 98-107.
12. Seshasai SR, Kaptoge S, Thompson A, et al. Diabetes mellitus, fasting glucose, and risk of cause specific death. N Engl J Med. 2011;364:829-41.
13. Nathan DM, Genuth S, Lachin J, et al. Diabetes Control and Complications Trial Research Group. The effect of intensive treatment of diabetes on the development and progression of long-term complications in insulin-dependent diabetes mellitus. N Engl J Med. 1993;329:977-86.
14. UK Prospective Diabetes Study (UKPDS) Group. Intensive blood-glucose control with sulphonylureas or insulin compared with conventional treatment and risk of complications in patients with type 2 diabetes (UKPDS 33). Lancet. 1998;352:837-53.
15. UK Prospective Diabetes Study (UKPDS) Group. Effect of intensive blood-glucose control with metformin on complications in overweight patients with type 2 diabetes (UKPDS 34). Lancet. 1998;352:854-65.
16. Gerstein HC, Miller ME, Byington RP, et al. Action to Control Cardiovascular Risk in Diabetes Study Group. Effects of intensive glucose lowering in type 2 diabetes. N Engl J Med. 2008;358:2545-59.
17. Patel A, MacMahon S, Chalmers J, et al. ADVANCE Collaborative Group. Intensive blood glucose control and vascular outcomes in patients with type 2 diabetes. N Engl J Med. 2008;358:2560-72.

18. Duckworth W, Abraira C, Moritz T, et al. VADT Investigators. Glucose control and vascular complications in veterans with type 2 diabetes. N Engl J Med. 2009;360:129-39.
19. Ohkubo Y, Kishikawa H, Araki E, et al. Intensive insulin therapy prevents the progression of diabetic microvascular complications in Japanese patients with non-insulin-dependent diabetes mellitus: a randomized prospective 6-year study. Diabetes Res Clin Pract. 1995;28:103-17.
20. Ray KK, Seshasai SR, Wijesuriya S, et al. Effect of intensive control of glucose on cardiovascular outcomes and death in patients with diabetes mellitus: a meta-analysis of randomised controlled trials. Lancet. 2009;373:1765-72.
21. Turnbull FM, Abraira C, Anderson RJ, et al. Control Group. Intensive glucose control and macrovascular outcomes in type 2 diabetes. Diabetologia. 2009;52:2288-98.
22. Gerstein HC, Miller ME, Byington RP, et al. Action to Control Cardiovascular Risk in Diabetes Study Group. Effects of intensive glucose lowering in type 2 diabetes. N Engl J Med. 2008;358:2545-59.
23. ACCORD Study Group. Nine-year effects of 3.7 years of intensive glycemic control on cardiovascular outcomes. Diabetes Care. 2016;39:701-8.
24. Duckworth W, Abraira C, Moritz T, et al. Glucose control and vascular complications in veterans with type 2 diabetes. N Engl J Med. 2009;360:129.
25. Hayward RA, Reaven PD, Wiitala WL, et al. VADT Investigators. Follow-up of glycemic control and cardiovascular outcomes in type 2 diabetes. N Engl J Med. 2015;372:2197-206.
26. Holman RR, Sourij H, Califf RM. Cardiovascular outcome trials of glucose-lowering drugs or strategies in type 2 diabetes. Lancet. 2014;383:2008-17.
27. John M, Gopalakrishnan Unnikrishnan A, Kalra S, et al. Cardiovascular outcome trials for anti-diabetes medication: a holy grail of drug development? Indian Heart J. 2016;68:564-71.
28. Nissen SE, Wolski K, Topol EJ. Effect of muraglitazar on death and major adverse cardiovascular events in patients with type 2 diabetes mellitus. JAMA. 2005;294:2581-6.
29. Nissen SE, Wolski K. Effect of rosiglitazone on the risk of myocardial infarction and death from cardiovascular causes. N Engl J Med. 2007;356:2457-71.
30. Dormandy JA, Charbonnel B, Eckland DJ, et al. PROactive Investigators. Secondary prevention of macrovascular events in patients with type 2 diabetes in the PROactive Study (PROspective pioglitAzone Clinical Trial In macroVascular Events): a randomised controlled trial. Lancet. 2005;366:1279-89.
31. Meinert CL, Knatterud GL, Prout TE, et al. A study of the effects of hypoglycemic agents on vascular complications in patients with adult-onset diabetes. II. Mortality results. Diabetes. 1970;19:789-830.
32. Goldner MG, Knatterud GL, Prout TE. Effects of hypoglycemic agents on vascular complications in patients with adult-onset diabetes. 3. Clinical implications of UGDP results. JAMA. 1971;21:1400-10.
33. Knatterud GL, Meinert CL, Klimt CR, et al. Effects of hypoglycemic agents on vascular complications in patients with adult-onset diabetes. IV. A preliminary report on phenformin results. JAMA. 1971;217:777-84.
34. UK prospective diabetes study (UKPDS) Group. Intensive blood-glucose control with sulphonylureas or insulin compared with conventional treatment and risk of complications in patients with type 2 diabetes (UKPDS 33). Lancet. 1998;352(9131):837-53.
35. Boussageon R, Supper I, Bejan-Angoulvant T, et al. Reappraisal of metformin efficacy in the treatment of type 2 diabetes: a meta-analysis of randomised controlled trials. PloS Med. 2012;9(4):e1001204.
36. Holman RR. Post trial monitoring results of the UKPDS sulfonylurea plus metformin substudy. Munich: EASD; 2013.
37. Ramachandran S, Anandan V, Kutty VR, et al. Metformin attenuates effects of cyclophilin A on macrophages, reduces lipid uptake and secretion of cytokines by repressing decreased AMPK activity. Clin Sci (Lond). 2018;132:719-38.

38. Frye RL, August P, Brooks MM, et al. BARI 2D Study Group. A randomized trial of therapies for type 2 diabetes and coronary artery disease. N Engl J Med. 2009;360(24):2503-15.
39. Raz I, Wilson PW, Strojek K, et al. Effects of prandial versus fasting glycemia on cardiovascular outcomes in type 2 diabetes: the HEART2D trial. Diabetes Care. 2009;32(3):381-6.
40. Ceriello A. Postprandial hyperglycemia and cardiovascular disease: is the HEART2D study the answer? Diabetes Care. 2009;32(3):521-2.
41. Raz I, Ceriello A, Wilson PW, et al. Post hoc subgroup analysis of the HEART2D trial demonstrates lower cardiovascular risk in older patients targeting postprandial versus fasting/premeal glycemia. Diabetes Care. 2011;34(7):1511-3.
42. Gerstein HC, Bosch J, Dagenais GR, et al. ORIGIN Trial Investigators, Basal insulin and cardiovascular and other outcomes in dysglycemia. N Engl J Med. 2012;367(4):319-28.
43. Epstein M, Sowers JR. Diabetes mellitus and hypertension. Hypertension. 1992;19:403-418.
44. The National High Blood Pressure Education Program Working Group. National High Blood Pressure Education Program Working Group report on hypertension in diabetes. Hypertension. 1994;23:145-58.
45. KDOQI. KDOQI clinical practice guidelines and clinical practice recommendations for diabetes and chronic kidney disease. Am J Kidney Dis. 2007;49:S12-54.
46. Bakris GL, Sowers JR; American Society of Hypertension Writing Group. ASH position paper: treatment of hypertension in patients with diabetes—an update. J Clin Hypertens (Greenwich). 2008;10:707-15.
47. U.S. Food and Drug Administration. Guidance for industry: diabetes mellitus-evaluating cardiovascular risk in new antidiabetic therapies to treat type 2 diabetes. [online] Available from www.fda.gov/downloads/Drugs/GuidanceComplianceRegulatoryInformation/Guidances/ ucm071627.pdf. [Accessed November, 2018].
48. Regier EE, Venkat MV, Close KL. More than seven years of hindsight: revisiting the FDA's 2008 guidance on cardiovascular outcomes trials for type 2 diabetes medications. Clin Diabetes. 2016;34:173-80.
49. Novo Nordisk. Novo Nordisk receives complete response letter in the US for Tresiba and Ryzodeg. [online]. Available from https://www.novonordisk.com/bin/getPDF.1676900.pdf. [Accessed November, 2018].
50. Leiter LA, Teoh H, Braunwald E, et al. Efficacy and safety of saxagliptin in older participants in the SAVOR-TIMI 53 trial. Diabetes Care. 2015;38(6):1145-53.
51. Scirica BM, Bhatt DL, Braunwald E, et al. Saxagliptin and cardiovascular outcomes in patients with type 2 diabetes mellitus. N Engl J Med. 2013;369(14):1317-26.
52. White WB, Cannon CP, Heller SR, et al. Alogliptin after acute coronary syndrome in patients with type 2 diabetes. N Engl J Med. 2013;369(14):1327-35.
53. Zannad F, Cannon CP, Cushman WC, et al. Heart failure and mortality outcomes in patients with type 2 diabetes taking alogliptin versus placebo in EXAMINE: a multicentre, randomised, double-blind trial. Lancet. 2015;385(9982):2067-76.
54. Green JB, Bethel MA, Armstrong PW, et al. Effect of sitagliptin on cardiovascular outcomes in type 2 diabetes. N Engl J Med. 2015;373(3):232-42.
55. Pfeffer MA, Claggett B, Diaz R, et al. Lixisenatide in patients with type 2 diabetes and acute coronary syndrome. N Engl J Med. 2015;373(23):2247-57.
56. Zinman B, Wanner C, Lachin JM, et al. Empagliflozin, cardiovascular outcomes, and mortality in type 2 diabetes. N Engl J Med. 2015;373(22):2117-28.
57. Marso SP, Daniels GH, Brown-Frandsen K, et al. Liraglutide and cardiovascular outcomes in type 2 diabetes. N Engl J Med. 2016;375:311-22.
58. Marso SP, Bain SC, Consoli A, et al. Semaglutide and cardiovascular outcomes in patients with type 2 diabetes. N Engl J Med. 2016;375:1834-44.

59. Marso SP, McGuire DK, Zinman B, et al. Efficacy and safety of degludec versus glargine in Type 2 diabetes. N Engl J Med. 2017;377(8):723-32.
60. Neal B, Perkovic V, Mahaffey KW, et al. Canagliflozin and cardiovascular and renal events in Type 2 diabetes. N Engl J Med. 2017;377(7):644-57.
61. Holman RR, Bethel MA, Mentz RJ, et al. Effects of once-weekly exenatide on cardiovascular outcomes in Type 2 diabetes. N Engl J Med. 2017;377(13):1228-39.
62. Holman RR, Coleman RL, Chan JCN, et al. Effects of acarbose on cardiovascular and diabetes outcomes in patients with coronary heart disease and impaired glucose tolerance (ACE): a randomised, double-blind, placebo-controlled trial. Lancet Diabetes Endocrinol. 2017: S2213-8587(17)30309-1.
63. Boden WE, O'Rourke RA, Teo KK, et al. Optimal medical therapy with or without PCI for stable coronary disease. N Engl J Med. 2007;356:1503-16.
64. BARI Investigators. The final 10-year follow-up results from the BARI randomized trial. J Am Coll Cardiol. 2007;49:1600-6.
65. Rutter MK, Nesto RW. The BARI 2D study: a randomised trial of therapies for type 2 diabetes and coronary artery disease. Diab Vasc Dis Res. 2010;7:69-72.
66. Onuma Y, Wykrzykowska JJ, Garg S, et al. 5-Year follow-up of coronary revascularization in diabetic patients with multivessel coronary artery disease: insights from ARTS (arterial revascularization therapy study)-II and ARTS-I trials. JACC Cardiovasc Interv. 2011;4:317-23.
67. Farkouh ME, Domanski M, Sleeper LA, et al. Strategies for multivessel revascularization in patients with diabetes. N Engl J Med. 2012;367:2375-84.
68. Kapur A, Hall RJ, Malik IS, Qureshi AC, Butts J, de Belder M, et al. Randomized comparison of percutaneous coronary intervention with coronary artery bypass grafting in diabetic patients. 1-year results of the CARDia (Coronary Artery Revascularization in Diabetes) trial. J Am Coll Cardiol. 2010;55:432-40.
69. Kaul U, Bangalore S, Seth A, et al. Paclitaxel-eluting versus everolimus-eluting Coronary Stents in Diabetes. N Engl J Med. 2015;373:1709-19.
70. Stone GW, Sabik JF, Serruys PW, et al. Everolimus-Eluting Stents or Bypass Surgery for Left Main Coronary Artery Disease. N Engl J Med. 2016;375:2223-35.
71. Borges N, Kapadia SR, Ellis SG. Unprotected Left Main Coronary Artery Disease: Management in the Post NOBLE and EXCEL Era. Interv Cardiol. 2017; 2:92-6.
72. Bundhun PK, Bhurtu A, Yuan J. Impact of type 2 diabetes mellitus on the long-term mortality in patients who were treated by coronary artery bypass surgery. A systematic review and meta-analysis. Medicine (Baltimore). 2017;96:e7022.
73. Liu Z, Matsuzawa Y, Herrmann J, et al. Relation between fractional flow reserve value of coronary lesions with deferred revascularization and cardiovascular outcomes in non-diabetic and diabetic patients. Int J Cardiol. 2016;219:56-62.
74. Kennedy MW, Hermanides RS, Kaplan E, et al. Fractional flow reserve-guided deferred versus complete revascularisation in patients with diabetes mellitus. Am J Cardiol. 2016;118:1293-9.
75. Cook CM, Jeremias A, Petraco R, et al. Fractional flow reserve/instantaneous wave-free ratio discordance in angiographically intermediate coronary stenoses. JACC Card Vasc Inter. 2017;10: 2514-24.

Index

Page numbers followed by *b* refer to box, *f* refer to figure, *fc* refer to flowchart, and *t* refer to table.

C

D

E

F

G

J

K

L

N

O

P

Q

R

S